About the Autho

JANE B. DONEGAN is a
of American History at Onondaga
Community College, Syracuse,
New York. Her articles have appeared in "REMEMBER THE LADIES"
and the ONONDAGA COUNTY MEDICAL
SOCIETY BULLETIN.

D0225538

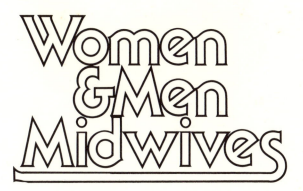

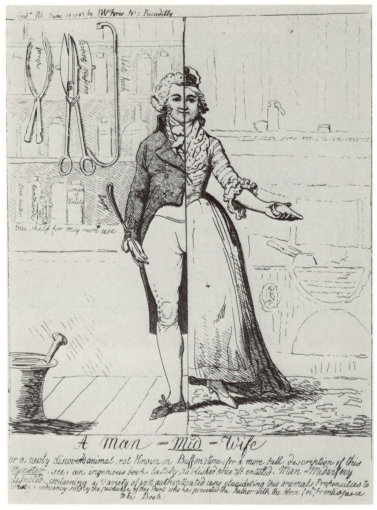

Cartoon of "A Man-Mid-Wife or a newly discovered animal," depicting a midwife bisected into male and female halves. Note the instruments, cantharides, and "love water" that allegedly comprised the man midwife's stock-in-trade.—From S. W. Fores, *Man-midwifery Dissected*, London, 1793. (Courtesy of the Wellcome Institute for the History of Medicine.)

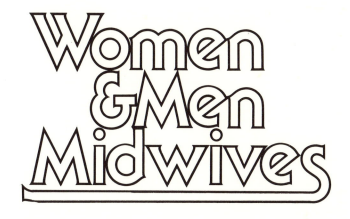

Women & Men Midwives

Medicine, Morality, and Misogyny in Early America

Jane B. Donegan

Contributions in Medical History, Number 2

GREENWOOD PRESS
Westport, Connecticut • London, England

MESABI COMMUNITY
COLLEGE LIBRARY
VIRGINIA. MINN

Library of Congress Cataloging in Publication Data

Donegan, Jane B
 Women and men midwives.

 (Contributions to medical history ; no. 2 ISSN 0147-
1058
 Bibliography: p.
 Includes index.
 1. Obstetrics—United States—History. 2. Midwives—
United States—History. 3. Women in medicine—United
States—History. 4. Sex discrimination against women—
United States—History. 5. Women—United States—
Social conditions. I. Title. II. Series: Contributions
in medical history ; no. 2.
RG518.U5D66   618.2   77-87968
ISBN 0-8371-9868-2

Copyright © 1978 by Jane B. Donegan

All rights reserved. No portion of this book may
be reproduced, by any process or technique, without
the express written consent of the publisher.

Library of Congress Catalog Card Number: 77-87968
ISBN: 0-8371-9868-2
ISSN: 0147-1058

First published in 1978

Greenwood Press, Inc.
51 Riverside Avenue, Westport, Connecticut 06880

Printed in the United States of America
10 9 8 7 6 5 4 3 2 1

Contents

17.95

B+T

5 F 81

38093

Acknowledgments

I am happy to acknowledge with gratitude the many debts I have accumulated in the completion of this book. Nelson Manfred Blake guided the work in its earlier stages and encouraged me all along the way. Lillie Kinney and Peter Uva suggested sources and located rare materials. The staff of the State University of New York Upstate Medical Center Library granted me free access to their collection, answered my questions with patience, and provided a congenial atmosphere for research. The following institutions provided materials: Bard College, the British Museum, the College of Physicians of Philadelphia, Columbia University, Cornell University, the Court of Appeals Library in Syracuse, Franklin D. Roosevelt Library, Harvard University, the Institute of the History of Medicine at the Johns Hopkins University, the Library of Congress, McGill University, the National Library of Medicine, the New York Academy of Medicine, the New-York Historical Society, Onondaga Community College, Onondaga Historical Association, Onondaga County Medical Society, Syracuse Public Library, Syracuse University, and the Wellcome Institute of the History of Medicine.

Anwar A. Al Mudamgha, Carol V. R. George, Dorothy L. Kelly, Hiram L. Smith, Verne L. Sugarman, and Nancy K. Weeks read all or portions of the manuscript and offered helpful criticisms. Photographic work was prepared by Gregg A. Texido. My colleagues and students at Onondaga Community College were supportive throughout. Jane Frost typed the manuscript with meticulous attention to detail.

The study was supported in part by a Summer Stipend from the National Endowment for the Humanities. Chapter 5 and a portion of chapter 8 constitute a slightly revised version of my essay published originally as "Man-Midwifery and the Delicacy of the Sexes" in *"Remember the Ladies"*: *New Perspectives on Women in American History,* edited by Carol V. R. George (Syracuse, N.Y.: Syracuse University Press, 1975), and appears with permission of the Syracuse University Press. A portion of chapter 7 was published originally as "Early Medical Coeducation in Central New York," Onondaga County Medical Society *Bulletin* (July 1976), and is used with permission of the editor.

Without the assistance of my mother, Mary Barlow Bauer, I would not have completed this book. "M" read every draft of the manuscript with enthusiasm and offered valuable criticism and needed encouragement. In addition, she cared for her grandchildren with unfailing good humor, creating the time for me to write. To "M" and to my children, Stuart and Jennifer, I dedicate this book with love and thanks.

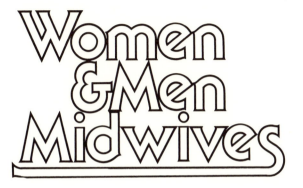

Introduction

In America today the term *midwife* suggests a variety of images. Some picture an ignorant, slovenly crone, whose ministrations luckless women were obliged to endure with the "agonies" of childbirth in the remote past. Those familiar with the highly skilled professional nurse-midwives of Great Britain, Europe, Africa, and Asia may regard them as exclusive inhabitants of foreign shores. Only a few realize that programs to train modern nurse-midwives in the United States have been available for nearly half a century. Increasingly, these specialists are being suggested as a viable solution to the current problems of inadequate health-care delivery and high medical costs.[1]

Very little has been written about the midwife and her work, in spite of the considerable and at times prominent role she has played in America's past. Standard histories of medicine fail to mention her at all or dismiss her as a relic discarded not a moment too soon in the name of medical progress. Such treatment ignores the fact that large numbers of Americans can recall having learned that a parent or grandparent was delivered by a midwife prior to World War I, and in the case of Southerners, as late as the 1940s. It is all the more surprising when one learns that as late as 1910, midwives reported approximately 50 percent of all births in the United States, and among city dwellers, the percentage was frequently higher.[2]

Within the past decade, feminists in particular have rediscovered the midwife. Some have seen her primarily as the victim of male bias and sexist aggression and glorify her past role as helper of women. Such an explanation for the decline of the American midwife requires research into primary source materials and more thorough documentation than has yet been offered. At present it leaves unanswered the interesting question of why female midwifery continued to thrive in cultures where deeply rooted machismo attitudes are known to be perpetuated.[3] Decisions by some contemporary women to bear their children at home, attended by unlicensed midwives, have led to the official condemnation and prosecution of "lay-midwives" for practicing without recognized credentials. One reaction has been to interpret the prosecution as persecution, a reenactment of earlier contests between the medical establishment and the midwives.[4]

A great deal of the renewed interest in midwifery has come about since 1970, when I first began to explore the heritage of American obstetrics. The late Richard Shryock's observation that Anglo-Saxon women had abandoned their midwives in favor of male physicians in an age of increasing prudishness[5] led me to wonder why historians had never attempted to explain this paradox in detail. This book is one such attempt. It is neither a history of obstetrics in the technical sense nor a history of the feminist movement, although it contains elements of both. Primarily, it is an examination of the development of male-dominated obstetrics against the background of middle-class concepts of morality, reform movements, and emerging feminism.

Historically, midwifery had been the unquestioned province of women. In the eighteenth century, significant advances in British medicine led to the development of the "new obstetrics," with its promise of greater safety for women and children. In the 1760s the new obstetrics spread to America, and traditional midwifery habits began to change along the pattern already evolving in England. By the early nineteenth century, male physicians had succeeded in replacing the midwives almost completely in their attendance on upper- and middle-class urban women. This study explores the evolution of this change, which was brought about by the technology developed by an emerging medical profession.

Leisure-class women were the first to give up the midwives. This study concentrates on the women in that class who lived in Philadelphia, Boston, and New York between the middle of the eighteenth century and the Civil War. An examination of the ramifications of the new obstetrics on a society that claimed to revere modesty and the concept of the "delicacy of the sexes" forms an integral part of the work. Throughout the period, critics of man midwifery attempted to return to the past by restoring obstetrics to the midwives. Their reactionary crusade began in the 1760s in England and continued without much success there or in the United States until the 1840s.

Then its direction modified as its goals became intertwined with those of other reform movements. Supporters of women's rights, seeking to expand opportunities for personal fulfillment and rebelling against the narrow confines of "woman's sphere," demanded that the medical profession be opened to women. Proponents of alternative medical systems, attacking the heroic practice of orthodox doctors, played an important role because they were reform-minded. These medical reformers, known as sectarians or irregulars, encouraged women to study medicine and admitted them to their colleges. Sectarian impact upon women was complex, and this book explores a portion of that contribution.

The response of orthodox physicians, or regulars, to attacks by reactionary critics, feminists, and irregular practitioners constitutes an essential ingredient of this study. With their grasp on lucrative obstetrics and the treatment of the diseases of women still tenuous, doctors tried to justify continued male dominance. They reinforced sexist stereotypes, promised safe and rapid deliveries that they could not guarantee, resulting in "meddlesome midwifery," and developed procedures calculated to avoid offending the sensibilities. In this way doctors designed a strategy that helped them retain control over a branch of medicine, the practice of which they themselves admittedly found embarrassing and frequently frustrating.

Although critics cited the need for trained midwives, it was not until the late 1840s that Samuel Gregory opened his "midwife manufactory" in Boston. By then, the doctors' potent argument that competence in obstetrics demanded thorough education in all branches of medicine contributed to the idea that women who wished to practice midwifery must first qualify as physicians. Thus, the reactionary goals of the anti-man midwifery forces merged with the radical objectives of feminists seeking to open the medical profession to women. The critics of man midwifery never reached their goal. Yet, their activities did focus attention on the incongruity of expecting women to accept the services of the accoucheur and at the same time observe the dictates of a rigid moral code.

In the 1850s, pioneering medical women began to move beyond traditional strictures and to redefine woman's sphere. The resistance they encountered while seeking "laurels in forbidden paths" radicalized some and gave them a sense of sisterhood, just as it discouraged others. The help and support this small band received from male feminists, and especially from sectarian reformers, gave them a sense of what the cooperative efforts of women and men could produce. Some of these women disclaimed identification with the far-reaching goals of hard-core feminists. Nevertheless, their actions and their writings reveal the determination to control their own destinies, which has been a hallmark of feminism from its inception.

NOTES

1. Discussions of programs for modern nurse-midwives are found today in lay periodicals as well as in professional journals. Examples of the former are: Carl M. Cobb, "Solving the Doctor Shortage," *Saturday Review* 53 (August 22, 1970):24-26; Nancy A. Comer, "Midwifery: Would You Let This Woman Deliver Your Child?" *Mademoiselle* (June 1973):134; B. Day, "Return of the Midwife," *Redbook* 132 (March 1969):72-73; D. C. Davis and L. Middleton, "Rebirth of the Midwife," *Today's Health* 46 (February 1968):28-31; Patrick Young, "The Thoroughly Modern Midwife," *Saturday Review* 55 (September 2, 1972):42-43; N. Ander, "Return of the Midwife," *Good Housekeeping* 183 (September 1976):198-200; H. Kaminetzky, "New Midwife—Sophisticated and Caring: Training Program at the College of Medicine and Dentistry of New Jersey," *Intellect* 104 (March 1976):417-418.

Discussions in the professional literature include *The Midwife in the United States. Report of a Macy Conference* (New York: Josiah Macy Jr. Foundation, 1968); Ruth W. Lubic, "Myths about Nurse-Midwifery," *American Journal of Nursing* 74 (February 1974):268-269; Janice T. Kuhlmann and Edward G. Kuhlmann, "Nurse-Midwifery: A New Concept for Middle-Class Americans," in Alice M. Forman, et al, eds., *16th Interna-*

tional Congress of Midwives, New Horizons in Midwifery (Baltimore: Waverly Press, 1973), pp. 107-110; Evelyn Hart and Teresa Marsico, "Creative Approaches to Nurse-Midwifery Education," *Journal of Nurse-Midwifery* 20 (Spring 1975:17-19; 20 (Fall 1975):24-26.

2. Most medical historians have been men, who were unconcerned with the midwives' role in medicine. Notable exceptions include Richard H. Shryock, especially his *Medicine in America: Historical Essays* (Baltimore: Johns Hopkins University Press, 1966) and John B. Blake, "Women and Medicine in Ante-Bellum America," *Bulletin of the History of Medicine* 39 (March-April 1965):99-123. A recent well-documented study is Judy Barrett Litoff's *American Midwives: 1860 to the Present* (Westport, Conn.: Greenwood Press, 1978). Ann H. Sablowsky, "The Power of the Forceps: A Comparative Analysis of the Midwife—Historically and Today," *Women and Health* 1 (January-February 1976):10-13, gives a brief summary of developing views. The early British scene is examined by Hilda Smith in "Gynecology and Ideology in Seventeenth Century England," in Berenice A. Carroll, ed., *Liberating Women's History: Theoretical and Critical Essays* (Urbana, Chicago, and London: University of Illinois Press, 1976), pp. 97-114. Martha H. Verbrugge, "Women and Medicine in Nineteenth-Century America," *Signs: Journal of Women in Culture and Society* 1 (Summer 1976):957-972, presents a useful overview but omits reference to midwives. On the training of midwives in post-World War II Mississippi, see James H. Ferguson, "Mississippi Midwives," *Journal of the History of Medicine* 5 (Winter 1950):85-95. The statistics cited above are drawn from Frances E. Kobrin, "The American Midwife Controversy: A Crisis of Professionalization," *Bulletin of the History of Medicine* 40 (July-August 1966):350. They reflect the fact that immigrant women, especially those from southern and eastern Europe, clung to their traditional female midwives.

3. See, for example, Adrienne Rich, *Of Woman Born: Motherhood as Experience and Institution* (New York: W. W. Norton & Company, Inc., 1976); G. J. Barker-Benfield, *The Horrors of the Half-Known Life: Male Attitudes Toward Women and Sexuality in Nineteenth-Century America* (New York, San Francisco, and London: Harper and Row, 1976); Barbara Ehrenreich and Dierdre English, *Witches, Midwives and Nurses: A History of Women Healers* (Old Westbury, N.Y.: The Feminist Press, 1973); Carol Somer, "How Women Had Control of Their Lives and Lost It," *The Second Wave: A Magazine of the New Feminism* 2 (1973):5-10, 28.

4. Becky Taber, "Midwives Reclaim Birth," *Plexus* (January 1976):6-7; David Talbot and Barbara Zhevtlin, "*California* vs. *Midwives:* The Legalities of Attending a Birth," *Rolling Stone* (May 23, 1974):12-13; Elizabeth Fishel, "Childbirth: A Feminist View," *Ramparts* 13 (September 1974):40-44.

5. Some of the current work on nineteenth-century woman's sexuality casts doubt upon the idea that prudishness actually increased. John S. Haller and Robin M. Haller, *The Physician and Sexuality in Victorian America* (New York: W. W. Norton & Company, Inc., 1977; Urbana, Chicago, and London: University of Illinois Press, 1974), argue that such prudery was a "mask" utilized by women seeking control over their bodies and resisting attempts to define them as sex objects. Carl N. Degler, "What Ought to Be and What Was: Women's Sexuality in the Nineteenth Century," *American Historical Review* 79 (December 1974):1467-1490, reviews standard assessments and shows the wide gap that existed between society's ideal and reality. Carroll Smith-Rosenberg, "Puberty to Menopause: The Cycle of Femininity in Nineteenth-Century America," *Feminist Studies* 1 (Winter-Spring 1973):58-72, shows how women's biological functions were used to keep them in traditional roles. Ben Barker-Benfield, "The Spermatic Economy: A Nineteenth Century View of Sexuality," *Feminist Studies* 1 (Summer 1972):45-74, contends that men feared woman's sexuality and devised means to avoid or destroy its effects.

1

The Mysterious Office of Women

These are to certify those whom it may concerne that Elizabeth Davis wife of Thomas Davis of the parish of St. Catherine Creechurch in London midwife is a woman that wee knowe very well to be of a good & honest life and Conversation, & very knowing skillful and expert in the practice of Midwifery wch office or ffunction of a midwife she has pformed for the space of eighteen yeares wth great care and good success, and in testimony herof we have subscribed our Names. —MIDWIFE'S LICENSE, 1661

For centuries the art of midwifery was the exclusive province of women. Childbearing was woman's essential, inescapable function, which some were known to have effected totally unassisted. Biblical references reinforced the view that such a feat was possible. In Exodus, the ancient midwives Shiphrah and Puah excused their failure to comply with the order to destroy all Hebrew male infants at birth by claiming that the Hebrew women were "lively, and . . . delivered ere the midwives came in unto them."[1]

Under ordinary circumstances, however, the English woman of the seventeenth century did not expect to deliver alone. Once labor had begun, one of the neighborhood midwives would be called in. These local women were empirics who gained their knowledge of the birth process through observation and personal experience. Then, as now, most births were normal. The midwife's role was confined primarily to offering comfort and reassurance to her patient, encouraging and supporting her without interfering in the normal process of parturition. Once the child had been born, she tied off the umbilical cord, supervised the expulsion of the placenta, and cared for mother and infant during the confinement.

Childbirth had not yet been labeled inherently traumatic and dangerous. The "good" midwife of the period, then, was pious, mature, kind, compassionate, and experienced. Those who wrote about the "mysterious office" stressed the value of emulating nature by permitting the birth to unfold with little or no interference. Percival Willughby, a seventeenth-century physician, advised midwives to "observe the waies and proceedings of nature for the production of her fruit on trees, or the ripening of walnutts and almondes, from theire first knotting to the opening of the huskes and falling of the nutt." Nature separated the fruit without any "enforcement," and so it was to be with the midwives. All of the signs of nature should "teach midwives patience, and persuade them to let nature alone to perform her own work, and not to disquiet women by their strugglings, for such enforcements," warned Willughby, "rather hinder the birthe than any waie promote it, and oft ruinate the mother and usually the childe."[2] Midwives were nature's servants and must ever bear this in mind.

In 1724, John Maubray summarized the ideal qualifications of the midwife in *The Female Physician:*

SHE ought not to be too *Fat* or *Gross,* but especially not to have thick or fleshy *Hands* and *Arms,* or large-*Bon'd Wrists*; which (of Necessity) must occasion racking *Pains* to the tender *labouring* Woman. . . . SHE ought to be *Grave* and *Considerate,* endued with *Resolutioñ* and *Presence of Mind,* in order to foresee and prevent ACCIDENTS. . . . SHE ought to be *Patient* and *Pleasant*; *Soft, Meek,* and *Mild* in her *Temper,* in order to encourage and comfort the *labouring* Woman. She should pass by and forgive her small *Failings,* and peevish *Faults,* instructing her gently when she *does* or says *amiss*: But if she will not follow *Advice,* and Necessity require, the MIDWIFE ought to reprimand and put her smartly in mind of her *Duty*; yet always in such a manner, however, as to encourage her with *Hopes* of a happy and speedy DELIVERY.[3]

In brief, the midwife was to be a paragon of virtue, a source of comfort and support to the woman in labor. In practice, no doubt, the midwives fell short of the ideal. Even so, Maubray's catalog of virtues demonstrates that the primary emphasis was placed on the general conduct of midwives, rather than on their skills. In the overwhelming majority of cases, where the presentation was normal and there were no complications such as hemorrhaging or tedious labor, the midwives could accomplish delivery without possessing specialized abilities or detailed anatomical information.

The definition of childbirth as a normal function of women explains in part the apparent general lack of concern about how the midwives practiced. There does not appear to have been any attempt to regulate English midwives until the middle of the sixteenth century. In 1547, the physician Andrew Boorde attributed prolapse of the uterus to the "evyl orderynge af a woman whan that she is delivered." Hoping to reduce the number of miscarriages and stillbirths, Boorde proposed that every midwife be presented to the bishop upon recommendation of "honest women" who were prepared to testify that she was "a sadde woman wise and discrete, havynge experience, and worthy to have ye office." The bishop of the diocese and a "doctor of physicke" would then examine her on technique, "instruct her in that thinge that she is ignoraunt" when necessary, and finally admit her to practice. Perhaps Boorde's suggestion that the "byshoppes . . . loke on this matter" had an effect; beginning with Edmund Bonner, Bishop of London at mid-century, the episcopacy began to license midwives.

The Church of England's interest in midwifery was twofold. Bishops wished to ensure that properly instructed midwives would baptize infants when time was a crucial element and a priest was not readily available. Then too, in an age when superstitions abounded the Church was apprehensive lest the midwives resort to witchcraft and magic in the course of their ministrations. These concerns are evident from the list of questions drafted by Bishop Bonner for use on episcopal inspection visits. Church inspectors were to inquire whether the practicing midwives in the region had been examined and licensed by the bishop. They were to determine if any of the women employed "witchcraft, charms, sorcery, [or] invocations," and to learn of cases in which the midwives, assistants, or

patients had exhibited signs of "disorder or evil behaviour." Queen
Elizabeth's representatives made similar inquiries, asking "whether
you knowe anye that doe use charmes, sorcerye, enchauntments,
inuocations, circles, witchcrafts, soothsayinge, or any lyke craftes
or ymaginations inuented by the Devyll and specyallye in the tyme
of women's travayle." Midwives found guilty of practicing without
a license were subject to fines and excommunication.[4]

Before the midwife could receive her license, she was required to
swear an oath, the contents of which changed little in more than a
century. The fifteen items separately detailed illustrate the stress
placed by the episcopacy upon character and moral conduct. The
midwife swore to be "diligent and faithful and ready to help every
woman labouring with child, as well the poor as the rich; and . . .
in time of necessity [not to] forsake the poor woman to go to the
rich." In the matter of assigning paternity, she was cautioned not
to "cause nor suffer any woman to name or put any other father to
the child, but only him which is the very true father thereof indeed."
It was the midwife's responsibility to see that children were properly
baptized into the Church of England according to the Book of
Common Prayer and, in the case of stillbirths, to see that the child
was properly buried and not "cast into the jaques [privy] or any
other inconvenient place." Midwives were enjoined from exercis-
ing "witchcraft, charm, or sorcery" and from administering "any
herb, medicine, or potion or any other things, to any woman being
with child" to shorten labor in exchange for a higher fee. If, having
exhausted her skill, the midwife suspected the life of either mother
or child to be in jeopardy, it was her duty to "thenceforth in due
time send for other midwives and expert women in that faculty and
use their advice and council in that behalf."[5]

Once the midwife had sworn the oath and paid the required fee
of eighteen shillings, she received her license to practice. Customar-
ily, licenses were witnessed by churchwardens, ministers, and licensed midwives, all of whom certified the woman's loyalty, piety,
and residency, as well as her "known & experienced ability in her
pfession of Midwifery" as determined by "sufficient testimony of
many persons she hath delivered." One license extant included
among its witnesses several women who had been delivered safely
by the midwife in question, and another license noted that the
candidate was "most apt and able through five years of practice."[6]

The bishops' emphasis upon conduct and character tells us little about contemporary expectations of medical competence for the obstetrical attendant. Although the individual items in the oath may be indicative of widespread abuses, it is not possible to determine accurately how much obstetrical skill these early midwives possessed. The testimonials on the licenses suggest that many women gained their experience by practicing midwifery unlicensed for years. It is doubtful that in so doing they were always or even often supervised by more experienced women. Perhaps licensing did tend to eliminate the grossly incompetent. This was the opinion of Samuel Merriman early in the nineteenth century. By 1815 the licensing requirement for midwives had been eliminated. According to Merriman, the result was that contemporary women, from whom an examination was "never required," had far less skill than did their seventeenth-century predecessors.[7]

Merriman's observations were made two decades after the Royal College of Physicians had officially recognized midwifery as a legitimate form of medical practice for its licentiates, all of whom were men. The candidate's qualifications for obstetrical practice were determined by an examination administered by the college.[8] To place the evolution of midwifery in clearer perspective, it is useful to review briefly the medical distinctions and licensing requirements that obtained in England by the eighteenth century.

In London, the nation's capital and by far its largest city, there were three distinct groups of medical practitioners, all of whom were licensed by the appropriate corporation and subject to some regulation. The midwives did not fall under the jurisdiction of any of these corporations. The physician, or Doctor of Physic, normally held a university medical degree from Oxford, Cambridge, or one of the continental universities, such as Leyden or Padua. He could be licensed in one of three ways: by an English university, by a bishop in whose diocese he planned to practice, or by the Royal College of Physicians, incorporated by Henry VIII in 1518.

Although degree requirements varied from university to university, training for the bachelor of medicine generally required a B.A. degree with emphasis on the Greek language, an M.A. degree with concentrated reading in Galen, Hippocrates, and some medieval authorities, plus an additional three years of study devoted largely to listening to lectures by the Regius Professor of

Medicine and attending (but not participating directly in) two anatomical dissections. Those who earned the degree of doctor devoted four more years to theoretical study and attended one or more additional "anatomies." Until the early 1700s, it was possible to obtain a license to practice physic without a degree by passing the extra-licentiate examination administered by the Royal College of Physicians in London. After 1750, however, a university degree was required. The extensive university training for physicians was costly in terms of both time and money. That physicians were an elitist group is therefore not surprising. Early in the eighteenth century, for example, the entire membership of the Royal College of Physicians totaled 114, about 80 of whom practiced in London.

By comparison the training of a surgeon required far less expenditure of time and money. In 1540 Henry VIII had formally united the barber-surgeons and the surgeons into a single corporation in which the role of each group was defined. The barbers were limited to the performance of minor surgery, such as extraction of teeth and venesection. All major surgery was in the hands of the surgeons, who obtained their training by apprenticing themselves to a practicing surgeon. The apprentice studied anatomy in some detail, and for the purpose of dissection fellows received the bodies of four felons yearly. Upon passing an examination administered by the surgeons, the apprentice was admitted to the company as a freeman and permitted to practice.

Apothecaries comprised the third formal group of medical practitioners. In 1607 they had been incorporated with the grocers, and shortly thereafter they received a monopoly on the purchase and sale of drugs. The activities of apothecaries in London were regulated by the College of Physicians and Surgeons.

An attempt to distinguish the practice of these three groups within London, where the jurisdiction of the Royal College of Physicians and Surgeons obtained, suggests itself as follows: Physicians were addressed as "Doctors," held medical degrees, enjoyed the greatest prestige, and treated members of the upper class. Their practice consisted largely of diagnosing and treating diseases and other nonoperative ailments. Surgeons, who were less prestigious than physicians, were engaged in what one practitioner termed "the most fatiguing part" of medicine. They treated ulcers, skin diseases, operated for hernia and stone in the bladder, performed amputations, and bled patients. Apothecaries compounded medicines and sold drugs prescribed by the physicians.

Within London these medical distinctions were maintained rigidly. In the provinces, however, rural conditions worked against specialization, especially in those areas where few medical practitioners of any sort were available. Moreover, the authority of the regulatory corporations did not extend into the provinces. As a result, the distinctive lines were blurred and the general practitioner was referred to as apothecary-surgeon, and later as "surgeon, apothecary and man-midwife." In the eighteenth century, a consensus developed that experience in both surgery and medicine was increasingly desirable for the apothecary-surgeon functioning as a general practitioner. This training could be obtained in a variety of ways. Walking the wards of a hospital, serving as a dresser to a surgeon, taking one or more courses of lectures in anatomy and related fields, and practicing surgery in the army or navy all provided opportunities for acquiring medical and/or surgical knowledge. In 1815 the trend toward upgrading the training for this group of practitioners was accelerated with the passage of the Apothecaries Act. This required that surgeon-apothecaries undergo a five year apprenticeship and also attend formal lectures in medicine and surgery.[9]

The contrast between the training available to male medical practitioners and that to women was greater under the Georges than under the Stuarts. Misogynists naturally denigrated the midwives, yet even allowing for their bias, it is virtually impossible to read the medical treatises, midwives' manuals, and recorded case histories without coming away with some impressions about the limitations of the midwives. Whatever skills and knowledge they had was acquired empirically. Some worked closely with experienced midwives and learned their craft well. Yet, even the midwives' staunchest defenders agreed that many in practice knew little or nothing of their field. Percival Willughby, whose daughter was a midwife, called for the "better educating of all, especially ye younger midwives," observing that "When ye meanest of ye women, not knowing how otherwise to live, for the getting of a shilling or two to sustain their necessities, become ignorant midwives, their travailing women suffer tortures.''[10]

Had all births been normal, the disparity among the midwives would have been less crucial. Regrettably, there was no guarantee that complications would not arise. As the midwife's oath indicated, practitioners were expected to recognize situations in which the patient's needs exceeded their midwifery abilities. The *"Sagacious* and *Prudent"* midwife, confronted with a difficult case, was not to rely solely upon her own judgment but rather should have "immediate *Recourse* to the ablest *Practiser* in the ART, and freely submit her Thoughts to the discerning *Faculty* of the more Learned and Skilful.''[11]

In a rare personal account, Alice Thornton graphically detailed the consequences that could befall a woman whose complicated labor demanded more than routine assistance. In 1647, six months into her fifth pregnancy, Mrs. Thornton suffered a serious fall. Premature labor resulted, and the midwife confidently predicted imminent delivery. Her optimism was unwarranted. Alice later recalled:

The child stayed in the birth [canal], and came cross with his feet first, and this condition continued till Thursday morning between two and three o'clock, at which time I was upon the rack in bearing my child with such exquisite torment, as if each limb were divided from other, for the space of two hours; when at length, being speechless and breathless, I was, by the infinite providence of God, in great mercy delivered.

Unfortunately, disappointment followed the conclusion of this preternatural labor. Thornton lamented:

But I having had such sore travail in danger of my life so long, and the child coming into the world with his feet first, caused the child to be almost strangled in the birth, only living about half an hour. . . . This sweet goodly son was turned wrong by the fall I had got in September before, nor had the midwife skill to turn him right, which was the cause of the loss of his life, and the hazard of my own.[12]

Had Mrs. Thornton's midwife acted in accordance with role expectations, she would have sent for a more expert woman whose greater experience and skill might have enabled her to turn the child and prevent the tragedy. In ordinary, then termed natural, births the fetus begins its passage through the birth canal with the head presenting. This presentation is called cephalic and is the most common. In some cases, however, another part of the fetus may present, such as a foot, an arm, a shoulder, or the buttocks. Of these preternatural positions, the footling presentation was the least likely to provoke serious complications, provided the attendant knew to take hold of the infant's feet and complete the delivery. Far greater risks for both mother and child were posed when a different part of the fetus presented. Then the well-informed and capable midwife might attempt to perform version. This operation consisted of turning the fetus and manipulating it either externally or internally into a podalic presentation so that the child could then be delivered footling.

There is evidence that some midwives performed podalic version. Jane Hawkins, the seventeenth-century midwife who attended Mary Dyer in New England, probably possessed this skill, for Governor John Winthrop recorded that the child "came hiplings till she turned it."[13] Nicholas Culpeper, a "gentleman student in physic and astonomy," believed that midwives should learn version. His *Directory for Midwives* included these directions for coping with the faulty presentation: "Let the Midwife reduce it into the Cavity of the Womb when it comes not forth right, and place it right. . . . When the Feet cannot be thrust upwards, let the Midwife supple the Parts with Oil, and take hold of the Part and help it and give Sneezings."[14] Culpeper's admonition to the midwife to "always labour to put the child in a right Posture" was easier to recommend than to accomplish. Apart from administering "Sneezings" to encourage the mother to bear down, the directions appear at first glance to be straightforward enough. Among women who had no opportunity to study anatomy formally, however, there was gross ignorance of the location and functions of the internal organs of the female.

Laboring to put the child in a right posture could take many forms among the uninitiated. A case described by Edmund Chapman in 1731 makes this point. An arm had presented and when Chapman arrived, it alone ". . . had been 18 hours in the world, and much swelled by the long Time and the Ignorance of the

Midwife, who pulled violently at the Arm every Pain; not knowing that it was altogether impossible to extract a full grown Infant by that Method." Other midwives employed equally useless tactics in cases of malpresentation. Commented Chapman, there was no "Excuse for the Folly of dipping the Infant's Hand, thus hanging out of the Womb, in *Cold Water,* rubbing it with Ice, or touching it with a wet Cloth, which some ignorant Midwives practice in hopes that the Child, upon perceiving the Cold, will presently draw it in again."[15]

Podalic version was always a difficult operation. It required the attendant to insert her hand into the uterus and turn the fetus while the patient's contractions exerted tremendous pressure on the operator's arm and hand. One eighteenth-century surgeon, describing the difficulties inherent in the procedure, wryly observed that "sometimes you will hardly be able to move a single Finger (and is it not amazing that some Authors have wrote about Turning Children with as much Ease as though they were upon a Table?)"[16]

Regardless of the degree of skill attained by midwives, for centuries considerations of propriety and tradition had dictated that men absent themselves from scenes of childbirth. As a general rule, no males, whether husbands, physicians, or surgeons, were welcome in the lying-in chamber. On the continent, the exclusion of men had led to amazing excesses. Howard Haggard cites the case of a German physician named Wertt, who in 1522 assumed a woman's dress so that he might attend and study a case of labor undetected. When his deception was discovered, authorities ordered that Wertt be burned to death. Less dramatic was the fate of Francis Rayus, arrested in Wells, Massachusetts, in 1646 and fined fifty shillings "for presuming to act the part of a midwife." For many years, midwives' oaths in England and the colonies admonished the midwife not to attend women in the presence of men "unless necessity or great urgent cause" compelled her to do so. One historical account from the early 1800s observed that for centuries

It was the fashion to employ women, and none but women, in the momentous process of child-birth. . . . Natural modesty, not always in league with fashion, gave additional force to the general custom, and imperious as was the call for the occasional employment of persons, who had been regularly taught at the schools of anatomy, and had hence acquired a scientific knowledge of the organs concerned in gestation and labour, and of the changes they undergo during these respective processes,—life was in general rather to be sacrificed, than a male practitioner of surgery to be resorted to.[17]

During the mid-seventeenth century, however, this taboo against men began to modify as the surgeon, or "man-midwife," slowly and tentatively opened the door to the lying-in chamber. The generally accepted explanation of the origin of man midwifery is that it began at the French court of Louis XIV. In 1663 Louise de la Vallière, then the king's mistress, is said to have been attended in childbirth by the surgeon Julien Clément; Louis' desire for secrecy about the birth led to the exclusion of the midwives, or sage-femmes. As a reward for his services the king conferred upon Clément the title of "Physician-Accoucheur." Gradually the French nobility began to emulate royalty by employing accoucheurs, and by the early 1700s the fashion had been adopted by some upper-class families in England.[18]

In his historical account of the evolution of man midwifery written in the mid-eighteenth century, William Smellie, probably the best known British accoucheur of his day, paid tribute to the French. In Paris during the time of the great French surgeon Ambroise Paré, explained Smellie, surgery was more advanced than elsewhere in Europe. This Smellie attributed to the opportunities afforded surgeons who worked at the Hôtel Dieu, that infamous institution founded in the seventh century to accommodate the indigent sick. Among the unfortunates admitted to the Hôtel Dieu were pregnant destitute women. There surgeons were afforded the opportunity to attend them, as the women were in no position to object. According to Smellie, the results were fortuitous, for the French surgeons were able to improve their knowledge through practical experience and consequently devise better methods of practice. Summarized Smellie: "The success that attended, which together with the progress of polite literature, that began to flourish about this time in *France,* got the better of those ridiculous prejudices which the fair sex had been used to entertain, and they had recourse to the assistance of men, in all difficult cases of Midwifery."[19]

As William Smellie well knew, however, the "ridiculous prejudices" against men midwives were not so easily overcome. For every English midwife sufficiently expert to cope successfully with the complications of abnormal presentations, there were many more women whose cursory knowledge limited the range of their usefulness to the normal cases that could be managed with little or no interference. Even so, the women's monopoly over midwifery had behind it the potent force of centuries of custom bolstered by deeprooted attitudes and assumptions about modesty, propriety, and appropriate sexual roles. Those who advocated displacing the midwives with trained surgeons would inevitably be compelled to find an effective method of dealing with these cultural tenets. These attitudes included sexist assumptions about the innate physical and intellectual limitations of women. Eighteenth-century Englishwomen and Englishmen alike, irrespective of class, accepted a maledefined view of women that held that however capable they might be in certain prescribed areas, women were neither emotionally, physically, nor intellectually suited to the discipline required in protracted formal study.

The historian who attempts to depict accurately the actual strengths and limitations of the midwives' practice is faced with a paucity of primary sources. Rarely did the women leave written accounts of themselves or of their patients. A few in the seventeenth and eighteenth centuries wrote midwifery manuals. From these we can glimpse their methods. Even here, however, it is not easy to separate the ideal techniques from those that really were employed. As women, most midwives were socialized to view themselves as innately inferior beings, that is, beings whose sexual natures assigned them positions and roles subordinate to those held by men. One consequence was that the literate women who could have left records were unlikely to consider their work worth reading.

Available sources fall into several categories: the complimentary and/or critical references to midwives found in cases reported by male surgeons and physicians; midwives' oaths and official licensing requirements drafted and enforced by an establishment, whether church or state, that was male-defined and controlled; accusations founded in male suspicion that the "mysterious office" of the midwives encouraged the practices of sorcery, witchcraft, abortion, and infanticide; and allusions to the midwives in the occasional autobiography. Particularly in the eighteenth century were added on the one hand exaggerated claims about the midwives' competence, made in defense of woman's domain against encroachments threatened by men midwives, and on the other hand equally unreliable accusations alleging the incompetence of midwives, made by those promoting the cause of the accoucheur. In weighing such evidence it is crucial to keep in mind the obvious limitations of these materials.

Discussing methodology and women's history, Hilda Smith noted the tremendous amount of seventeenth-century medical literature containing negative judgments about women's nature and status. She correctly classified this literature as misogynistic when it contained scurrilous attacks against women and also when it was based on presumptions of feminine incompetence and moral laxity.[20] The tone of English medical literature did not change perceptibly in the following century. Sexist assumptions about women's incompetence are evident in the translator's note inserted by Hugh Chamberlen, who indicated that since he had designed his translation of Mauriceau "chiefly for the Female Sex," he had not bothered "to oppose or comment upon any Physical or Philosophical Position my author proposeth." They are present as well in Edmund Chapman's observation that the value of eighteenth-century obstetric improvements lay in "preserving the FAIR in the time of their greatest Danger; and by that Means, of saving many great and eminent Men who otherwise" would never have been born to serve king and country.[21] It is not always clear when the medical literature cites the deficiencies of midwives whether the observation is based upon direct evidence obtained through interaction or upon a misogynistic position that automatically presumed a correlation between femaleness and incompetence. Cases reported by surgeons who preferred improving the quality of service provided by midwives to driving them from the field would seem to be more reliable assessments.

In early modern England widespread ignorance and misinformation existed in general about medicine, anatomy, physiology, and surgery. The teachings of Aristotle and Galen, which for centuries had held sway over medical thought, were only slowly discredited in the seventeenth century. The work of Thomas Sydenham on clinical observation and experience and that of William Harvey on anatomy, the circulatory system, and related physiological functions were major milestones. Gradually, as doctors began to rely less on medieval authorities and more on their own powers of observation, medical science, including obstetrics, profited.[22] At the same time, superstitions persisted and medieval notions regarding sorcery and witchcraft still were prevalent.

Historically these notions had been important in shaping definitions of women. Throughout the medieval period woman depicted as witch had been a common phenomenon. The classic witch-hunter's manual, *Malleus Maleficarum,* explicitly elaborated the supposed relationship between women's sexuality and their occult powers:

All witchcraft comes from carnal lust, which is in women insatiable. . . . There are three things that are never satisfied, yea a fourth thing which say not, It is enough; that is, the mouth of the womb. Wherefore for the sake of fulfilling their lusts they consort even with devils. . . . it is no matter for wonder that there are more women than men found infected with the heresy of witchcraft. . . . And blessed be the Highest Who has so far preserved the male sex from so great a crime.[23]

Thomas Forbes's fascinating account of British midwives, *The Midwife and the Witch,* details the relationship that existed in the seventeenth-century mind between midwifery and witchcraft. Exploring why women were targets of witch-hunts, Mary Nelson has observed that midwives were especially suspect because as "experts" in birth control, they were likely to cooperate in abortions and infanticides. Anglican church authorities retained these suspicions up to the eighteenth century, as the proscriptions in the midwife's oath clearly indicate. In the essay, "Anne Hutchinson and 'The Revolution that Never Happened'," Carol George noted that the controversial religious figure was another midwife whose activities were described in terms of her sexuality. In light of these perceived relationships it is not surprising to learn of Governor John Winthrop's allegation that

. . . it was known that she used to give young women oil of mandrakes and other stuff to cause conception; and she grew into great suspicion to be a witch, for it was credibly reported, that when she gave any medicine (for she practised physic), she would ask the party, if she did believe, she could help her, etc.[24]

The entire process of reproduction, from gestation to parturition, was still very imperfectly understood as late as the mid-eighteenth century. With so much unanswered, childbirth retained its mysterious aura. Beyond associating midwives with magic, this aura reinforced the view that midwifery really was a woman's office, the secret ministrations of which were best not revealed to men except in the most exceptional of circumstances. The cultural attitudes toward modesty and decorum that contributed to the exclusion of men from the lying-in chamber also tended to prevent the midwives from learning more about their work from the few obstetrical texts in print.

The first obstetrical work available to English midwives in the vernacular was Eucharius Roesslin's *Der Swangern Frawen und Hebammen Rosengarten,* translated by Richard Jonas and printed by Thomas Raynalde in 1540 under the title *The Byrth of Mankynde, Otherwise Named the Womans Booke.* The edition carried an acknowledgment of contemporary criticism:

Many think it is not meet ne fitting such matters to be intreated of so plainly in our mother and vulgar language, to the dishonoure (as they say) of womanhood, and the derision of their own secrets by the detection and discovering whereof *men it reading* shall be moved thereby . . . every boy and knave reading them as openly as the tales of Robin Hood.[25]

More than a hundred years later, Hugh Chamberlen's translation of Mauriceau's treatise (1672) omitted anatomical plates. Observed the translator, there were several such drawings already available in English and, moreover, there was "here and there a passage that might offend a chast English eye."[26] In his second edition (1683), however, Chamberlen "thought fit to add . . . with some little amendments" a section entitled "An Anatomical Treatise of the

Parts of a Woman destin'd to Generation" including four figures detailing the female reproductive system.[27]

This excessive prudery that prevented midwives from improving their knowledge of female anatomy was carried over into the eighteenth century. In the 1730s Edmund Chapman brought out his *Treatise on the Improvement of Midwifery,* written specifically for the edification of experienced midwifery attendants of both sexes. In view of the author's stated purpose, his failure to include either a description of the female reproductive system or a collection of plates is only slightly less remarkable than his explanation of the omissions. After observing that if the reader had not personally witnessed a dissection (a remote possibility for women, at best), written descriptions of anatomy would not be helpful. Chapman's primary concern, however, was one of modesty, for he elaborated his explanation in this amazing passage:

. . . much less would they receive any Advantage from the *Cuts* and *Figures* usually prefixed to Books of this Kind, which are generally but very indifferently done, and serve to raise and encourage *impure* Thoughts in the Reader's Mind, rather than to convey any real *Instruction.* . . . Authors on this Subject already extant in our Language have, in my Opinion, written in a very improper *Style,* and their works seem to be calculated at least, as much to please the Reader's *Fancy,* as to improve the *Operation.* My Design, on the contrary, was to compose such a Treatise as One of either Sex might read without a *Blush,* and to express myself in such a Manner as would not give the least Offence to the most modest Reader.[28]

Even if it were possible to attribute Chapman's position to a self-conscious defense against the critics of men midwives, the inescapable conclusion is that midwives who could not attend anatomical dissections could hardly improve their procedures by reading texts that deliberately omitted the kind of specific information they most needed to acquire.

When one encounters a reference to the "ignorant" midwife in medical literature, it is well to keep in mind realistic comparisons with the abilities of other medical practitioners of the period. To comment that the midwife knew little about anatomy and/or physiology in an age when these areas of knowledge were only then emerging into the world of modern medicine is less a condemnation of the midwife than it would be once the surgeons and anatomists had made their tremendous strides in the eighteenth century.

So long as childbirth continued to be defined as a normal process for women, society did not expect from the midwives a high degree of specialization, especially as the nuances of the process were generally unrecognized. As nature's assistant rather than as prime agent, the "good" midwife was the respectable woman who carried herself correctly, encouraged and supported her patient, and interfered as little as possible in the actual mechanics of the birth. The overwhelming majority of cases were uneventful, just as they are today, so that if she did not resort to meddling tactics through some misguided effort to shorten the duration of the labor or to ease the patient's travail, the midwife was on safe enough ground. She might well practice her art for many years without ever encountering a single case of malpresentation, tedious labor, or other abnormality. Usually she practiced her profession as an adjunct to other economic activities; in no sense was she a career-oriented medical expert. Moreover, regardless of licensing requirements or training—indeed even in the absence of both—her reputation among the local women would be the chief element in determining the size and the duration of her practice. This is not to deny that many of the women who practiced the craft were grossly incompetent, but merely to insist that those fortunate enough to learn from a competent and experienced midwife were capable of managing the normal childbirth despite a lack of formal training.

When the midwife did encounter the rare complicated case, she was expected to recognize this fact. Society then required that she seek assistance from those women who had a superior store of midwifery skills. Frequently in abnormal cases, infants and mothers were lost through the limitations even of those considered experts. It is useful to keep in mind that when midwives appealed to male surgeons, they did so only as a last resort. The surgeon, with no opportunity to attend normal childbirths, knew little about obstetrics, although his knowledge of anatomy was adequate. Usually he employed his surgical skill to save the mother at the expense of the child. Even in cases where the surgeon sacrificed the child, the mother's survival was a major victory when compared to the otherwise inevitable death of both.

As the eighteenth century progressed, abnormal cases received more attention than they had previously. They may in fact have increased in number, partly as the result of accelerated urbanization. Among its undesirable side effects were the unwholesome living conditions and the impoverished diets of the urban working classes. These led to the unfortunate increase in the number of infants and children who suffered from rachitis, or rickets. When the females among these rachitic children grew to womanhood, they were much more apt to suffer malformed pelvic structure. Such malformation produced complications at parturition. At the point where medical thought began to comprehend what constituted the normal female pelvic structure and to understand the normal parturient process, this information could be utilized in developing procedures to cope with abnormal cases. The disparity between those men who were able to obtain this knowledge and the women from whom it was kept would then be much more evident, and the midwives would indeed appear inadequate by comparison.

In Stuart England, long before such comparisons were viable, there were a few people who for various reasons displayed an interest in the midwives and their practice. Members of the Chamberlen family, with whom one associates the secret use of forceps, were well known to the midwives because of the assistance they occasionally gave in difficult cases. In 1616 Peter Chamberlen the Elder and his brother, known as Peter Chamberlen the Younger, petitioned James I to incorporate the midwives. By then, physicians, surgeons, and apothecaries all had their own corporations, which acted as regulatory bodies. James and his advisors referred the Chamberlens's request to the College of Physicians, which opposed it. A corporation for the midwives, ''a thing not exampled in any Commonwealth,'' observed the college, was neither necessary nor convenient.[29]

In the following generation, Dr. Peter Chamberlen III, apparently in a self-serving effort to make himself governor of the midwives, also attempted incorporation. Again the College of Physicians opposed the idea. Of even greater interest is the position taken by the midwives themselves, who were then under the jurisdiction of the episcopacy. The women's objections, which they sent to the bishops, clearly indicate how determined they were to maintain the distinction between midwifery and other aspects of medical practice. Chamberlen was a specialist from whom the midwives occasionally sought help "as a phisicion more peculiarly applying himself to the practise thereof than others," but they nevertheless denied absolutely any dependence upon him.[30]

Basically the midwives had three principal objections to his proposal. Dr. Chamberlen, they insisted, could not teach them the art of midwifery as it applied to normal births "because he hath no experience in itt but by reading." Women who desired to learn the craft needed the experience that could be gained only through "continual practise" in attending normal cases. They must be present at many deliveries and observe "the worke and behavior of such as be skilfull midwifes who will shew and direct them and resolve their doubts." Their work, they insisted, was "contrary" to that of Chamberlen. They did not use instruments, nor had they any desire to do so, having "neither parts nor hands for that art." Chamberlen, on the other hand, delivered "none without the use of instruments by extraordinary violence in desperate occasions." Evidently these women considered Chamberlen's instrumental approach far beyond the scope of normal midwifery requirements. As for his suggestion that he teach them more about anatomy, they rejected this as well. Anatomical demonstrations and lectures were of little value to the midwife, they maintained, unless the subject of the dissection were a pregnant or post-partum woman. The English law that made felons available for anatomical dissections exempted gravid women. Thus, reasoned the midwives, any possible anatomical demonstration Chamberlen could present would be irrelevant to their purposes. Added the women, books on anatomy were available in English and literate midwives could learn more from them than from Chamberlen's "learned lectures." In the end the bishops not only rejected the Chamberlen plan but also told him to apply to the Lord Bishop of London for a midwifery license![31]

Similar disdain for formal learning as a means to effective obstetrical performance appeared in *The Midwives Book* (1671). Authored by Jane Sharp after over thirty years in practice, the work was the first written by an English midwife. Sharp took note of the criticism some had leveled against the midwives and admitted that women lacked the theoretical knowledge available to men:

Some perhaps may think, that . . . it is not proper for women to be of this profession, because they cannot attain so rarely to the knowledge of things as men may, who are bred up in Universities, Schools of Learning or serve their Apprenticeship for that end and purpose, where Anatomy Lectures being frequently read the situation of the parts both of men and women . . . are often made plain to them.[32]

She maintained, nevertheless, that midwifery was legitimately woman's business. It was not necessary that midwives be given university educations nor be instructed in foreign languages in order that they might read the treatises of learned authorities.

It is not hard words that perform the work, as if none understood the Art that cannot understand Greek. Words are but the shell. . . . It is commendable for men to employ their spare time in some things of deeper Speculation than is required of the female sex; but the art of Midwifery chiefly concerns us.[33]

Even the name man-midwife, observed Sharp, was borrowed from the women.[34]

Sharp's book was one of several that appeared late in the seventeenth century in an attempt to instruct the women. Nicholas Culpeper's *Directory for Midwives,* according to its author, was a practical and easily comprehended text. He assured midwives that his "Rules . . . are very plain, and easy enough; neither are they so many, that they will burden your Brain, nor so few that they will be insufficient for your Necessity." Culpeper, far from an admirer of men in the birth chamber, hoped that his work would eliminate male surgeons from midwifery. He promised the women that if they followed his directions carefully, they would find their work easy, and they would not need to "call for the help of a Man Midwife, which is a Disparagement, not only to your selves, but also to your Profession." Unlike some of the manuals then available to women, this *Directory* contained specific anatomical detail of the female reproductive system. Culpeper believed strongly that women needed this information and hoped that they would profit from it.[35]

Claiming to be the "real friend" of the English "ladies and gentlewomen" to whom it was dedicated, the author of *Dr. Chamber-*

lains' Midwifes Practice [probably Dr. Paul Chamberlen (1635-1717)] explained his motivation for writing. "A great many Women," he charged, "(not wanting ignorance nor impudence) presume to take upon them this Mysterious Office." Lacking proper knowledge, these women "rashly" took on cases and in so doing endangered many lives. Chamberlen boasted that by leading the reader through nature's "most Meandering Labyrinths in the Conception, Procreation and Birth of Mankind, [his book] distinctly and plainly laid open the *Anatomicall* part thereof." Chamberlen was familiar with the rival *Directory* of Culpeper, which he characterized as "Carping Nonsense." He accused "quacking Culpeper" of wishing chiefly to "rail at the Learned, rather than any wayes to instruct the Ignorant," an attack motivated perhaps by Culpeper's opinion that doctors were lazy men, "most of whose Covetousness outweighs their Wits."[36] In any case, Chamberlen did agree with Culpeper's opinion that the midwives needed to know more about anatomy.

Hugh Chamberlen's edition of François Mauriceau's treatise also appeared late in the 1600s. Chamberlen had at first planned to bring out a "small Manual" of his own but decided instead to translate Mauriceau's *Traite des Maladies des Femmes Grosses* into English for the benefit of the midwives. Chamberlen was correct in his assessment of the work as far superior to all others, including Culpeper and Sharp. Mauriceau's treatise was unquestionably the most practical, explicit, and accurate of the obstetrical texts, and it enjoyed great popularity among English surgeons and physicians. The literate midwife who read it with care could learn much about her art. Yet, useful as this work was, Chamberlen realized that the mere reading of it could not alone produce a competent midwife. Books, however excellent they might be, could not substitute for training and experience. As Chamberlen made clear, he did not intend his work "to encourage any to practise by it, who were not bred up to it; for it will hardly make a Midwife, tho it may easily mend a bad one."[37]

Similar views were expressed early in the 1730s by Edmund Chapman, who after twenty-seven years as a surgeon and man-midwife published his *Treatise on the Improvement of Midwifery*. Chapman had designed his book "chiefly for the Use of the . . . [women] to whom the Majority of Practice in this important and difficult Profession is committed." He explained that his work was not for the novice but would be useful to experienced attendants "whose Profession has already led them to make some Progress in this Science."[38] Adding to the midwives' knowledge of anatomy was not among Chapman's purposes, however, for it will be recalled that he had deliberately omitted plates and descriptions to avoid embarrassment to his readers.

By the time Chapman's work appeared, some critics of the midwives had already suggested that the women be replaced. Chapman alluded to these critics but disclaimed any association with their position. "I am far from attempting or desiring, with some of my Brethren," he wrote, "that the Practice of *Midwifery* should be confin'd to my own SEX." The reasons he advanced are important, especially since Chapman was writing from long experience in a practice that gave him many opportunities to work with and to observe the midwives:

"First, Because among so great a Number of Child-bearing Women, of all Degrees, a much greater Attendance is required, than we alone could possibly give. Besides, where the Labour is natural, as it happens with most Women, there is seldom any greater Assistance necessary than what those of their own Sex, who have been bred up to it, are capable of affording; especially in this *Metropolis,* where I have met with several extremely well-qualified."[39]

It is interesting that although Chapman was one of the first to formally teach midwifery in London, nowhere in his book does he mention women among his students. As a specialist in difficult cases he expected that the male practitioners whom he trained would leave the normal cases to the midwives but be available to provide superior assistance when it was needed. Interested as he was in keeping the midwives in practice, he had not the slightest intention of turning women into practitioners capable of coping with cases other than normal.[40]

For over a century obstetrical practitioners had decried the general ignorance of the English midwives. Doctor Peter Chamberlen was appalled by the midwives he encountered in the course of his seventeenth-century London practice. These women, he opined, were "neither . . . sufficiently instructed in doing good, nor restrained from doing evil."[41] William Harvey, whose interest in midwifery is overshadowed by his contributions to our knowledge of the circulatory system, wrote several texts on obstetrics, the best known of which was *Exercitatio de Partu.* Harvey and his close friend Dr. Percival Willughby, author of the *Country Midwife's Opusculum,* commented on the methods employed by contemporary midwives. They found most reprehensible their attempts to shorten labor by resorting in desperation to the use of crude, makeshift instruments, such as pothooks and knives. "To save their credits and cloak their ignorances," charged Willughby, the midwives subjected their patients to grave hazards by refusing to send for help in complicated cases.[42] These lamentable conditions had not improved in the century that followed. In 1727 John Maubray, writing in *The Female Physician,* commented that male "extraordinary midwives," or, to use his preferred term, "Andro-Boethogynists," were "seldom or never called but in extraordinary cases of difficult or preternatural births." Even so, when they arrived it was not easy for them to get the desired cooperation from the midwives, to whom Maubray referred disparagingly as "such obstinate creatures."[43]

William Hunter (1718-1783), the anatomist and obstetrician, was no less critical of the midwives of his day. Extremely conservative in his own practice, he observed:

"[the midwives] cram their patients with cordials, keeping them intoxicated during the time they are in labour, driving poor women up and down stairs, notwithstanding their shrieks, and shaking them so violently as often to bring on convulsive fits on pretence of hastening their labours, laughing at their cries, and breaking wretched jests upon the contortions of the women, whose torments would make a feeling man shudder at the sight.[44]

The men were not alone in making these criticisms. Knowledgeable midwives were aware of the deficiencies of their sister practitioners. Sarah Stone, an experienced and respected midwife herself, had read anatomy and attended dissections. She wrote vividly of the blundering country midwife who had delayed so long in sending for help that when Mrs. Stone arrived, she found "the child with one eye out, and the whole face injured, having no skin left on it, and the upper lip tore quite hollow from the jawbone." Deploring such ignorance, she recommended a remedy that would require midwives to be employed "three years at least with some ingenious woman in practising this art." Reasoned Mrs. Stone, "if seven years must be served to learn a trade, I think three years as little as possible to be instructed in an art where life depends."[45]

In response to the critics who railed against "ignorant" midwives, John Douglas, a surgeon, published in 1736 *A Short Account of The State of Midwifery in London.* He proposed that the "midwomen" be given a means by which they might "qualify themselves thoroughly . . . at a moderate expense." The women, he thought, would readily agree to a "reasonable" expenditure of time and money in order "to be so thoroughly instructed." Such decisions, reflected Douglas, did not lie within the women's power. Succinctly he summarized the problem: "The midwomen cannot, and the midmen will not instruct them. The midmen will object and say that the midwomen want both capacity and strength (instruct them as ye please)."[46]

To these objections Douglas himself did not subscribe. He pointed out that French women trained in midwifery at the Hôtel Dieu in Paris exhibited ample ability both to learn and to perform their craft. It was absurd to argue that English women, given the same instruction, would demonstrate less "capacity, docility, strength, or activity" than did the sage-femmes. Douglas then set forth a proposal calling for regular and "proper instruction" of the women, to be followed by examinations conducted by two surgeons who had lectured to them, along with "six or seven other persons appointed by His Majesty, because I don't think it reasonable that so many people's bread should depend on the humour and caprice of two men only." If this scheme were executed, predicted this confident surgeon, within "a very few years there would not be an ignorant midwife in England, and consequently the great agonies most women suffer at the very sight of a man would be almost entirely prevented, and great expense and much life saved."[47]

This proposal, unfortunately never adopted, reveals one surgeon's insight, as perceptive as it was unusual, into the midwives' dilemma as it had evolved by the first quarter of the eighteenth century. The theoretical understandings and the practical obstetrical experience of the men- midwives was on the increase. By contrast, women continued to learn their craft on a catch-as-catch-can basis. When compared to the surgeons, even women formerly considered adequate to attend normal births would soon be regarded as deficient. The taboo against men in the birth chamber was still sufficiently strong to frighten and embarrass women forced to employ accoucheurs in abnormal cases. At the same time, however, society's male-oriented definition of women as innately inferior beings worked against solutions such as Douglas's that would have provided the midwives with the formal training necessary to upgrade their practice. In 1730 normal cases remained the province of women. In the next quarter century this monopoly would be threatened. Precluded by sexual definitions from attending universities, walking the hospital wards, or learning surgery in the military services, the women would need to find new definitions for themselves and for their art if they hoped to continue in their mysterious office.

NOTES

1. Exodus 1: 15-19.
2. Percival Willughby, quoted in Irving S. Cutter and Henry R. Viets, *A Short History of Midwifery,* 1st ed. (Philadelphia and London: W. B. Saunders Co., 1964), p. 7.
3. John Maubray, *The Female Physician,* quoted in Cutter and Viets, *Short History,* p. 13.
4. Andrew Boorde, *The Breviary of Helthe* (1547), quoted in Thomas R. Forbes, *The Midwife and the Witch* (New Haven and London: Yale University Press, 1966), pp. 140-150; Sophia Jex-Blake, *Medical Women: A Thesis and a History* (Edinburgh: Oliphant, Anderson & Ferrier, 1886; London: Hamilton, Adams and Co., 1886; New York: Source Book Press Reprint, 1970), pp. 16-17.
5. J. H. Aveling, *English Midwives: Their History and Their Prospects* (London: Churchill, 1872), pp. 90-93; Forbes, *Midwife and Witch,* pp. 146-147. The item dealing with paternity relates to the English common law that required mothers of children born out of wedlock to name the rightful fathers, who were then responsible for support. Edmund Morgan cites in-

stances in which women, unwilling to burden their lovers with financial obligations, falsely assigned paternity to another, often wealthier man. Similar cases in England would account for the inclusion of this item. See Edmund Morgan, "The Puritans and Sex," in Jean Friedman and William Shade, *Our American Sisters,* 2nd ed. (Boston: Allyn and Bacon, 1976), pp. 17-18. Forbes's version of the midwives' oath is taken from the anonymous Book of Oaths issued in 1649, whereas the eighteenth-century version is given in Aveling.

6. Aveling, *Midwives,* p. 93; Forbes, *Midwife and Witch,* plates 1-8, facing pp. 144-145.

7. Samuel Merriman, "On the Art of Midwifery as Exercised by Medical Practitioners in Reply to Dr. Kinglake," *London Medical and Physical Journal* 35 (April 1816):289.

8. William Nicholson, "Midwifery," *The British Encyclopedia or Dictionary of Arts & Sciences,* Vol. 8, 3rd American ed. (Philadelphia: Mitchell Ames and White, 1821), no pagination; Cutter and Viets, *Short History,* p. 186.

9. Medical licensing in London and the provinces underwent substantial alterations between the sixteenth and nineteenth centuries. The brief summary in this chapter was drawn primarily from the following sources: Wallace Notestein, *The English People on the Eve of Colonization, 1603-1630* (New York: Harper & Brothers, 1954), chapter 9; Joseph F. Kett, "Provincial Medical Practice in England, 1730-1815," *Journal of the History of Medicine and Allied Sciences* 19 (January 1964):17-29; Bonnie Bullough and Vern Bullough, "A Brief History of Medical Practice," in Elliot Friedson and Judith Lorber, *Medical Men and Their Work* (New York: Aldine-Atherton, 1972), pp. 86-102.

10. Percival Willughby, quoted in Cutter and Viets, *Short History,* p. 50.

11. John Maubray, *The Female Physician,* quoted in Cutter and Viets, *Short History,* p. 13.

12. Alice Thornton, "The Autobiography of Mrs. Alice Thornton, of East Newton, Co. of York," in Joan Goulianos, ed., *by a Woman Writt: Literature from Six Centuries By and About Women* (Baltimore: Penguin Books, 1974), pp. 45-46.

13. John Winthrop, *History of New England,* Volume 1, quoted in Frances R. Packard, *History of Medicine in the United States,* Vol. 1 (New York: Hafner, 1963), p. 45.

14. Nicholas Culpeper, *A Directory for Midwives: Or, A Guide for Women, In their Conception, Bearing, and Suckling their Children . . .* (London: Norris, Bettesworth, Ballard and Batley, 1724), p. 297.

15. Edmund Chapman, *Treatise on the Improvement of Midwifery . . . ,* 3rd ed. (London: L. David and C. Reymers, 1759), pp. 111, 113.

16. Benjamin Pugh, *A Treatise of Midwifery, chiefly with regard to the Operation, with several improvements in that ART . . .* (London: J. Buckland, 1754), p. 44.

17. Howard W. Haggard, *Devils, Drugs and Doctors,* 4th ed. (New York: Pocket Books, Inc., 1959), p. 30; Collections of the Maine Historical Society, in Samuel Gregory, *Letter to Ladies in Favor of Female Physicians* (New York: Fowler and Wells, 1850), p. 26; Aveling, *Midwives,* p. 93; Nicholson, "Midwifery," in *British Encyclopedia,* Vol. 8, no pagination.

18. See, for example, W. Goodell, "When and Why Were Male Physicians Employed as Accoucheurs?" *American Journal of Obstetrics and the Diseases of Women and Children* 9 (August 1876):381-390; H. D. King, "The Evolution of the Male Midwife with Some Remarks on the Obstetrical Literature of Other Ages," *American Journal of Obstetrics and Gynecology* 77 (February 1918):177-186; William F. Mangert, "The Origin of the Male Midwife," *Annals of Medical History,* n.s. 4 (September 1932):453-465; R. W. Johnstone, *William Smellie: The Master of British Midwifery* (Edinburgh and London: E. & S. Livingstone Ltd., 1952), p. 30. In a revision of this view, George Bancroft-Livingstone, "Louise de la Vallière and the Birth of the Man Midwife," *Journal of Obstetrics and Gynaecology of the British Commonwealth,* n.s. 63 (April 1956):261-267, suggests that it was a male surgeon by the name of Boucher, rather than Clément, who delivered the child.

19. William Smellie, *A Treatise on the Theory and Practice of Midwifery,* 3rd ed. (London: D. Wilson and T. Durham, 1756), pp. liv-lv.

20. Hilda Smith, "Feminism and the Methodology of Women's History," in Berenice A. Carroll, *Liberating Women's History: Theoretical and Critical Essays* (Urbana, Chicago, and London: University of Illinois Press, 1976), p. 375. On methodology and women's history in general, see Gerda Lerner, "Placing Women in History: Definitions and Challenges," *Feminist Studies* 3 (Fall 1975):1-14.

21. Hugh Chamberlen, "Translator to the Reader," in François Mauriceau, *Diseases of Women with Child, and in Child-bed,* 2nd ed., trans. Hugh Chamberlen (London: John Darby, 1683), no pagination; Chapman, *Treatise,* p. 68.

22. Arturo Castiglioni, *A History of Medicine,* 2nd ed., trans. E. B. Krumbhaar (New York: Knopf, 1958), Chapter 17; Johnstone, *Smellie,* p. 30.

23. Jacob Sprenger and Henry Krämer, *Malleus Maleficarum,* trans. M. Summers (Suffolk, England: John Rodker, 1928), quoted in Mary Nelson, "Why Women Were Witches," in Jo Freeman, ed., *Women: A Feminist Perspective* (Palo Alto, Calif.: Mayfield Publishing Co., 1975), p. 339.

24. Forbes, *Midwife and Witch,* Chapter 10; Nelson, "Why Women

Were Witches," p. 339; Carol V. R. George, "Anne Hutchinson and 'The Revolution that Never Happened,' " in Carol V. R. George, ed., *"Remember the Ladies": New Perspectives on Women in American History* (Syracuse, N.Y.: Syracuse University Press, 1975), pp. 15-17. The association between lay women healers and witchcraft allegations is also explored by Barbara Ehrenreich and Deirdre English, *Witches, Midwives and Nurses: A History of Women Healers* (Old Westbury, N.Y.: The Feminist Press, 1973), pp. 4-18. These authors suggest that the medieval church's attack on empiricist healers was an attempt to retain control over the general populace. "In the persecution of the witch," they assert, "the anti-empiricist and misogynist, anti-sexual obsessions of the church coincide: Empiricism and sexuality both represent a surrender to the senses, a betrayal of faith" (p. 13). Adrienne Rich asserts that this misogyny "attached itself to the birth-process, so that males were forbidden to attend at births" because the church fathers "saw woman—especially her reproductive organs—as evil incarnate." See Adrienne Rich, *Of Woman Born: Motherhood as Experience and Institution* (New York: W. W. Norton & Co., Inc., 1976), p. 134.

25. Castiglioni, *History of Medicine,* pp. 481-482; Cutter and Viets, *Short History,* p. 4; Jex-Blake, *Medical Women,* p. 17n.

26. Hugh Chamberlen, quoted in Hilda Smith, "Gynecology and Ideology in Seventeenth-Century England," in Berenice A. Carroll, ed., *Liberating Women's History: Theoretical and Critical Essays* (Urbana, Chicago, and London: University of Illinois Press, 1976), p. 111.

27. Mauriceau, *Diseases,* pp. 1-13.

28. Chapman, *Treatise,* pp. xx-xxi.

29. Aveling, *Midwives,* quoted in Cutter and Viets, *Short History,* p. 46.

30. Ibid., p. 49.

31. Cutter and Viets, *Short History,* pp. 46-49.

32. Jane Sharp, *The Midwives Book or the Whole Art of Midwifery,* quoted in Hilda Smith, "Gynecology and Ideology in Seventeenth Century England," in Carroll, *Women's History,* p. 112.

33. Ibid.

34. Jex-Blake, *Medical Women,* p. 19.

35. Culpeper, Directory, p. A-3.

36. [Paul Chamberlen?], *Dr. Chamberlain's Midwifes Practice: or a Guide for Women in the High Concern of Conception, Breeding, and Nursing Children* (London: Thomas Books, 1665), quoted in Cutter and Viets, *Short History,* pp. 52-53; Culpeper, *Directory,* p. A-2.

37. Hugh Chamberlen, "Translator to the Reader," in Mauriceau, *Diseases,* no pagination; Cutter and Viets, *Short History,* pp. 77-78.

38. Chapman, *Treatise,* p. viii.

39. Ibid., pp. x-xi.

40. Ibid., p. xxiv.

41. Quoted in Aveling, *Midwives,* p. 24.

42. Ibid., pp. 35-38.

43. Herbert R. Spencer, *The History of British Midwifery from 1650-1800* (London: John Bale Sons and Danielsson, 1927), pp. 7-8.

44. Aveling, *Midwives,* pp. 125-126.

45. Quoted in John Kobler, *The Reluctant Surgeon* (London: Heinemann, 1960), p. 31.

46. John Douglas, *Short Account of the State of Midwifery in London, Westminster, &c.* (1736), quoted in Jex-Blake, *Medical Women,* p. 22.

47. Ibid., pp. 22-23.

2

The "Seasonable Help" of the Men Midwives

The Improvements these great Men have made in MIDWIFERY, the Tenderness, the Compassion and Success with which they performed their Duty, have effectually removed that Load of Ignominy, with which this Profession was formerly branded.

—EDMUND CHAPMAN, *A TREATISE ON THE IMPROVEMENT OF MIDWIFERY*, 1759

When Hugh Chamberlen translated Mauriceau's treatise into English, he did so out of the conviction that the midwives needed to upgrade the quality of their practice. Admonishing the women to "learn from this what you should know," Chamberlen hoped that they would become sufficiently informed about their work so as to be capable of distinguishing accurately between what was "properly their Work" and what was not. Countless women and children perished every year, alleged the translator, from the failure of the midwives to make this distinction. The skillful midwife must separate those cases constituting "a right Labour" from the dangerous ones demanding a call for "seasonable help." As an aid to determining when they should "send for Physicians that are expert in this Practice," Chamberlen set these guidelines:

Most wrong Births, with or without Pain; all Floodings [hemorrhages] with Clods, tho little or no pain, whether at full time, or not: all Convulsions;

and many first Labours; and some others, tho the Child be right [not mal-positioned] if little or no pain after the breaking of the Waters, and the Child's not following them in some six or ten hours after.[1]

An experienced practitioner, Hugh Chamberlen was well aware of the then prevalent antipathy toward men midwives. Largely responsible for the aversion, he thought, was the surgeons' practice of using hooks to extract even the correctly positioned fetus whose birth was impeded by reason of some difficulty or disproportion in the mother. It was this operation, justified by Mauriceau and commonly employed in England, claimed Chamberlen, that had "very much caused the Report, that where a *Man comes one* or *both must necessarily die*; and is the reason why many forbear sending [for the surgeon] till the child is dead, or the Mother dying."[2]

A further contribution to the resistance was a fear among midwives that employing men would cause gossip, thus damaging their own reputation. Chamberlen vehemently denied the validity of this, urging "the good Women, not to be so ready to blame those Midwives, who are not backward in dangerous cases to desire advice." Continued criticism would be costly, he warned, discouraging the careful midwives and "forcing them to presume beyond their knowledge or strength, especially when there are but too-too-many overconfident." The principal duty of the midwife, he maintained, consisted not merely in "laying the Woman" but in doing so in a manner permitting "safety and convenient speed." When this was impossible for the midwife, yet "seasible by another," it was incumbent upon her to wave "her imaginary Reputation" and to send for help. It could not be nearly "so great a discredit to a Midwife (let some of them imagine what they please) to have a Woman or Child saved by a Man's insistance, as to suffer either to die under her own hand."[3]

That the resistance to men-midwives was not easily overcome is evident by the comments of surgeons in the next few decades. William Giffard was an innovative and experienced surgeon and man midwife. His *Cases in Midwifery,* published posthumously in 1734, described practical procedures clearly and succinctly. Case 46 is a description of a footling presentation that the midwife was unable to deliver. Commented Giffard, "This Case should be a Caution to Midwives, to send for help in time, when a Child comes Footling, and not to venture (unless they are very skilful) to bring it forwards."[4] Similar cautions were issued by Edmund Chapman, a contemporary of Giffard's, who like him practiced for many years in London. Chapman warned the midwives that the complications attending preternatural and tedious labors were so great that they must always be on the alert for them. He urged them to call upon men midwives for help even in cephalic presentations if the woman's contractions were not strong enough to accomplish the birth without some manual assistance. Other cases requiring male assistance were those of faulty presentation, where "the Child requires Turning," and all those accompanied by "Floodings" or hemorrhages, "a Rock on which many of the Sex are lost." Reiterating the theme elaborated by Chamberlen fifty years earlier, Chapman insisted that the best midwives were those who quickly recognized cases in which they would need "Superior Assistance" and called for help in sufficient time. In so doing they enhanced their own reputations as knowledgeable and responsible attendants. Chapman regretted that not all of the midwives were this amenable. Some "conceiving too favourable an Opinion of their own Judgment and Abilities, run great Hazards, or at the best, call us in too late, and thus lose their Reputation and Practice," lamented the surgeon.[5]

In 1733, when Chapman's first edition appeared, man midwifery was in its infancy and most birth attendants still were women. In nearly thirty years of practice, Chapman had seen and worked with many capable midwives whose work he admired. His avowed intention in producing his *Treatise* was to improve the skills of experienced practitioners, both male and female. Yet, in an interesting passage, he observed that version was a very difficult skill to acquire and counseled women not to attempt it:

I deny not, but that many Women-Midwives may know how to turn a Child, nor that they may, in some Subjects, perform it with Success. But then . . . [consider] the many unforseen Difficulties that may happen, especially the Head's sticking against the Bones of the Pelvis . . . in spite of the greatest Care and the most exact Position.[6]

Such skepticism concerning the abilities of midwives was very much in keeping with the sexist attitudes of the age. Some women might occasionally succeed in performing version, but these successes were due to chance. The inherent limitations imposed on women by their very femaleness would not allow them to cope with any unexpected crisis; women should, therefore, avoid placing themselves in situations with which they were unable to cope. In 1724 John Maubray, who was one of the first surgeons to teach midwifery to male students, openly expressed misogynistic opinions with his reservations. Arguing that men should be called in for abnormal cases, Maubray reasoned: "MEN . . . being better versed in *Anatomy,* better acquainted with *Physical Helps,* and commonly endued with greater *Presence of Mind,* have been always found readier or discreeter, to devise something more *new,* and to give quicker *Relief* in Cases of *difficult* or *preternatural* BIRTHS, than common MIDWIVES generally understand.[7]

Maubray's "common midwives" were continuing, of course, to dominate obstetrical practice, routinely delivering normal cases and caring for mothers and infants during the period of confinement. The male surgeon, whose assistance "was seldom solicited . . . till the last extremity,"[8] continued to be an unwelcome visitor to the lying-in chamber. With almost no opportunities to attend normal births, the men midwives understood little about the mechanics of labor; their assistance remained surgical. Those with the education and inclination to do so might have read the writers of antiquity, and therein discovered with William Smellie "several valuable jewels buried under the rubbish of ignorance and superstition." Soranus of Ephesus (second century A.D.) was the leading authority on obstetrics and gynecology in antiquity. Medical historians have traced to him many of the supposed innovations, such as the use of obstetrical chairs and podalic version, that appeared in Röesslin's *Rosengarten* (1513) and Raynalde's *Byrth of Mankynde* (1540). By the time the Byzantine physician Paul of Aegina (625-690) summarized what was then known about obstetrics and gynecology in his seven volume *Epitome,* podalic version had fallen into disuse and Paul made no reference to it. In the sixteenth century the French surgeon Ambroise Paré revised the technique and strongly recommended it in *De la Génération de l'Homme* (1550).[9] In the next century podalic version was employed in England by men midwives, and as we have seen, occasionally by women midwives. It was regarded generally as a surgical operation.

A knowledgeable attendant who recognized a case of faulty presentation but who was unwilling or unable to attempt the operation herself might then resort to a man midwife. He would try to turn the fetus and deliver footling. Podalic version remained a popular operation with the surgeons throughout the 1700s and after. One experienced and innovative operator at mid-century termed it "the best and surest Method of Relief." He recommended its use for all preternatural postures, for natural presentation accompanied by maternal hemorrhaging, convulsions, or excessive weakness that threatened either her life or that of the child, and for cases in which the operator found it necessary to extract a dead fetus.[10]

In view of the unsatisfactory alternatives available to treat laborious and preternatural cases, it is little wonder that the man midwife acquired and continued to carry with him the aura of death. If he were unable to turn an incorrectly positioned child, or if the mother's pelvis were malformed—too narrow, perhaps, to accommodate the fetal head—or if some other complication appeared, the surgeon would then resort to his bag of iron implements. This bag contained "a sharp-pointed extractor called the crotchets, together with a pair of long small scissars [sic] with stops in the middle of their blades, for drawing the child dead from the womb [and] a double blunt hook for assisting in the deliverying of the child, whether it be alive or dead in the womb." These instruments were designed to enable the operator to save the life of the mother by sacrificing that of the child. When protracted labor or some other cause resulted in the death of the fetus in utero—indeed even in cases where the fetus was not yet dead—the attending surgeon would perform an embryotomy—usually a craniotomy—to relieve the mother's suffering. Using these devices singly or in combination, he would decapitate the fetus in utero, perforate the skull, and empty it of its contents. Alternately, he might first amputate the protruding portion of the fetal anatomy that impeded progress through the birth canal before proceeding with the necessary reduction of the fetal skull.[11]

Embryotomies were terrifying, dangerous, and painful operations for women. Nor were they desirable from the viewpoint of the surgeon. They were, however, considered unavoidable at times. Because they called for surgical skill and a more accurate knowledge of female anatomy than the midwives were in a position to obtain, as well as courage and strength, which women were not expected to possess, these operations normally fell within the province of the men midwives. Hugh Chamberlen reported that some English midwives boasted of attempting embryotomies. He condemned this "rash presumption" among the women and pointedly noted that such action "in *France*, would call them in question for their Lives."[12]

William Smellie, whose many obstetrical contributions helped to reduce the number of infants sacrificed, nevertheless believed embryotomy at times was the only recourse. In the belief that all men midwives would be called upon to perform the operation at some time, he provided the student with explicit instructions. He was first to introduce his hand into the vagina and then:

> press two fingers against one of the sutures of the *Cranium*; then take out his scissars and guiding them by the hand and fingers till they reach the hairy scalp, push them gradually into it. . . . The scissars ought to be so sharp at the points, as to penetrate the integuments and bones when pushed with a moderate force; but no[t] so keen as to cut the operator's fingers, or the *Vagina*. . . .
> The scissars being thus forced into the brain, let them be kept firm in that situation . . . the operator must take hold of the handles . . . and pull them asunder . . . by which means the opening will be enlarged and sufficient room made for the introduction of the fingers.[13]

If the perforating scissors did not accomplish the task, the surgeon was then to introduce the crotchet within the opening in the skull. Having perforated the skull and destroyed the brain, the operator could then withdraw the instruments. Smellie warned of the importance of then inserting "two fingers into the opening which hath been made, that if any sharp splinters of the bones remain, they may be broken off and taken out; lest they should injure the woman's *Vagina,* or the operator's own fingers." The collapsed skull and the remainder of the fetus finally could be extracted.

The basic procedures in this operation remained largely unchanged well into the nineteenth century. The syllabus of lectures on midwifery delivered at Guy's Hospital in London in 1799 recommended using the perforator, crotchet, and blunt hook in essentially the same manner as that described by Smellie half a century earlier. There too the surgeon was cautioned about the necessity of "guarding against injury to the woman from the slipping of the instrument—in removing separated portions of the bone with care, etc."[14] The woman's anguish was heightened by the fact that the embryotomy was performed entirely without benefit of anesthesia, for chloroform and ether were as yet unknown in surgical operations. Authors on midwifery alluded often to the injuries the operator might inflict on the mother out of ineptness. The danger that the instrument would slip and rupture the vagina or other soft tissue was ever present. Given the limitations of surgery at the time, resultant injuries such as vesicovaginal or rectovaginal fistulas (tears between the bladder or the rectum and the vagina) were irreparable. Thus the woman who survived the operation but sustained an internal injury might be condemned to years of agony and embarrassment. Horrifying as we find these graphic descriptions even in the abstract, it is not difficult to imagine the terror with which the patient received the approach of the man midwife. Nor could it have been comforting to realize that the embryotomy he proposed was a final effort to save her own life. Little wonder that William Smellie advised young practitioners to conceal their instruments before they addressed their patients![15]

The most experienced of surgeons found these operations unsettling and exhausting. Smellie recounts that in some of his cases the mother's pelvis was so narrow or distorted that even after he had opened the fetal head and pulled at the bones during contractions, he was unable to extract the fetus. He then found it necessary to fix one crotchet, and occasionally a second, to the chin or base of the skull. "Using a good deal of force," he could then accomplish his aim. Particularly before the curved crotchets were developed to replace the straight models, the instruments continually slipped their hold and greatly "fatigued" the operator. In the aftermath of these especially rigorous embryotomies, Smellie reported, "I have scarcely been able to move my fingers or arms, for many hours . . . [yet] if this force had not been used, the mother must have been lost as well as the child."[16] Even so, Smellie was sensitive to the criticism of those who condemned as dangerous all use of the crotchet. Inclined to ascribe such charges to "ignorance, want of experience, or a worse principle," he insisted that he "never tore or hurt the parts of a woman with that instrument." By the same token he maintained, however, that he had "several times hurt the inside" of his own hand, such accidents occurring before he had begun to use the curved crotchet.[17]

Unwelcome and dangerous as embryotomies were, patients and surgeons unfortunately had almost no other recourse in treating preternatural and laborious cases. The cesarean section or cesarotomy, that is, removing the fetus from the uterus through an incision made in the lower abdomen of the mother, was a highly unsatisfactory alternative. This operation was almost never attempted while the mother was still alive. In an age lacking both anesthesia and a knowledge of aseptic and antiseptic techniques, the accompanying shock to the patient and the risks of infection were so horrendous as to cause all but the most foolhardy of surgeons to avoid proposing cesarotomy. Those cases of cesarean section alluded to in medical writings prior to the fifteenth century probably were performed on mothers already dead. A recent study reviewing the importance of the operation as a means of securing the fetus for baptism within the Roman Catholic Church cites a resurgence of interest in the eighteenth century. Between 1769 and 1833, according to the study, Franciscan Fathers in Alta California performed fourteen cesarean sections. In every case the mother had died before the operation had begun.[18]

According to Nicholas Culpeper's *Directory,* in seventeenth-century England cesarotomies were performed in three categories: when the child was dead and the mother alive, when the mother was dead and the child still living, and when both were living. He observes that the operation was "seldom" performed, however, and cautioned attendants to attempt it only in those cases where the lives of both mother and child were imperiled. In the following century, Edmund Chapman defined the procedure as "Cutting . . . [the child] out of the Womb of its Mother just expired." He advised against it regardless of circumstances, chiefly, it would seem, to protect the surgeon's reputation in a generally hostile climate. "What Man in his Senses," he asked, "would put his Character upon this Footing? It would be natural for the malicious World to say that, to save the Child, he killed the Mother; and the Friends and Others about the Deceased, either out of Fondness or Ignorance, might possibly imagine, that she was not quite dead before the Operation was Performed.''[19]

In sharp contrast, William Smellie did not rule out the operation absolutely. He termed the performance of a cesarotomy upon a living woman "certainly adviseable" when all other attempts to effect delivery had failed in preternatural and laborious labors. If the mother were still strong enough, he reasoned, "it is better to have recourse to an operation which hath sometimes succeeded, than to leave them both to inevitable death." His text supplied procedural details but counseled that in instances where the patient was weak, it was best to let her die before taking the child. Even at the close of the 1700s the syllabus for Guy's Hospital warned that, "In the living subject, the chances of complete success are but few: hence the expediency of the operation should be well ascertained." Even more cautious was Thomas Denman, an enormously successful and influential English man midwife whose writings were widely adopted by American medical schools in the early nineteenth century. Denman had never performed a cesarean operation himself, nor had he, despite his wide experience, even observed one. He could hardly have been more pessimistic than when he stated, "Every woman, for whom the caesarean operation can be proposed to be performed will probably die." Denman therefore confined its use to cases of absolute necessity when "there shall be no other way or method by which the life, either of the mother or the child, can possibly be preserved." Even at that, he insisted, consulting physicians must agree. One modern medical writer has stated that out of thirty-eight recorded cesarean operations performed in Great Britain between 1739 and 1845, only four women recovered.[20]

In light of the foregoing, it is understandable that throughout the eighteenth century British authorities preferred the embryotomy over the cesarean section while the mother remained alive. Yet during this period, some men midwives charged their colleagues with performing embryotomies routinely and unnecessarily. Edmund Chapman recalled Hugh Chamberlen's earlier criticisms and referred to the "barbarous Cruelty" of those men midwives who out of ignorance used the crotchet on "living Children." These men, in

Chapman's opinion, ought to be "utterly condemned and exploded by all fair and honest Practitioners." In a similar vein, Benjamin Pugh warned young men not to endanger their reputations by contributing to the high incidence of embryotomies without first consulting a more established obstetrician. He acknowledged that extraordinary cases demanded extraordinary methods but charged that very often surgeons excused murder by claiming that the fetal head had been too large to pass through the mother's pelvis when such was not the case. He insisted that there was "seldom a real Necessity" for resorting to embryotomy. "Never carry an Instrument of Death with . . . [you]," he cautioned the inexperienced man midwife, for the best "Means to avoid Temptation is to keep out of its Way." Predicted Pugh, "If every Operator would take care to qualify himself properly, the Art of Midwifery may no longer be looked on as cruel and terrible," and the happy result would be that "every ingenious Operator" would be "much esteemed and valued by all."[21]

The vehemence with which Edmund Chapman and Benjamin Pugh inveighed against some of their overzealous colleagues may be attributed in part to the fact that both men were early advocates of the forceps. This instrument, not generally known early in the 1700s but increasingly popularized in the second and third quarters of the century, helped to revolutionize obstetrics. It was the surgeons' possession of the forceps that enabled them to challenge directly the women midwives' traditional role as the attendants at all normal cases. Yet long before the full potential of the forceps was recognized, the surgeons were already attempting to escape from their reputations as murderers, or at the very least, harbingers of death. In 1724, for example, John Maubray, one of the first teachers of men midwifery in London, published *The Female Physician*. This work, despite its name, was an obstetrical and gynecological treatise for the edification of surgeons. The responsibilities of men engaged in midwifery were heavy ones, he insisted. Adopting an ultraconservative position that rejected the use of instruments "in all Conditions of Births, whether *Natural* or *Preternatural, Dead* or *Alive,*" Maubray maintained that the operator's hand alone "best serves, according to the Rules of his Profession to discharge the Duty of all Instruments in the Surgeon's Shop." The only exceptions he was willing to admit were "the Case of a *Monster*, or a very Hydropical Child."[22] Alleging the development of a recent, and in his view, fortunate trend, he asserted that parturient women had been taught finally "to lay aside all *childish Bashfulness* and *imaginary Modesty,* in order to secure their *Own* and their *Childrens* Safety, by inviting the *Assistance* of both SEXES."[23]

Maubray's optimism was premature, of course, and his death in 1732 prevented him from becoming embroiled in the bitter controversy that raged later over the increasing employment of men as obstetricians. Yet following his early lead, the surgeons continued to insist that midwifery was a suitably respectable employment for men and that the practice itself had risen to newer and higher ground precisely because of their participation. These self-conscious comments suggest at once the discomforting insecurity of the surgeons as they insinuated themselves further into a field that still retained its definition as primarily women's work. "Many great and famous Men," boasted Edmund Chapman, "have made Improvement of this Science the principal Business of their Lives." They had demonstrated the "eminent Usefulness of this Art" and had brought "Dignity" to it, both in England and in France. Chapman then pronounced midwifery "certainly One of the most noble and useful *Chirurgical* Operations in being."[24]

Benjamin Pugh prefaced his specialized treatise on midwifery operations by noting that the practice "is become almost as universal amongst Men in this Kingdom as ever it was *in France.*" According to Pugh, some people mistakenly believed that "because Midwifery has been hitherto chiefly in the Hands of Women . . . it is a trifling Affair." Nothing was further from the truth, he insisted, as "every Operator" could testify. It was true that the young, inexperienced surgeon might in the early days of his practice encounter only easy cases and from these assume that midwifery did not require special skills. Warned Pugh, these easy encounters were misleading; neither chance nor fortune could substitute for good instruction obtained from a skillful operator and combined with the experience gained from attending both preternatural and normal cases. He then pronounced the midwifery operation "one of the most difficult in all Surgery," an art that depended upon "as nice a Foundation as any." Reflecting his own experience in the profession, he concluded with the observation that "some Cases you will find will make you sweat plentifully in the coldest Day in Winter."[25]

In his historical survey of the profession, William Smellie was another who acknowledged the bad reputation of the surgeon. Its cause he attributed in part to the limited number of procedures then available. Smellie pointed out that the man midwife called to a laborious birth could usually bring the case to a satisfactory conclusion if podalic version were possible. In cases of protracted labor where version was not indicated, even if the fetus were extracted alive, the "long and severe compression of the head" bruised the soft tissue within the mother's pelvis. Sometimes the child died from the effects of this pressure; often the mother succumbed as well. As Smellie summarized: "If the child could not be turned, the method practised in these cases was to open the head and extract with the crotchet; and this expedient produced a general clamour among the women, who observed that when recourse was had to the assistance of a man-midwife, either the mother or child, or both, were lost." This "censure" was such a source of discouragement to male practitioners, maintained Smellie, that it served to stimulate the "ingenuity of several gentlemen . . . to contrive some gentler method of bringing along the head, so as to save the child, without any prejudice to the mother."[26]

The instrument that made possible this "gentler method of bringing along the head" was the obstetric forceps, several different types of which were designed and employed in the early decades of the eighteenth century. The forceps actually had been in limited use in the preceding century. Peter Chamberlen the Elder (1560-1631), a member of the Barber Surgeons' Company and one of the earliest of the English men midwives, is credited with inventing the short, straight forceps. Chamberlen's brother, Peter the Younger (1572-1626), also practiced midwifery in London. Succeeding generations of the family, Dr. Peter Chamberlen III (1601-1683), son of Peter the Younger, and his sons Hugh (b.1630), Paul (1635-1717), John (d.1700?), and Hugh Junior (1664-1728) all practiced midwifery. They kept the forceps a closely guarded family secret, utilizing the instrument as a nostrum and advertising that they could deliver women in tedious and difficult cases without resorting to embryotomies. Hugh Chamberlen, Junior, having no male heir to succeed him, let the general design of the family instrument be known before his death in 1728. Not until 1813 were the actual Chamberlen instruments accidentally discovered where they had been buried beneath the floor boards of a closet at Woodham, Peter Chamberlen's former country estate.[27]

Their possession of the obstetric forceps had enabled the Chamberlens to represent themselves as exceptional men midwives. Thus in 1672 Hugh Chamberlen, Senior, prefixed this claim to his translation of Mauriceau:

> My Father, Brothers and my Self (tho none else in *Europe* that I know), have, by God's Blessing, and our Industry, attained to, and long practised a way to deliver Women . . . without any prejudice to them or their Infants; tho all others (being obliged, for want of such an Expedient, to use the common way) do, and must endanger, if not destroy one or both, with Hooks. By this manual Operation may be dispatched, (when there is the least difficulty) with fewer pains, and in less time, to the great advantage, and without danger, both of Woman and Child.[28]

William Smellie later recalled that after the death of the Chamberlens, their forceps still were "so imperfectly known" that operators had difficulty using them with success. Consequently, "different practitioners had recourse to different kinds of fillets or lacks," as well as to blunt hooks.[29] These latter implements were imperfect and inefficient. Fillets had been developed initially as an aid to turning the fetus in utero. Edmund Chapman later claimed credit for devising a procedure to deliver the child in tedious labors by using the fillet as a noose, passing it over the infant's head, and pulling it along the birth canal.[30] The tool was not satisfactory. Surgeons found it difficult to introduce and even more difficult to use. Once applied, it had a tendency to slip off. In an effort to remedy this, Smellie mounted a piece of slender whale bone on the fillet to provide a firm support. Although this modification was easier to work with, he found it unacceptable, for it greatly increased the possibility of lacerating the mother. In cases where the head was low in the pelvis but contractions were not strong enough to effect delivery, in a final attempt to avoid embryotomy, Smellie would try "Mauriceau's fillet, which always failed, and another . . .

in form of a noose, which sometimes, though rarely, succeeded when the child was small."[31]

Benjamin Pugh termed all fillets except his own modified version "idle Things" applied only with great difficulty and seldom answering their intended purpose. Even when successful, the force necessary for their use caused them to pull to one side and cut the child. Pugh admitted the disadvantage of his own model was that it was useful "only" when the head lay very low.[32]

As the eighteenth-century men midwives continued their practice, they gradually comprehended more about the mechanism of labor. Greater knowledge, experimentation, and leaked bits of information from Chamberlen enabled some to deduce the general principle of the forceps. In 1733 Edmund Chapman exposed the Chamberlen nostrum by stating in the introduction of his treatise:

The Secret intimated by Dr. Chamberlen, by which his Father, two Brothers, and himself saved such Children as presented with the Head, but could not be born by natural Pains, was, as is generally believed, if not past all Dispute, the Use of the Forceps, well known to all the principal Men of the Profession, both in Town and Country.[33]

It was this passage that led Smellie later to attribute to Chapman the first "public . . . description of the forceps used by the Chamberlains."[34] Chapman did not accompany his description with an illustration, however, and this omission drew criticism from the "Learned Society established at Edinburgh for the Improvement of Physic and Surgery." In the revised editions of his work, Chapman responded by providing a drawing of his forceps which he described as "very little different from that used by the late Mr. *William Giffard.*" Giffard, another London practitioner, had openly used forceps, which he termed "extractors," seven years previous to Chapman's published description. Although he died in 1731, his *Cases in Midwifery* published posthumously three years later contained an illustration of the instrument he had developed.[35] In 1733 another surgeon, Alexander Butter, presented an original paper on the forceps before the Edinburgh Medical Society. Two years later the society published it in volume three of its *Medical Essays and Observations* under the title "The Description of a Forceps for extracting Children by the Head when lodged low in the Pelvis of the Mother.'' An engraving of Butter's forceps accompanied the essay.[36]

The models used by Butter, Chapman, and Giffard all were long, straight, and relatively crude instruments. Chapman mentioned the existence of ''several different Sorts of *Forceps*,'' some of which were useful and others ''faulty.'' Generally, however, even these early forceps were far superior to the fillet. Not only could they be introduced more easily into the pelvic cavity, but they permitted the operator to obtain ''a much stronger Hold of the Child'' and to draw it along the birth canal with ''more Ease and Security.''[37] Yet in 1737, while attending a case of ''laborious labor,'' William Smellie had ''tried to deliver the head with the French *Forceps,* recommended by Mr. Butter . . . but they were so long and ill formed'' that he could neither introduce them safely nor get a ''proper Hold.''[38] Within the next several decades, however, important modifications rendered the forceps more functional. A major improvement was the introduction of the pelvic curve, described by Benjamin Pugh, who claimed to have invented it circa 1740. Pugh accompanied the description of his instruments with plates showing two sizes of curved models, one fourteen inches in length and the other an eleven-inch model for use when the head lay ''low in the Passage.''[39] Although Pugh had also developed a ''Coronet, or Machine for extracting the Head when it lies low in the vagina,'' he preferred the curved forceps over all other available instruments.[40]

Forceps models differed, but innovative operators agreed that their use marked a major breakthrough in obstetrical practice. Chapman had avoided many embryotomies by employing them. He extolled their virtues, then added, ''All I can say, in Praise of this noble Instrument, must necessarily fall short of what it justly demands.'' Pugh was similarly enthusiastic. He hoped that ''every Operator'' would soon be ''sensible of their Advantages'' and claimed that in more than two thousand cases over a fourteen-year period, he had never again had to resort to craniotomy. William Smellie, whose contributions eventually surpassed those of all other man midwives, insisted that he had no wish to advance one method of practice over others. Yet, in his experience he too had found the

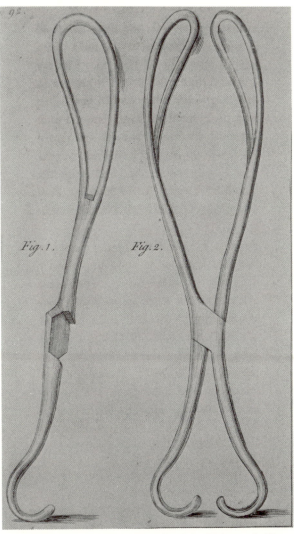

Early straight forceps first described by Edmund Chapman in 1733. In response to critics, Chapman included this drawing in subsequent editions.—From Edmund Chapman, *A Treatise on the Improvement of Midwifery,* London, 1759. (Courtesy of the State University of New York Upstate Medical Center Library.)

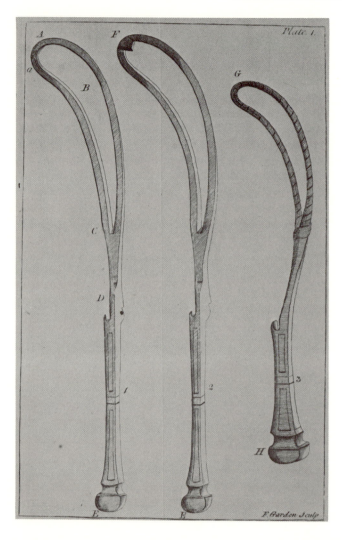

Benjamin Pugh was one of the earliest surgeons to develop forceps with a pelvic curve. His large forceps were fourteen inches
long, the smaller version eleven inches long. Note the small crotchet
attached to the top of the bow for use in craniotomies.—From
Benjamin Pugh, *A Treatise of Midwifery,* London, 1754. (Courtesy
of the State University of New York Upstate Medical Center Library.)

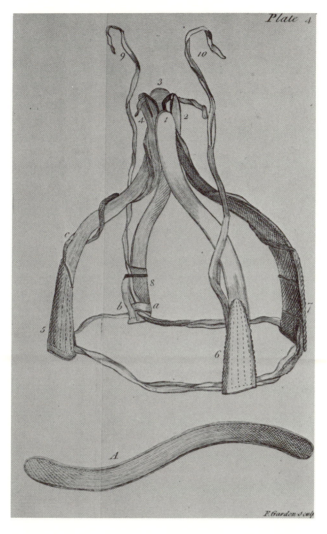

Benjamin Pugh's "Coronet, or Machine for extracting the Head when it lies low in the Vagina" consisted of S-shaped iron splints ten inches long and one-half inch wide inserted into pockets made of whale bone and cloth.—From Benjamin Pugh, *A Treatise of Midwifery,* London, 1754. (Courtesy of the State University of New York Upstate Medical Center Library.)

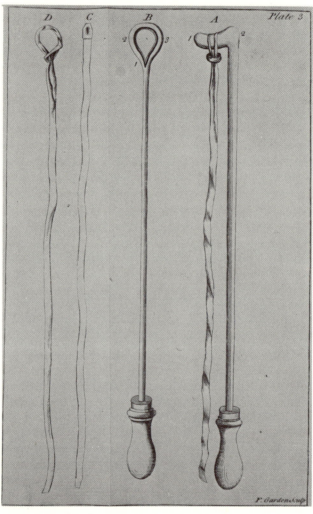

Innovator Pugh's instrument for "conveying a Noose over the
Child's foot in utero for turning." The operator was instructed to
make a noose in the fillet, place it over the instrument, and intro-
duce it "up the Arm to the Child's Foot."—From Benjamin Pugh,
A Treatise of Midwifery, London, 1754. (Courtesy of the State
University of New York Upstate Medical Center Library.)

forceps "more mechanically adapted, and easier applied than any other contrivance hitherto used." He urged their adoption, convinced that operators could then save "many Children, which otherwise must have been destroyed." Stressing the need for continued experimentation, improvement, and the sharing of advanced techniques, Smellie applied an obvious slap in the direction of the deceased Chamberlens when he added that he hoped "every Gentleman . . . [would] despise and avoid the character of a selfish secretmonger" in regard to any improvements or refinements he might develop.[41] Pugh was similarly critical of those who failed to share their new techniques, claiming, "It is much to be lamented, that the World has not the Advantage of every Man's Improvements; the Acquisitions of each Person added together, would amount to a large Sum, and consequently Arts wou'd flourish much more than they do."[42] Both these surgeons generously shared the results of their work. Pugh's *Treatise of Midwifery* contained drawings of the various instruments he had developed and supplied instructions on how they could be duplicated as well as how they were to be used. Smellie's elaborate *Treatise on the Theory and Practice of Midwifery* illustrated principles practically with reference to the normal and preternatural cases detailed in volumes two and three. A set of anatomical tables completed the work. Smellie was particularly critical of authors whose illustrations and examples referred only to successes; all surgeons had failures, and he was convinced that by presenting these, he could frequently provide young practitioners with badly needed cautions and suggestions on how to avoid similar mistakes.[43]

Physical possession of these instruments was merely the first step. Practitioners, whether experienced or novice, required instruction in their use. It is at once evident from the elaborate procedures described by Pugh and Smellie that they were addressing themselves to men midwives and definitely not to women midwives. The extensive knowledge of anatomy required to follow Pugh's rules on applying the forceps makes this evident, as is obvious in the following directions:

The Forceps must be introduced one Blade after another, in as private a Manner as possible, first introducing the Fingers of each Hand to carefully guard the Bows past the *Os Uteri,* and fairly over the side of the Head; for should the *Os Uteri* get between the Head and Forceps, it would at once prevent any firm Hold of the Head, and consequently fail you in the Attempt and also bruise the Part that intervenes, so as to endanger an Excoriation and great Inflammation. When both Blades are introduced, and the Head properly between the Forceps, they are to be brought close together, and the Nitches fixed into each other; taking Care, if the Nitches are within the *Vagina,* that none of the *Rugae* get between. You then take a clean Cloth, and turn about the Handles, which gives you much better Hold than you would otherwise have, and keeps your Hands from slipping, as likewise from being hurt by the Handles of the Forceps (for there is sometimes more Force required than possibly can be imagined, by a Person who is ignorant of the Operation) then firmly grasp them together with both Hands. . . . Then fixing one knee against the side of the Bedstead, the other upon a Cushion on the Ground, grasp the Forceps almost as tight as you can, or at least with sufficient Strength to keep them slipping over the Child's Head (and truly none but an Operator can conceive what a Child's Head will bear, without receiving any considerable Damage:) when the Pains come on, begin to pull the Head along from Side to Side, till you find it advance to the external Parts; then pull slowly, gradually dilating the Parts, which ought to have been lubricated well with Pomatum, raise the Handles of the Forceps, and pull the Head upwards, that it may turn out according to the Shape of the Curve Forceps, and prevent a Laceration of the *Perineum.* When I have brought the Head through the Bones of the *Pelvis,* so that I find it free and quite at the external Parts, I generally then unhitch the Forceps, and withdraw first one Blade, and then the other.[44]

Smellie's "General rules for using the Forceps" were considerably more detailed than were Pugh's and occupied nearly thirty pages of text.[45] His "minute directions in laborious and preternatural cases" occupy well over one hundred additional pages. Such detail, admitted Smellie, might be thought "idle and trifling by those practitioners, who without minding any stated rules, introduce the forceps, and taking hold on the head at random, deliver with force and violence; and who, in preternatural deliveries, thrust up their hands into the *Uterus,* and without considering the position, search for the feet, pull them down, and deliver in a hurry." These practices were wrong, warned Smellie; they might succeed occasionally but were more likely to destroy the child, bruise, injure, and endanger the life of the mother.[46]

Twenty years earlier, Edmund Chapman had been critical of surgeons who were ignorant of the forceps and continued to resort to the "most cruel unwarrantable Practice" of embryotomy.[47] Smellie's criticism was directed at the malpractice of those men midwives who had acquired a pair of forceps but not the expert knowledge required for their use. For the men, the acquisition of this information was within their grasp and merely had to be added to their considerable understanding of anatomy and physiology. The forceps were developed and improved upon by surgeons for their exclusive use in performing surgical operations in midwifery. They did not contemplate placing them into the hands of women, who were expected to continue to call upon surgeons for help in abnormal cases. It is impossible to overstress this point. The continuing development of improved procedures and equipment therefore widened the existing disparity between the midwives and the surgeons. The more sophisticated the technique, the greater the need for formal instruction of a type not available to women. Yet, so long as the surgeons limited their attendance to abnormal cases, the midwives could continue to deliver the normal cases that constituted the majority of the practice. In the second half of the eighteenth century, men midwives began to attend these normal cases, thereby posing a potentially serious threat to the women's domain. Many surgeons participated in these changes, but no figure looms so large as that of William Smellie. His work revolutionized Anglo-American obstetrics. The consequent effects upon the midwives were of enormous import.

William Smellie was born in Lanark, Scotland, at the close of the seventeenth century. At the local grammar school he acquired a good working knowledge of Latin and French. His interest in the medical field led to an apprenticeship, probably with Dr. John Gordon, a Glasgow surgeon especially interested in midwifery. When he had completed this training, Smellie returned to Lanark, establishing a general practice there that he continued from 1720 to 1739.[48] During the nineteen years of his general practice in Lanark, midwives called upon Smellie to assist in complicated cases. By 1722 he had become sufficiently interested in obstetrics to keep careful notes on those most "remarkable."[49] At that time he had no intention of making them public, but these cases later were used to illustrate some points in his *Treatise on the Theory and Practice of Midwifery*. These early records kept for personal use are especially valuable for the insight they provide into the limitations of both the midwives and the surgeons, upon whom the women were dependent in complicated cases. The antipathy that existed between them was frequently evident, as the following case recorded in 1724 and introduced by Smellie as an example of "The body pulled from the head, and left in the *Vagina*" amply illustrates:

A midwife, who never had any education, and who had formerly vaunted, that she always did her own work, and would never call in man to her assistance, was called to a case, in which the child presented wrong. After she had, with great difficulty, brought down the body, she could not deliver the head, from the woman's being of a small size, and the child large. During the time of her making these trials, the husband sent in great haste for me. In the meantime, when the midwife found that her endeavours were in vain, she rested, to recover from her fatigue, and told those who were present, that she would now wait for the assistance of the woman's pains. One of the servants seeing me at a distance, went in a hurry, and told her I was come. She not knowing that I was called, fell to work immediately, and pulled at the child with great force and violence. Finding, as she imagined, the child coming along, she called out, that now she had got the better of him. The neck at that instant separating, the body was pulled from the head, and she fell down on the floor. As she attempted to rise, one of the assistants told her that it wanted the head.[50]

The midwife was so overcome with shock at this discovery that she herself was "put to bed in another room." Smellie arrived and was "surprised to find the house in such confusion." He delivered the disembodied head with the crotchet and then revived the midwife. Smellie stated that the fetus appeared to have been dead for several days, and he was of the opinion that had it been less putrified, it could have been delivered with another of the midwife's pulls. The entire experience horrified Smellie less than it will the modern reader. A case such as this was not routine, yet he tersely remarked that the accident was "lucky" for him in that it "rendered the midwife more tractable for the future."

During the first year of his practice, Smellie later recalled, he was called to "lingering cases," which were prolonged by the "imprudent methods used by unskilful midwives to hasten labour, such as directing the patient to walk about and bear down with all her strength at every trifling pain, until she was quite exhausted, and opening the parts prematurely so as to produce inflammations, and torture the woman unnecessarily."[51] Smellie did not limit his criticisms of these practices solely to the women. On occasion he had been called in to remedy the malpractice of men midwives. In 1729, for example, he was asked to attend a woman who had been in labor for two days. When it became apparent to the attending midwife that the woman's case was complicated, a "gentleman famous in that part of the country for the practice of midwifery" had been called. This surgeon amputated one of the child's arms, as he stated, to make more room for the delivery. Yet when Smellie examined the amputated arm, he found it "not much swelled" and believed the operator guilty of malpractice. Although by this time the woman was so greatly exhausted from hemorrhaging that her death appeared imminent, her friends persuaded Smellie to make one last attempt at delivery. Motivated by a chance to be of service to the public by exposing "an ignorant pretender, who had acquired a great reputation, even in spite of several such blunders," Smellie managed to deliver her, although she died two hours later.[52]

In the early days of his practice, Smellie was extremely conscious of his own obstetrical limitations and felt "great uneasiness" when called too late or when presented with cases where version was not indicated and circumstances dictated embryotomy with its consequent sacrifice of the infant. As noted earlier, he had tried the forceps described by Alexander Butter but did not find them functional. He then read the treatises of Edmund Chapman and William Giffard, which extolled the virtues of forceps and contained directions for their use. Still dissatisfied, he journeyed to London "in order to acquire further information on this subject." There he "saw nothing was to be learned," and taking the advice of his friend Dr. Stewart, he proceeded to Paris and the courses on midwifery then given by Grégoire. Again Smellie was disappointed, for although he believed Grégoire's instruction "might be useful to young beginners," Smellie considered his mannequin too unsophisticated for an experienced surgeon.[52]

In 1739, having been unable to learn as much as he had hoped from these efforts, Smellie moved to London and established himself there as a surgeon and man midwife. At that time he was still following the forceps procedures recommended by Chapman, Giffard, and Grégoire. This consisted of "introducing each blade at random, taking hold of the head any how, pulling it straight along, and delivering with great force and violence." This method unfortunately tore the woman's tissue and bruised the child so frequently that many practitioners became discouraged and "altogether disused" the forceps, experimenting instead with different types of fillets.[54] Smellie's determination to improve both the forceps and the procedure had far-reaching results. He began by considering the parturient process "in a mechanical view," and according to his own account: "to reduce the extraction of the child to the rules of moving bodies in different directions: in consequence of this plan . . . [he] more accurately survey'd the dimensions and form of the Pelvis, together with the figure of the child's head, and the manner in which it passed along in natural labours."[55]

Thus after twenty years of experience attending tedious and preternatural cases, this logical and mathematically oriented surgeon determined to investigate scientifically the mechanical process that constituted normal childbirth. Smellie was the first to take careful, precise measurements of the normal female pelvis and investigate its shape and dimensions. He also studied the external shape of the fetal head. This information enabled him to arrive at an accurate explanation of the manner in which the head passes through the pelvic basin in normal childbirth. Further studies revealed the presence of various types of malformed pelvises among women. Since the distorted pelvic basin was a cause of many cases of preternatural births, this information was requisite for an operator faced with these complicated cases. As Smellie explained, "the danger in all such Cases must increase or diminish, according to the degree of distortion." He therefore alerted men midwives to the necessity of acquiring "an accurate knowledge of the figure, shape, and dimensions of the *Pelvis,* together with the shape, size, and position of the child's head." This information would then enable them to proceed correctly with the delivery.[56]

The results of Smellie's work were of incalculable importance to the development of scientific midwifery. Supplied with this new knowledge, he not only was able to deliver "with greater ease and safety than before," but he also had the "satisfaction to find in teaching, that . . . [he] could convey a more distinct idea of the art in this mechanical light than in any other; and particularly, give more sure and solid directions for applying the forceps." Subsequently he utilized this information to improve upon the design and the dimensions of the forceps. He further discovered that "mechanics applied to midwifery" could be useful when performing podalic version, which required that the operator consider uterine contractions, the child's position, and the "method of moving a body confined in such a manner."[57]

Had William Smellie's contributions been limited to the above, he would still be deserving of a major place in the annals of obstetrical progress. It is important to note, however, that in addition to his "pretty extensive" private London practice, which continued for nineteen years, he soon became England's leading midwifery instructor.

Smellie was not the first to teach midwifery in England through formalized courses. John Maubray, author of *The Female Physician,* is believed to have been the earliest surgeon to offer an organized series of lectures on this specialty. Maubray's instruction consisted of two courses of twenty lectures each that he gave at his house in New Bond Street. He advertised that with these "students and dutiful hopefuls . . . in four or five months' time could . . . perfect" themselves in "this our noble art of midwifery."[58] He did not stress the use of instruments, which he regarded as dangerous as well as unnecessary in most cases.

Sir Richard Manningham (1690-1759) was another early teacher. In 1739 Manningham established the first lying-in ward for women on public charity by providing a few beds for them in a house near his own residence in St. James, Westminster, and maintaining the facility out of public subscriptions. He was motivated in part by a desire to make clinical training available to his students, who included women as well as men. The disparity between fees charged was great; women paid ten guineas for the course, the men twenty.[59] This suggests that women were given a different, probably less complete course limited to normal births and omitting instrumental instruction. Manningham's teaching included demonstrations of the mechanism of labor utilizing a mannequin that he had devised.

In 1744 his midwifery manual was published, and its full title suggests the content of his course: *An Abstract of Midwifry* [sic], *for the Use of the Lying-in Infirmary; which with Due Explanations by Anatomical Preparations, etc., the Repeated Performances of all Kinds of Deliveries, on our Great Machine, with Ocular Demonstration of the Reason and Justness of the Rules to be Observed in all Genuine and True Labours, in the Lying-in Infirmary, on our Glass Machine, makes a Complete Method of Teaching Midwifry, by giving the Pupils the Most Exact Knowledge of the Art, and Perfectly Forming their Hands, at the Same time, for the Safe and Ready Practice of Midwifry.*[60] Manningham's private practice was fashionable and extensive; unfortunately it is impossible to determine the number of students he trained in midwifery.

Edmund Chapman also trained students at his house in Red Lion Square, Holborn. Chapman referred in his *Treatise* to having instructed ''several Gentlemen in the Art,'' some of whom he mentioned by name. In 1734 John Page wrote to his former instructor to report his success. After completing his course, he had used forceps on a case without injuring either mother or child. As a consequence, Page continued happily, he had ''come into such Credit, that . . . [he was] frequently called in twice or thrice a Week; and . . . [had] not yet met with the least Mishap.'' Continued Page, ''Our Midwifes here are pretty dexterous; but when the Head falls so as to require the Use of the Forceps, they are at a loss.''[61]

Successes such as these described by Page and other men midwives served to slightly erode some of the deeply ingrained fear of male attendants still so prevalent among women and thereby to encourage other surgeons to improve their midwifery techniques. It was by the examples of Maubray, Chapman, and Manningham before him that William Smellie embarked upon his teaching. He did not begin this phase of his career until he had amassed considerable experience by practicing midwifery for ''a long time in the country,'' that is, during his nineteen years at his Lanark practice. To the carefully recorded case histories he had kept during that period, he added those of his London practice, of which he was ''more careful and minute in forming a collection.''[62] These along with his lively and inquisitive mind, enthusiasm, and willingness to admit personal error combined to qualify him eminently for teaching. There is no doubt as to his success, which greatly extended his influence. By the time the first volume of his *Treatise* appeared, he had given in excess of 280 midwifery courses "for the instruction of more than 900 pupils, exclusive of female students."[63] He did not indicate the number of women he taught, and it is impossible to arrive at any estimate.

An advertisement in the *London Evening Post,* announcing his lectures on the theory and practice of midwifery to be delivered at his house in the New Court, Pall Mall, indicates that the course was segregated. Smellie instructed women at eleven o'clock in the morning and men at three in the afternoon.[64] As was the case with Manningham, the women probably received instruction in normal deliveries and were taught to recognize those cases calling for more expert assistance. Despite the later allegations of some of his contemporaries that he wished to drive women from the practice, this charge is not supported by the evidence. Throughout his writings are found references to skillful women, whose work he praised. He did criticize bunglers and meddlers but was equally as critical of the malpractice of men as of women midwives. His goal was to upgrade the entire practice, thereby eliminating the tragedies and gross malpractices to which he had so often been witness. It was the pursuit of this goal that caused him to include women among his pupils.

A 1742 brochure circulated by Smellie indicated that his course was a thorough one and included "The Structure of the *Pelvis* and *Uterus*; Of the *Foetus* in *Utero*, and after Parturition; The Management of Child-bearing Women, during Pregnancy, in Time of Labour, and after Delivery; The Manner of Delivering Women, in all the Variety of natural, difficult, and preternatural Labours, perform'd on different Machines made in Imitation of real Women and Children."[65] Smellie outlined the conditions of the course and the schedule of fees and clinical opportunities in the brochure:

I. The Course is divided into Twelve Lectures, and no more than four Persons can attend at once, each paying Two Guineas at the First Lecture.

II. They who come on purpose from the Country, and cannot wait 'till the Number of Subscribers is complete, pay Three Guineas.

III. The Expence of being present at a real Labour is One Guinea; but such as contract for Two Courses and Four Labours, pay only Five Guineas, and perform the last Delivery themselves.

IV. Pupils who engage for a Year pay Fifteen Guineas, and are intitled to attend all the Courses and Labours of that Time, whereby they will have the Opportunity of Seeing and Performing in several difficult Cases.

V. By paying Twenty Guineas they are admitted to this Course, with all the forementioned Advantages, for Two Years.

N.B. The Men and Women are taught at different Hours.[66]

From the above it is evident that Smellie's students varied widely in ability. Some were very advanced and specialized by studying with him for an entire year, or even two. Others took the shorter single course, in which they received rudimentary training. The women who studied with Smellie probably fell into the latter category. As working-class women, it was unlikely that they had access to the large sums required for the multiple courses, even if they had the time. Then too, Smellie's definite ideas about the qualifications of the good midwife, while admittedly comprehensive, were nevertheless a far cry from his expectations for the accoucheur. The woman, he believed, should be middle-aged, sensible, decent, and able to withstand fatigue.

[she] ought to be perfectly well instructed with regard to the bones of the *Pelvis,* with all the contained parts comprehending those that are subservient to generation; she ought to be well skilled in the method of touching pregnant women [that is, giving digital examinations] and know in what manner the womb stretches, together with all the different kinds of labour, whether natural or preternatural, and the methods of delivering the Placenta.[67]

Women who had acquired this degree of training certainly would have been competent to manage the normal birth without untoward incident. They also would have had the ability to recognize the symptoms that signaled danger and/or abnormality; significantly, they were not taught the skills needed to cope with such cases. Nor is there evidence to suggest that Smellie attempted to teach women to use either the forceps or other instruments. No less a sexist than his contemporaries, he pointedly stated that he did not expect midwives to be able to meet the qualifications one had a right to expect in the male attendant.

In this regard one can liken Smellie's attitude to those of other surgeons and teachers desirous of upgrading the quality of the midwives' practice. John Memis, for example, "one of the first of many male and female pupils" instructed in midwifery by Thomas Young in Edinburgh, taught midwifery to women students. He published a manual specifically designed to make the subject "intelligible" to women, substituting common lay terms for the medical terminology he believed the midwives would not understand. His list of knowledge appropriate for the women was similar to Smellie's in that it consisted of an understanding of the anatomy of the pelvis, the technique of touching, familiarity with the different types of births, and the methods that might be employed to deliver the placenta. Memis's abbreviated coverage of symptoms and simplified instructions were adequate for attendants who were expected to call upon the more knowledgeable male practitioners in the event of complications.[68]

Edmund Chapman was another surgeon who noted the differences in the duties and training of male and female operators. The men, he insisted, must learn to use fillets and forceps in preference to the hook. "How necessary it is then," he stressed, "that Men, who profess *Midwifery*, should make themselves Masters of either the Forceps or Fillet? For I now once for all declare, I have no Design of Putting them into the Hands of Female Practitioners."[69] It was unnecessary for Chapman to elaborate this point; to have trained women as instrumentalists would have required an admission that women were capable of comprehending technical anatomical and physiological details as competently as could the surgeon, an admission that Chapman was not prepared to make. Yet, there was at least one midwifery teacher who chafed against the male-defined assessments of women that kept such information beyond their reach. This was Margaret Stephen, the midwife who usually attended Queen Charlotte. Author of *The Domestic Midwife,* Stephen taught her women pupils principles of anatomy and the use of obstetric instruments and criticized those who did not. "It has been alleged," she complained, "that women's understanding does not admit of receiving such knowledge as is necessary in the practice of midwifery. I only wish that those who teach midwifery would give them as clear a knowledge of that science as they are capable of receiving."[70]

Certainly William Smellie's precise summary of the training requisite for the man midwife goes far beyond that which he believed women were capable of attaining. First, maintained Smellie, the man midwife must master anatomy and acquire a "competent knowledge of surgery and physick because of their connexions with the obstetric art." Following such acquisition:

He ought to take the best opportunities he can find, of being well instructed; and of practising under a master before he attempts to deliver by himself.

In order to acquire a more perfect idea of the art, he ought to perform with his own hands upon proper machines, contrived to convey a just notion of all the difficulties to be met with in every kind of labour; by which means he will learn how to use the forceps and crotchets with more dexterity, be accustomed to the turning of children, and consequently, be more capable of acquitting himself in troublesome cases.[71]

As an aid to teaching all of his students, male and female, Smellie had developed several different types of mannequins. He may have seen Sir Richard Manningham's model; he definitely had seen that used by Grégoire in Paris. The latter did not impress him favorably, for he characterized it as "no other than a piece of basketwork, containing a real pelvis covered with black leather, upon which he could not clearly explain the difficulties that occur in turning children, proceeding from the contractions of the *Uterus, Os Internum and Os Externum.*" For his own part, Smellie considered the possibility of forming machines "which should so exactly imitate real women and children as to exhibit to the learner all the difficulties that happen in midwifery."[72] That his "uncommon labour and application" were amply rewarded is seen in this description provided by Peter Camper, a Dutch student who studied with Smellie in the early 1750s:

He explains the osteology of the pelvis in both a healthy and in a morbid and misshapen state. He explains both their external and internal parts by using the dead bodies of women but much more clearly in other exhibits specially prepared for the purpose. He also shows his listeners an almost complete series of foetuses.

He demonstrates parturition in models of women of which the pelvis and spine of a well-modelled woman are the starting point. Both the abdominal and extra-abdominal parts have been made out of leather with such remarkable skill that not only is the structure as natural as possible but the necessary functions of parturition are performed by working models. For example, the contraction of both the internal and external os, the generation of water in parturition and dilatation of the os uteri are so natural that hardly any difference is to be noticed between these, and those in natural women.

The foetuses which he uses in the machines are all artificially made of wood according to the natural dimensions, shapes and methods of jointing. The bones of the head work just as in the actual living foetuses, the nose is inset and the jaw is movable. Likewise the afterbirth is made out of various leathers.[73]

Such then was the remarkable complexity of the mannequins Smellie had "contrived to resemble and represent real women and children and on which all kinds of different labours . . . [were] demonstrated and even performed by every individual student."[74]

Yet, extraordinary as these models were, Smellie realized the value of clinical training. He therefore devised a plan under which he agreed to deliver indigent women without charge provided they permit his students to observe, examine them, and assist at the deliveries. By 1751 Smellie, accompanied by students, had delivered 1,150 women, all of whom were "supported in their lying-in" by the small additional sums the instructor charged his pupils for the privilege of attending these births. This figure apparently consisted primarily of normal cases; it did not include "those difficult cases" that he and his students were called to by the midwives "for the relief of the indigent."[75] If the experience recorded by Peter Camper is any criterion, Smellie's students received a great deal of experience in return for their tuition. Camper noted that one day late in July 1752, he "attended Smellie's lesson and examined twenty-one pregnant women between seven and nine months."[76]

Smellie awarded a certificate to each male student who completed his course. This testified that he had carefully attended the midwifery lectures, thereby receiving an "Opportunity of being full instructed in all the different Operations and Branches of that

Art.''[77] The certificate, impressively embellished with a bust of Hippocrates and signed by Smellie, was, as Henry Viets has remarked, the eighteenth-century equivalent of a university diploma; those who possessed it were well credentialed and advantageously positioned to attract antepartum women to a private practice. Smellie claimed to have instructed over nine hundred men in the first decade of his teaching.[78] By conservative estimate, in the London years remaining to his retirement, he could have trained several hundred more. As these graduates swelled the ranks of practicing men midwives, they challenged more directly the women's traditional monopoly over normal deliveries. Smellie and his students had already intruded upon this domain by delivering indigent parturient women. A passage in his second volume stating that within his private practice he had "very seldom occasion for the assistance of . . . [the forceps] or any other instrument"[79] indicates not only his conservatism when treating private patients but also suggests that by mid-century Smellie was attracting some private normal midwifery cases.

However extensive and lucrative Smellie's private practice was, it never included large numbers of upper-class women. It was William Hunter (1718-1783), the celebrated anatomist and former student of Smellie, who eventually became London's most fashionable midwifery practitioner. In comparison with that of his brother, the surgeon John Hunter (1728-1793), William's career is less well known. Yet no account of eighteenth-century obstetrics is complete without discussion of Hunter and his contribution to our knowledge of the human gravid uterus. Originally destined for an ecclesiastical career, William Hunter decided instead upon medicine. Accordingly he apprenticed himself to fellow Scot William Cullen, with whom he studied surgery for three years. A short period of study in Edinburgh followed. He then accepted his preceptor's advice and moved to London. There he studied with Smellie, residing at his home from Fall 1740 until the following August. He then became anatomical assistant to James Douglas (1675-1742), the surgeon whose *Description of the Peritonaeum* (1730) first detailed the pouch that bears his name. Douglas died in 1742 but not before his own anatomical studies had kindled still further Hunter's already keen interest in anatomy.[80]

In 1746 Hunter began to deliver his own course of anatomical lectures in Little Piazza, Covent Garden. They were well received, and he continued to conduct courses in anatomy over the next several decades.[81]

Hunter's midwifery career began in 1748, when he was selected to act as deputy to Daniel Peter Layard, then Man Midwife in Ordinary at Middlesex Hospital, where a part of the institution was reserved for the reception of married lying-in women. No teaching was done there, and no women were permitted to act as midwives. When Layard and the Man Midwife in Extraordinary at Middlesex, Francis Sandys, joined the staff of the new Lying-in Hospital for Women in Brownlow Street [British Lying-in Hospital], William Hunter joined the staff as surgeon and man midwife. There his duties included teaching small groups of women pupils who paid twenty guineas each for six months of midwifery instruction.[82] Hunter remained at British Lying-in until July 1759. An extremely conservative obstetrician, his reputation and private practice grew prodigiously. Through a combination of good fortune, personal charm, and impressive connections he succeeded to the fashionable practice of Sir Richard Manningham and Francis Sandys. In 1762 he attended Queen Charlotte in her first confinement, waiting in the anteroom against the event of an emergency, while the queen's midwife, Mrs. Draper, delivered her of a son, the future George IV. Two years later Hunter was appointed Physician Extraordinary to Her Majesty.[83]

William Hunter's private practice was confined chiefly to clinical midwifery, yet his most important contributions to obstetrics lay in his anatomical studies of the gravid uterus. He had begun the work in 1750, and more than twenty years later it culminated in the publication of his brilliant work, *The Anatomy of the Human Gravid Uterus* (1774). The importance of this work in the advancement of scientific midwifery may be appreciated when one realizes that until Hunter began his investigations, few anatomists had ever had opportunities to dissect the bodies of pregnant women. Their knowledge of the human uterus was based largely, therefore, upon what they knew to be true of lower animals. In the preface to his work, Hunter explained how his project had begun. Originally he had been studying anatomy in "brutes." Then,

A woman died suddenly, when very near the end of her pregnancy, the body was procured before any sensible putrefaction had begun; the season of the year was favourable to dissection; the injection of the blood-vessels proved successful; a very able painter . . . was found; every part was examined in the most public manner, and the truth was thereby well authenticated.[84]

Hunter decided to publish an anatomy of the gravid uterus based upon this dissection and began to sell subscriptions to the work. In the interim, however, he obtained a second subject for dissection, "which . . . afforded a few supplemental figures of importance enough" to be included in the work. Before the engravings had been completed, a third subject came into his possession, and this "cleared up some difficulties, and furnished some useful additional figures."[85] The acquisition of these three bodies within so short a period of time caused Hunter to amend his original design, and he postponed publication of the planned work. As he later explained, speaking of himself in the third person, he had realized that "in the course of some years, by diligence he might procure in this great city [London], so many opportunities of studying the gravid uterus, as to be enabled to make up a tolerable system; and to exhibit, by figures, all the principal changes that happen in the nine months of utero-gestation."[86] The delay in publication was admittedly extensive yet unquestionably warranted by the superior quality of the final product.

In an introductory lecture to the last course of anatomical lectures William Hunter delivered before his death in 1783, he summarized for his pupils his most significant findings in obstetrics:

The gravid uterus is a subject . . . which has afforded me opportunities of making considerable improvements; particularly one very important discovery; viz. that the internal membrane of the *uterus,* which I have named *decidua,* constitutes the exterior part of the *secundines,* or after-birth; and separates from the rest of the uterus every time that a woman bears a child or suffers a miscarriage. This discovery includes another, to wit, that the placenta is partly made up of an excrescence or efflorescence from the *uterus* itself.[87]

In order that his students would grasp the significance of his work, Hunter pointed out that "these discoveries are of the utmost consequence, both in the physiological question about the connection between the mother and child; and likewise in explaining the phaenomena of births and abortions, as well as in regulating our practice."[88]

As the culmination of more than twenty years of study and investigation, Hunter's *Anatomy of the Gravid Uterus* illuminated the clinical midwifery contributions of William Smellie. Taken together, the work of these two figures was primarily responsible for effecting the revolution that produced the "new obstetrics." As the art of midwifery continued its transformation into a science, it was brought into the medical orbit and legitimized as a practice for men. Indicative of this was the decision by the Royal College of Physicians of London in 1782 to establish a distinct category of licentiates in midwifery, whereby men who passed the examination were licensed as duly qualified practitioners of the specialty.[89]

Another major element in the rapidly developing science of obstetrics was the trend promoted by the medical profession between 1749 and 1765 toward establishing hospitals to receive parturient women. During this period five lying-in hospitals were founded in London: The British Lying-in Hospital (1749), The City of London Lying-in Hospital (1750), Queen Charlotte's Hospital (1752), Royal Maternity Hospital (1757) and the General Lying-in Hospital (1765).[90] These institutions provided care for women while at the same time affording men midwives greater opportunities to attend normal childbirths. How important such experience could be to them was illustrated well by William Smellie in the final volume of his work. A "Mr. W." had once taken a course of lectures from Smellie but had omitted the optional attendance at labors, believing that "every thing in midwifery [was] trifling and that the lectures on the extraordinary cases were sufficient." He subsequently had gained some following among the midwives, who called upon him often in preternatural cases. Late in 1748 he was retained to attend the normal case of thirty-eight-year-old primipara. Owing to his inexperience with the normal, he did not realize the advantages of permitting nature to advance the labor. He proceeded therefore to manual dilatation of the os uteri. Despite the woman's powerful and frequent contractions, she remained undelivered. Finding himself "foiled and at a loss how to manage the labour," Mr. W. asked that his former teacher be called. Instead, the patient's friends sent for another accoucheur, who according to Smellie's account had "by art and cunning . . . got a name among the lower sort of patients." The two accoucheurs soon fell into a violent disagreement about the presentation of the fetus, Mr. W. maintaining correctly that it was cephalic, and the new man insisting that a shoulder presented. During the ensuing debate the patient slept soundly. A nurse, alarmed lest her mistress be endangered by the quarreling "obstetric adversaries," advised the husband to seek still more help. When Smellie arrived, he prevailed upon both accoucheurs to wait, and the following morning Mr. W. "received" rather than delivered the child. This experience convinced both accoucheurs of their need to learn more about normal cases. They later enrolled with Smellie for "several courses" of lectures and seized every opportunity to be present at all of the "publick labours that happened during their attendance."[91]

Smellie protected the reputations of these accoucheurs out of a belief that it was "always" his duty to "make up such breaches for the general good of society, as well as for the honour of the profession." Yet, he claimed that he had seen a good deal of malpractice perpetrated by incompetent, competitive, and pompous men. Once, for example, he had been called in to see a woman who had been in labor for two days. Her attendant, a man "of no education or practice in midwifery," noted that the membranes had broken and "imagined it was his business to promote the delivery with all possible expedition; and with that view, fatigued the patient excessively, by ordering her to walk about and bear down with all her force at every inconsiderable pain."[92] Smellie put the woman to bed, leaving her with one of his students and a midwife. Two days later, well rested, she fortunately had a normal delivery. On another case, Smellie encountered incompetence of a different sort when a "lady" requested that he look in on her former servant. Smellie's arrival outraged the attending operator, who was pacified only when Smellie explained that he had not realized there was a man midwife on the case. He invited Smellie to observe the delivery, which he announced must take place at once, inasmuch as he had been "waiting two days on this case," had lost one case because of the delay, and was about to lose another. It developed that the delay was attributable to the massive doses of opium the accoucheur had prescribed to gain him some time to determine the presentation, the nature of which had puzzled him. The patient had become convulsed, had fallen into a stupor, and her contractions had ceased. After some insistence by Smellie, the accoucheur became convinced that the case was "not barely a case in midwifery" and agreed to send for a physician. The accoucheur and the apothecary disagreed on the size of the opium doses prescribed, and the former finally left the case. The patient slept off the effects of her overdose, but her child when eventually delivered was stillborn.[93]

Smellie chronicled other cases of malpractice and incompetence. By undercutting other's fees, one man midwife had acquired "a considerable share of low and middling practice." He habitually abused and was in turn abused by the midwives. Having built up a reputation by exaggerating the importance of his contribution in cases less difficult than he claimed, the long-range effect was damaging to man midwifery, for he "frightened many midwives from calling in men practitioners." Ultimately he was found out, but before he lost his following many patients suffered unnecessarily because of their refusal to have any assistance when he was proposed.[94]

If the presence of one man midwife could excite suspicion, large numbers of accoucheurs might provoke a riot. Smellie recalled that with the end of the War of the Austrian Succession in 1748, his lectures attracted an unusually large number of men from the army and navy. Called to one of the narrow lanes in Broad St. Giles to attend a preternatural case, the master accoucheur was accompanied by twenty-eight pupils! The presence of this army of men midwives caused a disturbance in the neighborhood, where a rumor quickly circulated that the men were experimenting upon the patient. The neighbors sent for the parish officers, and Smellie, anxious to conclude this particular delivery before the officers arrived, inadvertently broke one of the child's thighs.[95] By thus proceeding too hastily, Smellie had violated one of his cardinal obstetric rules. His works are replete with repeated cautions against hasty judgments and actions. He counseled operators confronted with the laborious case on the importance of proper timing by illustrating the dilemma they must face:

If we attempt to succour too soon, and use much force in the operation, so that the child and mother, or one of the two are lost, we will be apt to reproach ourselves for having acted prematurely. . . . On the other hand, when we leave it to nature, perhaps by the strong pressure upon the head and brain, the child is dead when delivered, and the woman so exhausted with tedious labour, that her life is in imminent danger: in this case we blame ourselves for delaying our help so long.[96]

Some practitioners were so excessively conservative that they eschewed the use of instruments entirely. It will be recalled that John Maubray had taken a position against the instrumentalists early in the 1700s, when forceps deliveries were first finding favor among the men midwives. Half a century later it was William Hunter who emerged as the arch-conservative. Displaying his own set of forceps covered with years of rust, he would lecture his students on the virtues of permitting their forceps to develop similar evidence of disuse. Alluding to the harm that forceps could do, he lamented, "I am sorry they were ever invented. Where they save one they murder 20."[97]

Smellie, who had greatly improved the forceps and popularized their use, acknowledged and addressed this criticism directed against men midwives:

A general outcry hath been raised against gentlemen of the profession, as if they delighted in using instruments and violent methods in the course of their practice; and this clamour hath proceeded from ignorance of such as do not know that instruments are sometimes absolutely necessary, or from the interested views of some low, obscure, and illiterate practitioners, both male and female, who think they find their account in decrying the practice of their neighbours. It is not to be denied, that mischief has been done by instruments in the hands of the unskilful and unwary, but I am persuaded, that every judicious practitioner will do every thing for the safety of his patients before he has recourse to any violent method either with the hand or instrument.[98]

Nevertheless, Smellie continued, cases did occur in which all other methods failed. Thus practitioners needed to learn correct instrumental procedures. He recommended that they be resorted to only when the life of the mother or child was evidently endangered; then they must be used only with "utmost caution." Offered Smellie, "I have always avoided them as far as I thought consistent with the safety of my patients, and strongly inculcated the same maxim upon those who have submitted to my instructions."[99] In the first collection of cases Smellie published to illustrate his theory and practice, he observed that the forceps had been developed as a more acceptable alternative to embryotomy. Yet when the nature of the case did not absolutely dictate their use, he warned, "The mischief that may ensue will often overbalance the service for which they were intended."[100]

Benjamin Pugh, an accomplished and inventive instrumentalist, preferred to use podalic version wherever possible. "This Practice of Turning," he wrote, "is of the utmost Importance; it is the grand Pillar of Midwifery; and Operators that are well versed in it, will very seldom need the Help of Instruments." On those rare occasions, however, when it was impossible to perform the operation manually and delay would endanger lives, Pugh declared instrumental interference "not only warrantable but commendable."[101] In the next decade John Memis reiterated the conservative position. He insisted that the attendant must always examine the patient first to determine whether it was essential to use forceps. "We never use instruments but in absolute necessity,"[102] he cautioned.

In 1800 Thomas Denman, writing with the authority of an experienced and successful accoucheur, reminded students that there would be occasions on which their patients would urge premature intervention. "Women, impelled by their fears and their sufferings in difficult labours," he wrote, "will very generally implore you to deliver them with instruments long before you will be convinced of the necessity of using them." The best course to follow in these cases, he advised, was to hold out some hope to the patient for possible future relief by suggesting that instruments might be used much later in the delivery.[103]

On the whole, male operators would have agreed with Smellie's statement that man midwifery had in England been "brought to perfection in this [more] than in any other kingdom."[104] Yet the fact remained that women continued to regard men midwives with suspicion. Some women midwives so resented male intruders that they rushed to complete deliveries before the accoucheur could arrive. Pugh, illustrating the consequences that could follow the failure of the midwife to catheterize a patient before attempting to perform podalic version, introduced his readers to such a midwife. Pugh had been called to help a woman who lived about eight miles from his home. While he was enroute to the patient, "the Midwife made such Haste to deliver the Woman before I came, and used such Force (the Bladder being distended with Water), that she certainly did deliver the Woman just before I got to her; but the consequence was the bursting of the Bladder and the Vagina," leaving the mother with a three-inch laceration that eventually developed into a small irreparable fistula.[105]

Cataloguing the virtues of the good midwife, Smellie insisted that she ought to avoid "all reflections upon men-practitioners." For their part, the men were told to encourage the confidence of the midwife by not openly condemning her methods, even when they were obviously faulty. Rather, thought Smellie, men ought to "make allowance for the 'weakness of the sex,'" correcting without exposing. Such conduct would have the advantage of safeguarding the patient's welfare while at the same time serving to build up the man's credits with the midwife. Well treated in this way, she might be more willing to have him called in future cases.[106]

Yet professional competition was strong, and men and women practitioners behaved badly toward each other. One stated that he would not be concerned with "such gossips" and "damned all midwives for ignorant b___s." Another, arriving after the midwife had completed the delivery, falsely accused her of malpractice in tearing the woman. Whan a patient of his suffered the same fate, the midwife learned of it, "hunted him out, and attacked him every where." In other cases, the "artful insinuations" of midwives terrified their patients with "dreadful accounts of the use of instruments," thus forestalling efforts to call upon an accoucheur.[107]

The man midwife's reputation as an instrumentalist needlessly inflicting pain and death was a major obstacle to his acceptance. Women, wrote Smellie, were "commonly frightened at the very name of an instrument." He therefore advised young practitioners to conceal their instruments, at least until they had established themselves. Carefully he outlined the procedure that would guarantee the desired secrecy:

[Once the patient had been positioned properly for the forceps delivery,] the blades ought to be privately conveyed between the feather-bed and the cloaths . . . that this conveyance may be the more easily effected, the legs of the instrument ought to be kept in the operator's side pockets. Thus provided, when he sits down to deliver, let him spread the sheet that hangs over the bed, upon his lap, and under that cover, take out and dispose the blades on each side of the patient; by which means he will often be able to deliver with the forceps, without their being perceived by the woman herself, or any other of the assistants.[108]

Smellie reiterated his warnings about the need for secrecy. To neglect this was to openly invite the "calumnies and misrepresentations of those people . . . apt to prejudice the ignorant and weak-minded against the use of any instrument" and of those who would accuse accoucheurs of malpractice whenever unforeseen "accidents" occurred.[109] Although Memis agreed that when instruments were used it was desirable to conceal them "all the time" if possible from patient and bystanders, Thomas Denman advised a more open policy. When it was necessary to use forceps, he insisted, the attendant ought to explain this to both the patient and those about her.[110]

The alarm that such an announcement could produce may be glimpsed from a touching entry written in Elizabeth Drinker's journal in 1799. The Drinkers were a well-established Philadelphia family, and their thirty-eight-year-old daughter, Sally Downings, in labor with her sixth child, had a celebrated accoucheur to attend her. William Shippen, Jr., held the M.D. from Edinburgh and had studied in London with Smellie's assistant, Colin MacKensie, and with William Hunter. Sally Downings's labor was protracted because the child presented abnormally. Shippen, an advocate of conservative midwifery, finally decided that he must intervene. As Sally's mother later recalled:

—he went out, which he had not done before, that he was going for instruments occur'd to me but I was afraid to ask him, least he should answer in the affirmative—toward evening I came home as usual, and after seeing all things in order, was getting ready to depart, when little Dan enter'd, the sight of him flutter'd me, yet I had a secret hope that it was over, when Dan told us that his Mistress had a fine boy and was as well as could be expected— . . . Dr. Shippen told me that he thought he should have had occasion for instruments, which s.^{d} he I have in my pocket, claping his hand on his side, when I heard them rattle, but sometime after you went away, I found matters were chang'd for ye better.[111]

Although William Smellie was more reluctant to discuss cases with the involved persons, he admitted that there were occasions when wisdom demanded that the accoucheur forewarn patient and relatives. When "violent flooding" [hemorrhaging] occurred during the last four months, he advised the attendant to "pronounce the case dangerous and prudently declare to the relations of the patient that unless she is speedily delivered, both she and the child must perish, observing at the same time, that by immediate delivery they may both be saved." He also proposed a consultation with an eminent person in the profession "to satisfy the patient's friends," thereby safeguarding the accoucheur's reputation.[112]

Then as now an attendant's reputation was crucial to success, and ethical considerations presented some men with problems. Edmund Chapman insisted that the accoucheur accept even the hopeless case and do what he could to assist the woman. He faulted John Maubray for advancing what seemed to Chapman an unnecessarily obdurate position. Maubray had stated that because his own character was well established, he would consent to go to desperate cases; yet he cautioned young practitioners against *"going headlong to Work in Cases of the greatest Danger,* and would have him *decline the Office, because if the Woman dies under his Hands, he may perhaps be blamed for the errant Midwife's Faults; or at least he will scarce avoid the Censure of the Ignorant and Malevolent. . . ."* It was unfortunately true, admitted Chapman, that the surgeon called too late or to a case admitting of "no Relief" would reap "malicious Reflections, and very foul Language, by the Ignorant and Passionate, who will make no Allowances for Circumstances." The practitioner must realize nevertheless that this was an occupational hazard. Any possible undesirable effects his actions might have on his reputation must not deter him from doing "what the Dictates of Conscience and the Rules of Art require."[113] Unquestionably the surgeon's skills were put to the test when he was, as Benjamin Pugh put it, called to help a patient "after a Midwife . . . [had] kept the poor Woman a long Time (perhaps some Days) . . . till her strength . . . [was] almost exhausted . . . the Parts also dry, and the Womb tightly compressing the Child."[114] In resolving the dilemma, William Hunter was more inclined toward Maubray's position than that of Chapman. Although he did not refuse to attend cases, he avoided interference almost at all costs. His rusty forceps, unused for many years, and his "great rule . . . to do nothing" in abnormal presentations were products of his conviction that "if any misfortune happens, the accoucheur may entirely lose his credit."[115] Most responsible accoucheurs in the eighteenth century counseled a conservative position that allowed for no interference in the absence of abnormal complications. On balance, this was infinitely preferable to the almost routine interference that came to characterize the "meddlesome midwifery" practices of later generations.

The determination of men midwives to increase their acceptability among the women led to stipulations in the manuals regarding ethical conduct. Benjamin Pugh reminded operators that they must never drink too much liquor, lest in a drunken state they commit "Monstrous Blunders and Mischiefs." Regardless of the provocation, he continued, they must not speak harshly to their patients nor display bad temper. Significantly, Pugh warned the men that they must "Never on any Account discover any thing relating to the Fair-Sex in Company, or suffer any Discourse concerning it, to be set on Foot, as has been too often very foolishly done by some of the Profession."[116] Chapman reminded men that their duty as accoucheurs extended to those not enrolled in the "List of Fortune's Favourites" as well as to those more affluent. All patients, he insisted, deserved to be treated with tenderness and compassion. Parturient women suffered greatly; Chapman observed perceptively, "Their Pains, both in regard of the *Mind* and *Body* are at that time very hard upon them, and their Condition calls for the softest Manner in the necessary Assistance."[117] Education, wisdom, resolution, prudence, and humanity all were required but not always found in the man midwife. Smellie reminded the student of the constant demand to "act and speak with the utmost delicacy of decorum." The man midwife must never violate the trust placed in him nor "harbour the least immoral or indecent design; but demean himself in all respects suitable to the dignity of his profession."[118]

In accordance with this principle of assuming a demeaning posture, Smellie advanced very definite views on what the man midwife should wear. While relating case histories, occasionally he mentioned the ludicrous costumes accoucheurs affected out of their misguided attempts to impress patients and friends. In 1745, for example, he was asked for a consultation by a gentleman "of very little experience in midwifery." His appearance amazed Smellie, who termed his "apparatus . . . very extraordinary. . . . His arms were rolled up with napkins, and a sheet was pinned round his middle as high as his breast." On another occasion Smellie encountered a man midwife dressed in a manner as "forbidding as his countenance." He wore "an old greasy matted wrapper, or nightgown, a buff broad sword-belt of the same complection round his middle: napkins wrapped round his arms, and a woman's apron before him to keep his dress from being daubed." This costume by itself was not sufficiently impressive, apparently, for the accoucheur had completed it with the addition of a "large tie periwig."[119]

To Smellie such attire was too formal, and he thought it more likely to frighten the women than to create the desired atmosphere of trust and confidence. Aprons and sleeves might be used in hospital settings, he conceded, but private patients should be spared such spectacles. "The more genteel and commodious dress," he favored, was a "loose washing night-gown," which the operator should always don immediately before delivery. He suggested that a waistcoat without sleeves be worn, so that the operator's arms would have more freedom "to slide up and down under cover of the wrapper"; his shirt sleeves could be "rolled up and pinned to the breasts of his waistcoat." Modesty and decorum demanded that the accoucheur never gaze upon his exposed patient; therefore all obstetric operations were of necessity performed under covers and blankets. In natural labors the sheet that hung over the side of the bed could be laid in his lap to keep the accoucheur sufficiently clean and dry. Abnormal cases that required the accoucheur to alter his position could be conducted decorously if the sheet were "tucked round him, or an apron put on," but the latter must be worn only when he was actively engaged.[120]

Despite William Smellie's meticulous attention to what he perceived to be appropriate attire, behavior, and attitudes for obstetricians, he more than any other practitioner of the age attracted the criticism of those who resented the intrusion of the men midwives. Benjamin Rush, lecturing to medical students early in the nineteenth century, acknowledged that the most able practitioners were not always those to reap the greatest rewards. Pointing to Smellie as an example, Rush faulted him for his lack of "popular and engaging manners." It was this deficiency, according to Rush, that consigned him to the second rank of business in London and prevented the acquisition of a fashionable practice. The illustrious career of William Hunter stood in sharp contrast. Younger and less experienced, Hunter nevertheless succeeded where Smellie had failed, observed Rush, chiefly because his talents and knowledge were accompanied "with agreeable and insinuating manners."[121]

Rush's assessment was accurate. William Smellie was a brilliant theorist and a creative technician. Moreover, it was his teaching and practice more than that of any other that emphasized the importance of attending normal cases, thus permanently opening the door of the lying-in chamber to men. Although very successful, ironically he never did develop a fashionable practice. Instead, long after his death in 1763, William Smellie was vilified and ridiculed. He had become the symbol of the new obstetrics, and as such his name aroused the ire, scorn, and wrath of all those men and women who rejected out of hand the "seasonable help" of the men midwives.

NOTES

1. Hugh Chamberlen, "Translator to the Reader," in François Mauriceau, *The Diseases of Women with Child, and in Child-bed,* 2nd ed., trans. Hugh Chamberlen (London: John Darby, 1683), no pagination.
2. Ibid.
3. Ibid.
4. William Giffard, *Cases in Midwifery* (London: B. Motte, T. Wotton, & L. Gulliver, 1734), quoted in Irving S. Cutter and Henry R. Viets, *A Short History of Midwifery* 1st ed. (Philadelphia and London: W. B. Saunders Co., 1964), pp. 18-20.
5. Edmund Chapman, *A Treatise on the Improvement of Midwifery . . . ,* 3rd ed. (London: L. Davis and C. Reymers, 1759), pp. xi, 139, 142.
6. Ibid., p. xii.
7. John Maubray, *The Female Physician . . .* (London: James Holland, 1724), quoted in Cutter and Viets, *Short History,* p. 12.
8. William Smellie, *A Treatise on the Theory and Practice of Midwifery,* 3rd ed. (London: D. Wilson & T. Durham, 1756), p. lxx.
9. Ibid.; Fielding H. Garrison, *An Introduction to the History of Medicine,* 4th ed. (Philadelphia: W. B. Saunders, 1929), pp. 111, 124, 226.

10. Benjamin Pugh, *A Treatise of Midwifery, Chiefly with Regard to the Operation, with Several Improvements in that ART* . . . (London: J. Buckland, 1754), pp. 37-38, 64-65.

11. John Memis, *The Midwife's Pocket-Companion: or a Practical Treatise of Midwifery on a New Plan* . . . *adapted to the Use of the Female as well as the Male Practitioner in that Art* (London: Edward and Charles Dilly, 1765), pp. 91-92; I. Snapper, "Midwifery, Past and Present," *Bulletin of the New York Academy of Medicine,* n.s. 39 (August 1963):507.

12. Hugh Chamberlen, "Translator to the Reader," in Mauriceau, *Diseases of Women,* no pagination.

13. Smellie, *Theory and Practice,* pp. 297-298.

14. Guy's Hospital, London, *Syllabus of Lectures on Midwifery Delivered at Guy's Hospital & at Dr. Lowder's & Dr. Haighton's Theatre, Southwark* (London: Guy's Hospital, 1799), pp. 52-54.

15. Smellie, *Theory and Practice,* p. 296.

16. Ibid., p. 304.

17. Ibid., p. 303.

18. Cutter and Viets, *Short History,* p. 154; Rosemary Keupper Valle, "The Cesarean Operation in Alta California During the Franciscan Mission Period (1769-1833)," *Bulletin of the History of Medicine* 48 (Summer 1974):266-269.

19. Nicholas Culpeper, *A Directory for Midwives* . . . (London: Norris, Bettesworth, Ballard and Batley, 1724), p. 300; Chapman, *Treatise,* pp. xiv-xv.

20. Smellie, *Theory and Practice,* pp. 375-379; Guy's Hospital, *Syllabus of Lectures,* p. 71; Thomas Denman, *An Introduction to the Practice of Midwifery,* Vol. 2 (New York: James Oram, 1802), pp. 103-104; 106; 111-112; Alan Guttmacher, *Pregnancy and Birth* (New York: New American Library, 1962), p. 190.

21. Chapman, *Treatise,* p. 72; Pugh, *Midwifery,* pp. v, 88-89, 121.

22. Maubray, *The Female Physician,* quoted in Chapman, *Treatise,* pp. 89-91.

23. Maubray, *The Female Physician,* quoted in Cutter and Viets, *Short History,* p. 11.

24. Chapman, *Treatise,* pp. xv-xviii.

25. Pugh, *Midwifery,* p. viii.

26. Smellie, *Theory and Practice,* pp. 248-249.

27. Arturo Castiglioni, *A History of Medicine,* 2nd ed. trans E. B. Krumbhaar (New York: Knopf, 1958), p. 554; Cutter and Viets, *Short History,* pp. 44-50, 191-192.

28. Hugh Chamberlen, "Translator," in Mauriceau, *Diseases,* no pagination.

29. Smellie, *Theory and Practice,* p. 250.

30. Chapman, *Treatise,* p. 81.

31. Smellie, *Theory and Practice,* pp. 253-256; William Smellie, *A Collection of Cases and Observations in Midwifery to Illustrate His Former Treatise, or First Volume on that Subject* (London: D. Wilson and T. Durham, 1754), p. 352.

32. Pugh, *Midwifery,* p. 91.

33. Chapman, *Treatise,* p. 69.

34. Smellie, *Theory and Practice,* pp. lviii, lxvi.

35. Chapman, *Treatise,* pp. 91-92; Smellie, *Theory and Practice,* p. 251; Guttmacher, *Pregnancy and Birth,* p. 6; Cutter and Viets, *Short History,* pp. 18-19, 193.

36. Cutter and Viets, *Short History,* p. 60.

37. Chapman, *Treatise,* p. xxv.

38. Smellie, *Cases and Observations,* pp. 352-353.

39. Pugh, *Midwifery,* pp. 132-133, vii.

40. Ibid., pp. 135, 75.

41. Chapman, *Treatise,* pp. 82, 86; Pugh, *Midwifery,* p. iv; Smellie, *Theory and Practice,* pp. lxv, 255-257.

42. Pugh, *Midwifery,* p. v.

43. Smellie, *Theory and Practice,* p. lxiii.

44. Pugh, *Midwifery,* pp. 83-84.

45. Smellie, *Theory and Practice,* pp. 261-289.

46. Ibid., pp. 357-358.

47. Chapman, *Treatise,* pp. xxi-xxiv.

48. Robert W. Johnstone, *William Smellie: The Master of British Midwifery* (Edinburgh and London: E. & S. Livingstone Ltd., 1952), pp. 1-15. Johnstone notes that in this early period, organized medical training was not yet available. In centers like Edinburgh, Leyden, and Paris, teachers offered separate courses in botany, anatomy, chemistry, and physic. Students could take these courses independently and bypass a university degree, which was expensive and not required for practicing either physic or surgery. Medical practitioners were licensed by the Royal Colleges of Physicians and Surgeons in London and in Edinburgh. In Glasgow, the Faculty of Physicians and Surgeons were empowered to examine and license. It was twelve years before Smellie became a freeman of that corporation and was licensed; in 1733 he became a member of the Faculty of Physicians and Surgeons of Glasgow. In 1745 Smellie received the Doctorate in Medicine from the University of Glasgow. See also A. H. McClintoch, "Memoir of William Smellie," in A. H. McClintoch, ed., *Smellie's Treatise on the Theory and Practice of Midwifery,* Vol. 1 (London: The New Sydenham Society, 1876), 1-23.

49. *Cases and Observations,* p. iii.

50. William Smellie, *A Collection of Preternatural Cases and Observations in Midwifery,* 2nd ed. (London: D. Wilson and T. Durham, 1766), pp. 320-322.

51. Smellie, *Cases and Observations,* p. 351.

52. Smellie, *Preternatural Cases,* pp. 179-182.

53. Smellie, *Cases and Observations,* pp. iii-iv, 352-353.

54. Smellie, *Theory and Practice,* p. 253.

55. Ibid., pp. 251-252. In 1742 the Dublin surgeon Fielding Ould published his *Treatise of Midwifery,* in which he presented a detailed description of the mechanism of labor. See Cutter and Viets, *Short History,* p. 182.

56. Johnstone, *William Smellie,* pp. 42-45; William Smellie, *A Set of Anatomical Tables with Explanations, and an Abridgement of the Practice of Midwifery* . . . (Worcester, Mass.: Isaiah Thomas, 1793), pp. 8-9; Smellie, *Theory and Practice,* pp. 78-82, 281-282.

57. Smellie, *Theory and Practice,* pp. 252-253.

58. Cutter and Viets, *Short History,* pp. 13-15.

59. M. Dorothy George, *London Life in the Eighteenth Century* (New York: Harper and Row, 1965), pp. 48, 335n.

60. Cutter and Viets, *Short History,* pp. 15-16, 181.

61. Chapman, *Treatise,* pp. 87-88.

62. Smellie, *Cases and Observations,* pp. iii-iv.

63. Smellie, *Theory and Practice,* p. v.

64. Johnstone, *William Smellie,* p. 22.

65. Ibid., fig. 1, facing p. 24. This page of the brochure is reproduced in Johnstone from the only known copy, now in the National Library of Medicine.

66. Ibid., fig. 2, facing p. 25.

67. Smellie, *Theory and Practice,* p. 442.

68. Memis, *Pocket-Companion,* pp. v-vi, 1-2.

69. Chapman, *Treatise,* p. xxiv.

70. Quoted in Sophia Jex-Blake, *Medical Women: A Thesis and a History* (Edinburgh: Oliphant, Anderson & Ferrier, 1886; London: Hamilton, Adams and Co., 1886; New York: Source Book Press Reprint, 1970), pp. 24-25.

71. Smellie, *Theory and Practice,* pp. 440-441.

72. Smellie, *Cases and Observations,* pp. 353-354.

73. Journal of Peter Camper, quoted in Johnstone, *William Smellie,* pp. 26-27.

74. Smellie, *Theory and Practice,* p. 1.

75. Ibid., p. iv.

76. Camper, quoted in Johnstone, *William Smellie,* p. 28.

77. Henry R. Viets, "The Medical Education of James Lloyd in Colonial America," *Yale Journal of Biology and Medicine* 31 (September 1958):10.

78. Smellie, *Theory and Practice,* p. v.

79. Smellie, *Cases and Observations,* p. v.

80. K. Bryn Thomas, *James Douglas of the Pouch and his Pupil William Hunter* (Springfield, Ill.: Charles C. Thomas, 1964), pp. 24-25.

81. The earliest notes on William Hunter's lectures are contained in the manuscript recorded by one of his students for the year 1752 and reproduced as Hunter's *Lectures of Anatomy* (Amsterdam: Elsevier Publishing Company, 1972).

82. George C. Peachey, "William Hunter's Obstetrical Career," *Annals of Medical History,* n.s. 2 (September 1930):477-478.

83. John L. Thornton and Patricia C. Want, "William Hunter's 'The Anatomy of the Human Gravid Uterus,' 1774-1974," *Journal of Obstetrics and Gynaecology of the British Commonwealth,* n.s. 81 (January 1974):1-3; Cutter and Viets, *Short History,* pp. 33-37; John Kobler, *The Reluctant Surgeon* (London: W. Heinemann, 1960), p. 67.

84. Quoted in Thornton and Want, "Anatomy," p. 2.

85. Ibid.

86. Ibid.

87. William Hunter, *Two Introductory Lectures Delivered by William Hunter To His Last Course of Anatomical Lectures, at His Theatre in Windmill-Street . . .* (London: J. Johnson, 1784), p. 61.

88. Ibid.

89. William Nicholson, "Midwifery," *The British Encyclopedia or Dictionary of Arts & Sciences,* Vol. 8, 3rd American ed. (Philadelphia: Mitchell, Ames and White, 1821), no pagination.

90. J. H. Aveling, *English Midwives: Their History and Their Prospects* (London: Churchill, 1872), pp. 124-125.

91. Smellie, *Preternatural Cases,* pp. 482-486.

92. Smellie, *Cases and Observations,* pp. 255-256.

93. Smellie, *Preternatural Cases,* pp. 486-490.

94. Ibid., pp. 291-492.

95. Ibid., pp. 456-457.

96. Smellie, *Theory and Practice,* pp. 246-247.

97. Kobler, *Reluctant Surgeon,* p. 148.

98. Smellie, *Theory and Practice,* pp. 242-243.

99. Ibid.

100. Smellie, *Cases and Observations,* p. v.

101. Pugh, *Midwifery,* pp. 56-57.

102. Memis, *Pocket-Companion,* p. 96.

103. Thomas Denman, *Aphorisms on the Application and Use of the*

Forceps and Vectis; on preternatural Labours, on Labours attended with Hemorrhage, and with Convulsions (Philadelphia: Benjamin Johnson, 1803), pp. 16-17.

104. Smellie, *Theory and Practice,* p. 249.

105. Pugh, *Midwifery,* pp. 41-42.

106. Smellie, *Theory and Practice,* pp. 442-443.

107. Smellie, *Preternatural Cases,* pp. 487, 491; Smellie, *Cases and Observations,* p. 351.

108. Smellie, *Theory and Practice,* pp. 264-265.

109. Ibid., p. 271.

110. Memis, *Pocket-Companion,* p. 99; Denman, *Aphorisms,* p. 16.

111. Journal of Elizabeth Drinker, quoted in Cecil K. Drinker, *Not So Long Ago: A Chronicle of Medicine and Doctors in Colonial Philadelphia* (New York: Oxford University Press, 1937), pp. 60-61.

112. Smellie, *Theory and Practice,* p. 328.

113. Chapman, *Treatise,* pp. 159-161.

114. Pugh, *Midwifery,* p. 74.

115. Quoted in Kobler, *Reluctant Surgeon,* p. 148.

116. Pugh, *Midwifery,* pp. ix-x.

117. Chapman, *Treatise,* pp. 262-263.

118. Smellie, *Theory and Practice,* p. 441.

119. Smellie, *Cases and Observations,* p. 257; Smellie, *Preternatural Cases,* p. 486.

120. Smellie, *Theory and Practice,* pp. 335-336.

121. Benjamin Rush, "On the Means of Acquiring Business and the Causes Which Prevent the Acquisition, and Occasion the Loss of It, In the Profession of Medicine," *Sixteen Introductory Lectures, to Courses of Lectures Upon the Institutes and Practice of Medicine* . . . (Philadelphia: Bradford and Innskeep, 1811), p. 251.

3

"Churgeons," Midwives, and Physicians in English America

no Person or Persons whatsoever, Employed about the Bed of Men, women, or Children . . . for the preservation of Life or health . . . [should] presume to exercise or put forth any Acte Contrary to the known approved Rules of Art in each mistery or Occupation.

—THE DUKE'S LAWS, NEW YORK, 1665

The practice of midwifery in England's North American colonies was based on the prevailing tradition introduced from home and modified by the frontier environment. Just as in England during the seventeenth century, women controlled the field and men were excluded from the birth chamber. Those midwives whose names are found in the early New England town records generally were highly regarded. Bridget Fuller (d. 1664) practiced her art in Massachusetts Bay colony for many years. It is not known where she learned her skills; as the third wife of Deacon Samuel Fuller, who had studied medicine at the University of Leyden before emigrating to Plymouth on the *Mayflower,* she may have acquired some of her medical knowledge from her husband. When she was widowed in 1663, the magistrates of Rehobeth, anxious to have a midwife for their town, invited her to settle there, but she declined.

Another woman, identified only as Mrs. Wiat of Dorchester (d. 1705), attended over one thousand births, according to her epitaph. Ruth Barnaby (1664-1765) practiced the art for more than forty years. Remarkably alert, at the age of one hundred she had herself inoculated against the smallpox. Elizabeth Phillips (1685-1761) was born in London. In 1718 she received a midwifery license from the lord bishop of that city. The following year she came to Boston with her husband, John, and began to practice midwifery. Her practice, too, extended beyond a forty-year period. Phillips's epitaph indicated that she had "by the blessing of God brought into this world above 3,000 children." Ann Eliot, married to the missionary and physician John Eliot, was another prominent midwife who may have acquired some medical skills from her husband. The survivors of Mrs. Thomas Whitmore, of Marlboro, Vermont, claimed that she had never lost a patient in the course of attending over two thousand births.[1]

Many of these early midwives were incredibly hardy. The Boston *Weekly News-Letter,* in what may have been the first newspaper reference in North America to a midwife reported, "Yesterday was interred here [Philadelphia] the body of Mary Bradway, formerly a noted Midwife. She was born on New Years Day 1629-30, and died on the second of January, 1729-30, aged One hundred years and one day. Her constitution wore well to the last, and she could see to read without spectacles a few Months since." This undoubtedly was the Mary Broadwell for whom there was composed *An Elegy on the death of that Ancient, Venerable and Useful Matron and Midwife, Mrs. Mary Broadwell, who rested from her labours, January 2, 1730. Aged a hundred years and one day.*[2]

In the Dutch colony of New Netherland, women controlled midwifery. In 1633, just a few years after they had planted the settlement, the Dutch built a "small house for the midwife" in New Amsterdam. Usually the colony had an official midwife. Mrs. Trynje Jonas held this post in 1644, and in 1655 midwife Hellegond Joris received an annual salary of one hundred guilders for her attendance on poor women. In 1658 the councillors of New Amsterdam appointed midwife Hilletje Wilbruch matron of a proposed new hospital. Residents completed the building shortly before the English captured New Netherland in 1664 and renamed the colony in honor of Charles II's brother James, Duke of York. Under English control, midwifery practices in New York changed little, and women continued to dominate the field.[3]

Despite the laudatory comments lavished on some of the colonial midwives, several practitioners ran into serious trouble. In New England, church and civil authorities evinced the same propensity to equate midwifery and witchcraft exhibited by their English brethren. Anne Hutchinson practiced midwifery in Massachusetts Bay until her controversial challenge to Puritan orthodoxy led to her trials and subsequent expulsion from the colony. Although she did not deliver her friend Mary Dyer of the stillborn "monstrosity" that became the subject of curiosity and speculation among witch-conscious New Englanders, Hutchinson was present when Jane Hawkins performed the delivery. Hawkins was another well-known midwife, of whom one contemporary wrote, she was "notorious for familiarity with the devil." The suspicion that she was a witch led magistrates in 1638 to forbid her to practice medicine. Three years later the General Court finally threatened her with severe punishment unless she left the colony. Still another midwife, Margaret Jones, was accused by Charlestown authorities of practicing witch-craft. Continued speculation about her activities led to her execution in 1648, thereby awarding her the dubious distinction of becoming the first person executed in the colony of Massachusetts Bay.[4]

In general, at least until the middle of the eighteenth century, attempts to license any medical practitioners or to regulate their activities were rare in the still comparatively unstructured world of English America. The Anglican Church had not extended its episcopal supervision of midwives to the colonies. It is therefore of considerable interest that early in the 1700s the responsibility fell to local civil authorities. The models followed appear to have been the regulations then in force in both England and Scotland. The first town in the British Isles to draft regulations for midwives was Edinburgh, Scotland. The town council minutes for May 4, 1694, claimed that "many women take upon them the office of medwifs who are nowayes qualified for the Imployment and that others take up that profession unduly and for sinister ends." At this meeting the council adopted a plan designed to eliminate such abuses. "Persons declared fit by the magistrates" were to certify midwives only after examining them to determine the extent of their skills. After giving satisfactory responses to the examiners, the midwives were sworn to uphold specified ethical rules of conduct. As did their counterparts in England, the Scottish midwives swore to minister to the poor when necessary, to refrain from administering "drogs inwardly" to pregnant women, except upon the advice of a physician, not to conceal illegitimate births, and finally to report to the magistrates the names of those women who practiced without first obtaining the proper certification.[5]

In both its phrasing and in the abuses it addressed, the Edinburgh oath developed by the magistrates is similar to the oath administered by the English bishops since the sixteenth century. In 1716 the New York common council enacted "A Law for Regulating Midwives Within the City," containing an oath obviously based on those used in the British Isles. The law did not require any examination of skills, but compelled the midwife to swear before the mayor, recorder, or an alderman:

she will be diligent and ready to help any woman in labor, whether poor or rich; that in time of necessity she will not cause or suffer any woman to name or put any father to the child . . . but the very true father thereof . . . that she will not suffer any woman to pretend to be delivered of a child who is not . . . that she will not suffer any woman's child to be murdered or hurt . . . and as often as she shall see any peril, or jeopardy, either in the mother or child, she will call in other midwives for counsel; that she will not force a woman to give more for her services than is right: that she will not collude to keep secret the birth of a child [and] will be of good behaviour; will not conceal the births of bastards, &c.[6]

In its initial version, this ordinance, which the common council reenacted repeatedly between 1716 and 1763 with only slight modifications, contained no references to prohibiting men from entering the lying-in chamber. It is clear, nevertheless, that women attended ordinary cases, as indicated by a provision inserted in the 1730s requiring that the midwives swear not to "open any mystery appertaining to . . . [their] Office, in the presence of any Man." The exception to this rule was the difficult or abnormal birth that threatened life. Indeed, even after men midwives had begun to practice in

New York, the prohibition against them remained in the oath.[7] Curiously, as one historian has pointed out, the provision excluding men was introduced so late that it came only a decade or so before men midwives had invaded the field.[8]

As in England, the qualifications desired of colonial midwives stressed character rather than obstetric proficiency. Any examination to test midwifery skills would have been quite out of place in the first half of the eighteenth century, given the characteristic colonial laxity concerning medical licensing in general. Colonists had made a few local attempts to regulate medical practices at various times. The Massachusetts law of 1649, one of the earliest examples, was intended by its framers "not . . . to discourage any from all use of their skill, but rather [to] incourage & direct them":

Foreasmuch as the Law of God allows no man to impair the life or limbs, of any person, but in a judicial way. It is therefore ordered, That no person or persons whatsoever imployed at any times, about the bodyes of men, women or children for preservation of life or health, as Chirurgeons, Midwives, Physicians or others, presume to exercise or put forth, any act, contrary to the known approved rules of art, in each mistery or occupation, nor exercise any force, violence, or cruelty upon, or towards, the body of any, whether young or old (no not in the most difficult and desperate cases) without the advice and consent of such as are skilful in the same art (if such may be had) or at least of some of the wisest and gravest then present and consent of the patient or patients if they be mente compotes, much less contrary to such advice and consent upon such severe punishment, as the nature of the case may deserve.[9]

Despite its stated intention, this law strongly suggests a lack of public confidence in medical practitioners and served as the model for others. In 1665 the Duke's Laws in New York, written primarily for the English population of Westchester and Long Island in the colony so recently won from the Dutch, borrowed heavily from Massachusetts Bay. They contained a provision directed at "Churgeons, Midwives and Physicians" and warned:

no Person or Persons whatsoever, Employed about the Bed of Men, women, or Children . . . for the preservation of Life or health . . . [should] presume to exercise or put forth any Acte Contrary to the known approved

Rules of Art in each mistery or Occupation, or Exercise any force, violence, or Cruelty upon [patients] . . . without the advice and consent of
such as are Skillful in that same Art.[10]

By and large, however, statements such as these were rare, and this
background of laissez faire must be kept in mind in discussing the
whole question of medical regulation in colonial America.

All medical practitioners, that is, physicians, surgeons, apothecaries, and midwives, practiced with minimum supervision. William
Smith, the eighteenth-century historian, called attention to the need
for medical regulation with his observation that in New York,
"Quacks abound like locusts in Egypt, and too many have recommended themselves to a full practice and profitable subsistence."[11]
Critics charged that laxity in New York had led to a situation in
which "far the greatest Part of them [doctors] are meer pretenders
to a Profession, of which they are entirely ignorant,"[12] even to the
degree that they misspelled their newspaper advertisements.

In 1760 the New York assembly enacted its first law calling for an
examination of persons undertaking to practice "Physick and
Surgery" within the city of New York. It empowered a board
representing the provincial and city governments to examine and
license physicians. Those who practiced without first obtaining the
proper license might be fined £5 for each offense. The legislators
omitted all reference to the midwives; presumably they continued
to practice unlicensed.[13]

American physicians varied widely in their knowledge of medicine, surgical techniques, and their ability to implement what
they knew. The first medical schools in the colonies dated from the
decade immediately preceding the American Revolution. Those
who sought formal medical training before the 1760s of necessity
studied abroad. A few immigrants to the colonies had attended the
English universities; others had studied medicine at Leyden, Rheims,
or other schools on the Continent. After the medical school was
organized at Edinburgh in the 1720s, some of its students subsequently settled in the colonies. William Hunter (1729-1777) had
studied with the anatomist Alexander Monro *primus* (1697-1767) at
Edinburgh and had been at Leyden as well. When he emigrated to
Newport, Rhode Island, in 1752, he lectured on both anatomy and

midwifery, thus reflecting in his own successful practice the growing interest across the Atlantic in the new obstetrics that would eventually influence American medicine.[14] Beginning with the 1740s some young men traveled from the colonies to these centers of learning. As affluence and filial expectations grew, the number of these increased, but they always remained in the minority.

The vast majority of the estimated 3,500 colonial doctors in practice in 1775,[15] if they had any medical training at all, had acquired it through the apprentice system. A young man wishing to enter the medical field would serve as an apprentice to an established practitioner for a specified number of years. The "Articles of Agreement" concluded in 1736 between Zabdiel Boylston, of smallpox inoculation fame, and Joseph Lemmon, Sr., for the education of Joseph Lemmon, Jr., illustrate the system. As preceptor Boylston agreed to instruct young Lemmon in "the Arts Businesses or Mysterys of Physick and Surgery" and to provide food and lodging for a two-year period. In exchange, Lemmon Sr. agreed to pay Boylston £200 to furnish the boy's clothing and provide for his laundry.[16] The fees paid for such training appear to have varied as much as the duration and the quality of the training itself. An irate critic of preceptors writing in the *Boston Gazette* in 1766 declared that physicians would not accept apprentices for less than eighty to one hundred pounds.[17] Yet twenty years earlier Henry Lloyd paid £400 to John Clark, preceptor to his brother James in Boston.[18]

Working with a preceptor often became more a matter of working for him as general servant, groom, and fee collector. Still, in the period of apprenticeship ranging from two to seven years, the pupil did have opportunities to compound medications, observe a variety of cases, and even assist his mentor at his patient's bedside. Generally the apprentice augmented his empirical training by reading from the few medical books in his preceptor's library, snatching bits of time early in the day and late in the evening to absorb some medical theory from the works of Sydenham and Boerhaave, to which later in the century were added those of William Cullen and John Brown. Apprenticeship to an able practitioner could mean the opportunity to acquire valuable clinical training. Much depended, of course, on the method in which the preceptor himself had been trained. A poorly prepared apprentice, who in later years trained others, had little of value to impart and must have perpetuated ignorance, whereas those well trained by competent preceptors or through more formal study abroad were in an excellent position to advance the knowledge of their own pupils. There is a tendency to downgrade the quality of this type of apprentice training, yet lengthy service and association with a skillful mentor was more beneficial than attendance at an inferior medical college would have been.[19]

An example of the efficacy of the apprentice system functioning at its highest level may be seen in the successive medical careers of John Kearsley (1685-1772), John Redman (1722-1808), and Benjamin Rush (1745-1813). Kearsley, an able surgeon with a liberal English education, emigrated to Philadelphia. There he established an enviable reputation and a successful general practice. Among his gifted apprentices were such outstanding practitioners of later years as John Redman, Thomas Cadwalader (1707-1799), John Bard (1716-1799), and William Shippen, Sr. (1712-1801). All of these men, in turn, trained accomplished students, including in Bard's case his son, Samuel (1742-1821) and in Shippen's, William Shippen, Jr. (1736-1808). John Redman followed his Kearsley years with study at Edinburgh, attending the lectures on anatomy and physiology by Alexander Monro *primus* and those on materia medica offered by Charles Alston. From Edinburgh, Redman went on to Leyden, where he studied medicine with Boerhaave's successor, Jerome David Gaubius, and anatomy, surgery, and midwifery with Boerhaave's gifted student Bernhard Siegfried Albinus. After successfully defending his dissertation on spontaneous abortion, Redman observed in the Paris hospitals and walked the wards of St. Guy's in London.[20] Returning to Philadelphia, he established himself in practice and became one of the city's busiest and most respected physicians. In turn, Redman served as preceptor to such promising young students as John Morgan, who was to found the first American medical school, Caspar Wistar, who followed William Shippen, Jr., as Professor of Anatomy, Surgery, and Midwifery at the University of Pennsylvania, and Benjamin Rush, who became the most celebrated of all these early American doctors.

From the *Autobiography* of Benjamin Rush, we can gain first-hand appreciation of the hard work and long hours required to be apprenticed to the eminent Dr. Redman. Rush began with Redman in February 1761 and stayed with him until July 1766.

During this period, I was absent from his business but eleven days, and never spent more than three evenings out of his house. . . . In addition to preparing and compounding medicines . . . a little time and habit soon wore away all that degree of sensibility which is painful, and enabled me to see and even assist with composure in performing the most severe operations in surgery. The confinement and restraint . . . gave me no alternative but business and study . . . I read in the intervals of my business and at late and early hours, all the books in medicine that were put into my hands by my master, or that I could borrow from other students of medicine in the city.[21]

Since Redman was one of the physicians attached to the Pennsylvania Hospital, Rush was admitted to view the practice of five other physicians there; somehow he found time to attend Shippen's anatomy lectures in 1762 and 1765 as well as Morgan's materia medica lectures in 1765.

A substantial number of practitioners were at the other extreme from Rush, Shippen, and Wistar, for they had no medical training of any type. They simply fell into the medical field because they fancied it and had happened to have one or two successes, from which their reputations stemmed. In this respect these empirics were no different from the vast majority of women midwives, who were not formally apprenticed either. For the women, of course, their sex precluded attendance at universities, regardless of all other circumstances. In any case, given the general absence of medical licensing, any men or women who wished to do so could call themselves doctors. Dr. Alexander Hamilton related having met a former shoemaker in Connecticut, who by curing an old woman had acquired a physician's reputation. Thus "finding the practice of physick a more profitable business than cobling," remarked Hamilton dryly, "he laid aside his awls and leather, got himself some gallipots, and . . . fell to cobling human bodies."[22]

Similarly illustrative of the casual manner in which one could fall into medical practice was the case of one Dr. Avery of Dedham and Boston. Avery, described by a contemporary as "a man of pretty ingenuity," had acquired "some notable skill in physick and midwifery" as the result of his veterinary experiences. Before his death in 1687 he had developed some useful midwifery instruments.[23] Under such permissive conditions some women were practicing medicine along with midwifery in colonial America. This certainly was true of Anne Hutchinson early in the seventeenth century. There are good reasons to suggest that other women whose less spectacular lives were not sufficiently noteworthy to merit comment from their contemporaries also engaged in medical practice. Although women were not considered man's equal in colonial America, the favorable sex ratio and the frontier environment combined to create a fairly tolerant attitude toward women. This allowed them in practice, if not always in theory, to engage in a wide variety of occupations that included printer, tanner, blacksmith, and merchant.[24] There is no reason to suspect that the medical field was different from any other in this respect. Then too, colonial women and their English counterparts were the principal cooks and nurturers of the sick within their families. Cookbooks available on both sides of the Atlantic contained myriad recipes for the preparation of tonics and curatives of all types.[25] The women who successfully treated sick members of their own families might easily have turned to doctoring on a larger scale.

The absence of medical licensing had the additional effect of protecting, if not promoting, quackery, and practitioners of the period frequently were suspect. When Colonel Barré wrote to John Watts seeking support for a physician who planned to deliver a series of anatomical lectures in New York, Watts received the information without enthusiasm. He doubted there would be much interest in the lectures, but the thought did not disturb him. He offered the opinion that in New York there were "so many of the Faculty allready destroying his Majestys good Subjects, that in the humour people are, they had rather One half were hangd that are allready practicing, than breed up a New Swarm in addition to the old."[26]

Yet, the eighteenth century was a turning point for British medicine generally and for midwifery in particular. The effects of the dramatic changes taking place in British obstetrics were not long in spreading to the colonies. By the middle of the century a new group of young men intent on medical careers had appeared. Unlike the majority of apprentices, these sons of affluent and often influential families found the means to augment their apprenticeship with medical study abroad. With neither medical schools nor hospitals open to women students, daughters were excluded from such ventures, even in the unlikely event that parents would have approved or invested in daughters the considerable sums required to obtain formal medical education. Among the growing list of colonials to receive training abroad were John Van Brugh Tennent (1737-1770), James Lloyd (1728-1810), and John Jones (1729-1791), all of whom, along with Samuel Bard, William Shippen, Jr., John Morgan, and others would play key roles in the upgrading of American medical practice.

The first stop on their journey ordinarily was London. At mid-century this city presented the visitor with amazing contrasts. Capital of a proud and growing empire, it was the hub of social, cultural, and scientific life. The great and the hopeful from the world of art, letters, and science were drawn to its coffee houses and salons. Politicians, wits, artists, writers, aristocrats, and upwardly mobile members of the middle class were attracted to its world of fashion, high life, and culture. Its bustling wharves, the thriving international trade that daily increased the merchants' fortunes, and the busy shops were all a part of the city of which Ben Jonson would write, "When a man is tired of London he is tired of Life."

Yet there was the other side of London depicted so vividly in the works of Hogarth. Massive unemployment created by the seemingly ceaseless flow of men and women from the country to this urban center, incredibly low wages and impossible working conditions, washerwomen paid half a crown for laboring from two or three in the morning until nine or ten o'clock at night, laboring classes seeking solace in gin, beggars, prostitutes, abandoned children, disease, sickness, and poverty almost beyond belief—all these, too, were part of London life.[27]

Into this setting of poverty and wealth, fashion and degradation, came young Americans seeking to build upon the medical knowledge acquired from their preceptors. James Lloyd served his apprenticeship in Boston under the successful and fashionable Dr. John Clark (1698-1768). He thought of going on to Paris but decided instead on London, for which he sailed in the late summer of 1750. That winter he presented a letter of introduction to William Cheselden (1688-1752), the renowned surgeon who had perfected the perineal technique for extracting stone from the bladder. Semi-retired by then, Cheselden had left his surgical post at St. Thomas' Hospital, but Lloyd could frequent his clinic at the Royal Hospital in Chelsea. More important to his clinical training was the year he spent at St. Guy's Hospital in Southwark, attending lectures on anatomy and surgery and serving as dresser to Joseph Warner (1717-1801).[28]

For his teacher in midwifery he chose William Smellie, then at the height of his career. Lloyd enrolled for two complete courses with Smellie, receiving his certificate of attendance from the master in March 1752. In his selection of anatomy instructor he was no less fortunate, for he attended not only William Hunter's regular anatomical and surgical lectures in the Great Piazza, Covent Garden, but added to this a private course from Hunter in "Dissections and Operations of Surgery."[29] In spring 1752 the twenty-four-year-old Lloyd returned to Boston, his formal medical training completed. His two years abroad had cost his father several hundred pounds sterling. Yet with his exposure to Smellie, Hunter, Warner, and Cheselden, Lloyd could well claim value received. His superior training soon placed him in the forefront of those who within the following two decades would establish themselves as men midwives in colonial America.

In late summer 1758 William Shippen, Jr., left his father's comfortable Philadelphia home and thriving medical practice to board "Capt. Dingo's fine ship" for the seven and one-half week journey that would take him to Liverpool and thence to London. His object was to spend the winter "with the finest Anatomist for Dissections, Injections, &c. in England; at the same time visit the Hospitals daily, to attend Lectures of Midwifery with a Gentleman who will make that branch as familiar to him as he can want or wish to have it."[30] A graduate of the College of New Jersey in Princeton, young Shippen had studied medicine for three years under his father, William Shippen, Sr., once John Kearsley's apprentice. Philadelphia was the scientific capital of colonial America, yet the opportunities it offered for the training of medical students were limited. His bachelor's degree, the years of apprenticeship, and even his special opportunities to observe the practices of able physicians in the area were insufficient. As his father explained, still unavailable at home were the "variety of operations and those frequent dissections which . . . [were] common in older countries," and for which, added Shippen, "I must send him to Europe."[31]

Shippen arrived in London in the fall and soon moved into John Hunter's house in the Great Piazza, Covent Garden. There he resided, attending William Hunter's anatomical lectures and demonstrations, performing his own dissections, and learning the art of injecting the blood vessels for the purpose of preparing anatomical specimens. John Hunter especially had brought this latter, creative work to a high level. By injecting the vessels with various colored pigments mixed with warm liquid, cooling the specimens and immersing them in acid baths to destroy surrounding tissue, the anatomist produced a cast of the finer vessels that were ordinarily destroyed in dissections. This skill was immensely valuable to Shippen in his future teaching career.[32] In Summer 1759 Shippen, determined to learn all he could about the "new obstetrics," enrolled in Colin MacKensie's midwifery lectures. MacKensie (d. 1775), a close friend of John Hunter, had been William Smellie's assistant for several years. In 1754, after he and Smellie had fallen out, MacKensie began to offer his own midwifery course in the borough of Southwark, where he continued to perpetuate Smellie's teachings.[33]

Shippen's diary of 1759 to 1760 makes evident the enthusiasm and diligence he brought to his studies. On one Friday in July he "Spent the afternoon and Evening at 3 labours" and attended a lecture and an operation for a leg fracture at St. Guy's Hospital. On another day he rose at six to attend a labor that "lasted till night," visiting the patient periodically throughout the day. After attending MacKensie's lecture at eight o'clock in the evening, he returned to the woman and stayed with her until she delivered the next morning at five.[34] Several of Shippen's patients lived on Crucifix Lane, the site of a small lying-in hospital maintained for clinical teaching by MacKensie in a manner reminiscent of that of Richard Manningham and William Smellie. It is worth noting that when Shippen returned to Philadelphia and began to offer his own course in midwifery, he opened a similar establishment for poor lying-in women on Letitia Lane, near the waterfront.[35]

By summer 1760, when Shippen prepared to move northward to Edinburgh Medical School for his work in theory, he had attended many labors and had gained valuable experience. His interest in midwifery continued at Edinburgh as indicated by the subject of his medical thesis, "De Placentae cum Utero nexu," presented in 1761.[36] Following his studies with William Cullen, Alexander Monro *primus,* and his son, Alexander Monro *secundis,* and the others on the faculty of this dynamic and distinguished medical institution, Shippen traveled briefly in Europe. The Seven Years War precluded extended travel, and soon he returned to London for his marriage to Alice Lee of Virginia. The new couple sailed to Philadelphia several months later. By November 1762 Shippen already had begun to teach anatomy, the first of his many courses on anatomy and midwifery that comprised part of his legacy from the Hunters and MacKensie.

The war between France and England had influenced William Shippen's decision to study at Edinburgh rather than at Leyden. The Seven Years War intruded even more directly into the life of Samuel Bard. Bard, a graduate of King's College, had studied medicine under John Bard, his father, the highly esteemed New York doctor. Keenly interested in his son's medical career, the elder Bard encouraged him to pursue further study abroad. In early autumn 1761 Samuel boarded a vessel for London, thinking "of nothing but the advantages . . . [he] should reap, & the Pleasures . . . [he] should enjoy in London."[37] Three weeks out of New York, however, the French captured his ship on the high seas. Samuel was conveyed to France and imprisoned in Bayonne Castle. Benjamin Franklin, his father's influential friend in London, finally secured his release, but not before Samuel had spent several months and a considerable amount of his London fund on this French adventure.

In April 1762 Bard informed his parents of his safe arrival in London.[38] He had missed William Hunter's fall and winter lectures, as well as those of Colin MacKensie. MacKensie and John Fothergill, the Quaker physician and scientist who befriended so many American students abroad, advised Samuel on how to make up for the time lost. Accordingly Samuel immediately enrolled as a physician's pupil at St. Thomas' Hospital with Dr. Russell. Concurrently he enrolled as a "perpetual pupil" with MacKensie.[39] He regularly attended the operations performed both at St. Thomas' and St. Guy's, where he had "frequent opportunity's of seeing Dead Body's opened." MacKensie's midwifery lectures followed closely the theory and practice of William Smellie, and Bard usually read from Smellie the topic upon which MacKensie had lectured in the morning. As a physician who had been denied the advantages of study abroad, John Bard followed his son's progress with avidity, and Samuel carefully recorded for him the manner in which Mac-Kensie proceeded:

his Method was first to give a History of Midwifry, then the Description of the Pelvis, and Parts of Generation, and . . . some hints on Conception; he then procedes to an account of the Gravid Uterus and the Disorders of Women During pregnancy; after Discribes the true signs of labour and the requisites to a natural one, after this he gives a practical touching Lecture, and another upon the Various Instruments, of which he shows a great Collection; points out the different improvements, & mentions their Inventors, he intirely Discards many from practice, and recommends but few, and those to be used with the greatest Caution; only in Cases of Necessity—he next procedes to the Delivery of Both natural and preternatural Cases upon Machinery [that is, mannequins], then gives Directions for the management of the Patient in Labour, & During the Month, Discribes the Dissorders Incident to them at this time, and the Method of Cure, and Concludes his Course with the Dissorders Insident to the Infant, & some Directions, with regard to the choice of a Nurse.[40]

At MacKensie's lying-in house, where students delivered indigent parturient women under his supervision or that of a "very good Midwife" he retained for that purpose, Bard successfully attended a woman who had miscarried. To his great satisfaction she recovered well, and he admitted to his father that he could have had cases earlier, but his "timorousness" had at first prevented him from taking advantage of the opportunity to acquire this valuable clinical training.[41]

Bard had planned to stay on in London through the following winter, continuing with MacKensie's courses and hospital practice under Russell and adding anatomy with William Hunter. He asked whether his father wished him to enroll only in Hunter's lectures or to become a "dissecting pupil" as well, a difference of sixteen pounds sterling.[42] Bard replied that he thought it wiser for Samuel to begin at Edinburgh in the fall and to complete clinical training and the London lectures at a later date. Although this advice conflicted with that of the London doctors who believed it important to acquire clinical experience before delving deeply into theory, Samuel bowed to his father's wishes and moved north in the late summer.

Soon he had settled into a small room at one half crown per week. Taking his meals at an "ordinary," he made the valuable acquaintance of John Morgan, a former Philadelphia classmate of William Shippen's. The two Philadelphians had discussed the possibility of founding an American medical college and had been encouraged by John Fothergill. Morgan later seized the initiative in this, provoking bitter professional rivalry and personal antagonism between him and Shippen. But all this lay in the future. In the fall and early winter of 1762, Bard was delighted that John Morgan, "a person of distinguished merit," had taken notice of him.[43] He too had walked the wards of St. Thomas' in London and could describe to Bard his anatomical studies with the Hunters.[44] It is easy to imagine the two young men exchanging their anecdotes and hopes for the future of American medicine. Morgan shared with Bard his ideas on the projected medical college. Writing to his father, Samuel confessed to feeling "a little jealous of the Philadelphians," adding that he entertained similar ambitions for the establishment of a medical college in New York.[45]

At Edinburgh Samuel Bard proved to be a clever and diligent student. He studied anatomy under Alexander Monro *secundus,* whom he pronounced "a very good demonstrator, and a pretty orator." Bard had lost his opportunity to study with William Hunter and was less than enthusiastic about the "scull and . . . few old bones" he had been able to secure in Edinburgh. Chemistry under William Cullen (1712-1790) was challenging and stimulating. Describing Cullen's "new way of examining his pupils," Samuel reported that Cullen had begun with him. This was an honor, he confessed, from which he "would as lieve have been excused, for . . . [he] was not a little confused to be thus questioned before above a hundred students who all had their eyes fixed upon" him.[46]

Continuing to build his practice at home, John Bard received great pleasure from his son's narratives of life and work at Edinburgh. Expenses were heavy, but these he bore "chearfully" in anticipation of the day when Samuel would return to join him.[47] Analyzing the medical prospects in the city, the father optimistically predicted a bright and successful future.[48] For his part Samuel, with a mixture of pride and diffidence, presented his father with a copy of the "first Fruits of . . . [his] medical labours." This was a botanical paper read before the local medical society in the winter 1764, for which he was awarded a gold medal.[49] Upon his graduation in 1765[50] Samuel Bard returned to London to obtain additional clinical experience before sailing to New York and the already well-established practice that awaited him there.

One investigation of "Philadelphia Medical Students in Europe, 1750-1800," revealed that within this period 117 Americans had taken the doctor of medicine degree at Edinburgh, while many others had studied there for a term or two without taking the degree. By the time of the American Revolution, the steady flow of American medical students to England, Scotland, and the Continent had provided medical educations for about 400 of an estimated 3,500 practitioners in the colonies. Nor did this exodus to Great Britain end with the opening of hostilities in 1775. Indeed, the flow of Americans abroad actually increased after the Revolution.[51]

Walking the wards of the London hospitals, studying as private pupils with the celebrated London practitioners, and attending the lectures of the equally eminent physicians at Edinburgh or the Continent, the young Americans were thrust headlong into the dynamic medical revolution of the eighteenth century. They returned home representing all that was fresh, innovative, and progressive. Priceless opportunities to study with such distinguished and creative figures as William and John Hunter, Colin MacKensie, William Cullen, and the Alexander Munros sparked the desire to emulate their teachers. In so doing they would contribute directly to upgrading the quality of medical practice at home. Their exposure to the dynamic climate of scientific inquiry then fostering the development of the new obstetrics made it natural for them to fix on this field once they had returned. Midwifery would become, then, the branch of medicine most immediately affected by British trends. Those graduates who settled in the major northern cities found among their older colleagues persons of ability and experience who eagerly shared their enthusiasm for the improvement of American medicine. Significantly, as in England, women midwives in America would soon find their practices adversely affected.

NOTES

1. Francis R. Packard, *History of Medicine in the United States,* Vol. 1 (New York: Hafner, 1963), p. 44; Kate Campbell Hurd-Mead, *Medical Women of America* (New York: Froben Press, 1933), p. 17; Rhoda Truax, *The Doctors Warren of Boston: First Family of Surgery* (Boston: Houghton Mifflin, 1968), p. 5; Irving S. Cutter and Henry Viets, *A Short History of Midwifery* (Philadelphia and London: W. B. Saunders Co., 1964), pp. 143-144.

2. The Boston *Weekly News-Letter* January 6, 1730. No known copy of this elegy is extant, but it was advertised in the *Pennsylvania Gazette,* January 20, 1730.

3. I. N. Phelps Stokes, *The Iconography of Manhattan Island,* Vol. 4 (New York: Dodd, 1915-1928), pp. 79, 206, 193; Claude E. Heaton, "Obstetrics in Colonial America," *American Journal of Surgery,* n.s. 45 (September 1939):607; Packard, *History* 1, p. 51.

4. Packard, *History* 1, pp. 45-49; Cutter and Viets, *Short History,* p. 144; Howard W. Haggard, *Devils, Drugs and Doctors,* 4th ed. (New York: Pocket Books, Inc., 1959), p. 73.

5. R. E. Wright-St. Clair, "Easy Essays at Regulating Midwives," *New Zealand Medical Journal* 63 (November 1964):724-25.

6. *Minutes of the Common Council for the City of New York, 1675-1776,* Vol. 3 (New York: Dodd, Mead & Co., 1905), pp. 121-123.

7. *Laws, Orders and Ordinances of the City of New York* (New York: Bradford, 1731), pp. 27-29; *Laws, Statutes, Ordinances and Constitutions . . . of the City of New York . . .* (New York: Holt, 1763), pp. 34-36.

8. Richard H. Shryock, *Medical Licensing in America, 1650-1965* (Baltimore: Johns Hopkins Press, 1967), p. 16.

9. *The Colonial Laws of Massachusetts,* pp. 137-138, quoted in Henry B. Shafer, *The American Medical Profession, 1783-1850* (New York: Columbia University Press, 1936), p. 205.

10. *The Colonial Laws of New York from the Year 1664 to the Revolution,* Vol. 1 (Albany: Lyon, 1894), p. 27.

11. William Smith, *The History of the Province of New York* (London: Thomas Wilcox, 1757), reprinted in the *Collections of the New-York Historical Society,* Vol. 1 (New York: for the Society, 1929), p. 278-279. In *Medical Licensing,* pp. 8-9, Richard Shryock compared the American colonial experience to that of the English provinces, where the medical practitioner was required to administer to the needs of a broad range of cases. Far from London and the narrow restrictions imposed by the guilds and societies, the distinctions between physician and surgeon lost their meaning, with the result that the terms were used interchangeably in the

provinces. In America, "physician," "doctor," and "surgeon" were used interchangeably, and they are so used in this work. A more complete discussion of the breakdown in distinctive meaning of these terms is found in Joseph F. Kett, "Provincial Medical Practice in England, 1730-1815," *Journal of the History of Medicine and Allied Sciences* 19 (January 1964): 17-29. Kett mentions the common designation often used in the eighteenth century of "surgeon, apothecary, and man midwife." A useful collection of essays on the British experience is F. N. L. Poynter, ed., *The Evolution of Medical Practice in Britain* (London: Pitman Publishing Co., Ltd., 1961). Daniel J. Boorstin, observing that the American experience did not breed awe for the learned specialist in anything, reinforced the view that professional subdivisions had little practical significance among American colonial practitioners. See *The Americans: The Colonial Experience* (New York: Random House [Vintage Books], 1964), pp. 205, 230.

12. A., "The Use and Importance of the Practice of PHYSIC; together with the Difficulty of the Science, and the dismal Havock made by Quacks and Pretenders," *The Independent Reflector* (February 15, 1753):49.

13. *The Colonial Laws of New York from the Year 1664 to the Revolution,* Vol. 4 (Albany: Lyon, 1895), p. 455.

14. Cutter and Viets, *Short History,* p. 147.

15. See Whitfield J. Bell, Jr., "A Portrait of the Colonial Physician," in Whitfield J. Bell, Jr., *The Colonial Physician & Other Essays* (New York: Science History Publications, 1975), p. 6.

16. Articles of Agreement between Zabdiel Boylston and Joseph Lemmon for the education of Joseph Lemmon, Jr., 1736, quoted in Henry R. Viets, "The Medical Education of James Lloyd in Colonial America," *Yale Journal of Biology and Medicine* 31 (September 1958):6.

17. *Boston Gazette,* December 15, 1766, quoted in Martin Kaufman, *American Medical Education: The Formative Years, 1765-1910* (Westport, Conn.: Greenwood Press, 1976), p. 12.

18. Viets, "Education of James Lloyd," p. 7.

19. See Carl Bridenbaugh and Jessica Bridenbaugh, *Rebels and Gentlemen: Philadelphia in the Age of Franklin* (New York: Oxford University Press, 1962), p. 277.

20. Bell, *Colonial Physician,* pp. 28-29.

21. Benjamin Rush, *The Autobiography of Benjamin Rush: His "Travels Through Life" together with his Commonplace Book for 1789-1813,* ed. George W. Corner (Princeton: For the American Philosophical Society by Princeton University Press, 1948), pp. 38-39.

22. Quoted in Whitfield J. Bell, Jr., "Medical Practice in Colonial America," *Bulletin of the History of Medicine* 31 (September-October 1957):445.

23. Heaton, "Obstetrics in Colonial America," p. 606.

24. See Elisabeth A. Dexter, *Colonial Women of Affairs: A Study of Women in Business and the Professions in America Before 1776* (Boston and New York: Houghton Mifflin, 1924), especially pp. 180-194.

25. For an account of these recipes see John B. Blake, "The Compleat Housewife," *Bulletin of the History of Medicine* 49 (Spring 1975):30-42.

26. Quoted in John Duffy, *A History of Public Health in New York City, 1625-1866* (New York: Russell Sage Foundation, 1968), p. 64.

27. See M. Dorothy George, *London Life in the Eighteenth Century* (New York: Harper and Row, 1965) for an unparalled study of this city.

28. In the 1750s surgeon's dressers ranked below apprentices. They carried instruments and dressings but did not perform the minor operations they were permitted later in the century. See Betsy Copping Corner, *William Shippen, Jr., Pioneer in American Medical Education* (Philadelphia: American Philosophical Society, 1951), p. 51.

29. Viets, "Education of James Lloyd," pp. 7-11.

30. William Shippen, Sr., to Edward Shippen, Philadelphia, September 1, 1758, in Corner, *Shippen,* p. 7.

31. Whitfield J. Bell, Jr., "Philadelphia Medical Students in Europe, 1750-1800," in Bell, *Colonial Physicians,* p. 44.

32. See Corner, *Shippen,* p. 68.

33. According to John Hunter, the cause of the break between Mac-Kensie and Smellie was an incident in which MacKensie had procured and dissected the body of a pregnant woman without Smellie's knowledge. In 1780 John Hunter, who had broken with his brother years earlier, presented a paper to the Royal Society on the structure of the placenta, in which he took full credit for having discovered the anatomical and physiological role of the placenta. In his *Anatomy of the Gravid Uterus* (1774), William Hunter had mentioned John's help but had not credited his brother with any specific discovery. According to John's version, during the course of dissecting the body he had obtained in May, 1754, MacKensie had invited John to examine the uterus. It was then that John discovered the function of the placenta and communicated his findings to William. See George C. Peachey, *A Memoir of William and John Hunter* (Plymouth, Eng.: William Brendon and Son Ltd., 1924), pp. 177, 175.

34. William Shippen, Jr., *London Diary, 1759-60,* reproduced in Corner, *Shippen,* pp. 11, 19-20. Notes on other deliveries appear on pp. 14, 16, 24, and 27.

35. Corner, *Shippen,* pp. 37, 53.

36. Shippen's dissertation has been translated from the Latin by George W. Corner as *An Anatomico-Medical Dissertation on the Connection of the Placenta with the Uterus* and is printed in ibid., pp. 128-145.

37. Samuel Bard to John Bard, Bayon[ne] Castle, France, November 28, 1761, Bardiana Collection, Bard College, Annandale-on-Hudson, New York.

38. Samuel Bard to his parents, London, April 27, 1762. Bardiana Collection.

39. Samuel Bard to John Bard, June 22, 1762 quoted in John M'Vickar, *A Domestic Narrative of the Life of Samuel Bard* (New York: A. Paul, 1822), p. 24.

40. Samuel Bard to John Bard, Edinburgh, November 14, 1762, Bardiana Collection. The "practical touching Lecture" referred to the techniques employed by the physician in digital vaginal examination to determine pregnancy and the progress of labor.

41. Ibid.

42. Samuel Bard to John Bard, London, June 12, 1762, Bardiana Collection.

43. Samuel Bard to John Bard, Edinburgh, September 25, 1762, Bardiana Collection.

44. See Whitfield J. Bell, Jr., *John Morgan, Continental Doctor* (Philadelphia: University of Pennsylvania Press, 1965), especially pp. 45-50, for a discussion of Morgan's London training.

45. Samuel Bard to John Bard, Edinburgh, December 29, 1762, quoted in M'Vickar, *Narrative*, p. 37.

46. Samuel Bard to John and Susanna Bard, Edinburgh, December 5, 1762, quoted in M'Vickar, *Narrative*, pp. 35-36.

47. John Bard to Samuel Bard, New York, December 24, 1763, Bardiana Collection.

48. John Bard to Samuel Bard, New York, January 1, 1764, Bardiana Collection.

49. Samuel Bard to John Bard, Edinburgh, February 16, 1764; Samuel Bard to John Bard, Edinburgh, April 9, 1764, Bardiana Collection. No known copy of this paper exists.

50. Bard's medical diploma bears the signatures of the renowned physicians of the University of Edinburgh and is preserved in the Bardiana Collection.

51. Bell, "Philadelphia Medical Students," p. 1.

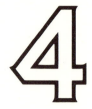

The Growth of Man Midwifery in America

It was one of the first and happiest fruits of improved medical education in America, that . . . [women] were excluded from practice; and it was only by the united and persevering exertions of some of the most distinguished individuals our profession has been able to boast, that this was effected. —[W. CHANNING], 1820

The first practitioner in America publicly referred to as a man midwife was John Dupuy of New York. In 1745, when he died at the age of only twenty-seven, his obituary read: "Last night died in the Prime of Life, to the almost universal Regret and Sorrow of this City, Mr. John Dupuy, M.D., Man Midwife; in which last Character, it may be truly said here, as David did of Goliath's Sword, there is none like him."[1] The positive tenor of this notice is remarkable for the period, considering the fact that midwifery in America definitely was a woman's uncontested stronghold.

It is probable that Dupuy, about whom little is known except that he was educated in France, was regarded as a surgical specialist who could be called upon for attendance at tedious and preternatural births. His early interest in obstetrics may be traced, perhaps, to his French training. It will be recalled that beginning in the mid-sixteenth century with the work of Ambroise Paré (1510-1590),

Jacques Gillemeau (1550-1612), and Louise Bourgeois (1563-1636), the French had revived podalic version and authored several important obstetrical texts. In the years that followed, practitioners such as François Mauriceau (1637-1709), Paul Portal (1630-1703), Guillaume Mauquest de la Motte (1655-1737), and Jean Astruc (1684-1766) continued to pioneer in the development of midwifery techniques, gradually popularizing the role of the accoucheur.[2] Thus, Dupuy would have been exposed to the works and to the improved procedures of the French school, where both men and women practitioners were recognized as having legitimate association with midwifery.

In America, other male practitioners were associating themselves with obstetrics. Benjamin Rush (1745-1813), comparing medicine in the new republic with that of the pre-Revolutionary generation, noted that in the 1760s the practice of physic and surgery were "united." Physicians practiced both and "were seldom employed as man-midwives except in preternatural and tedious labours."[3] In Philadelphia, a Dr. Spencer may have been the first accoucheur. Thomas Cadwalader (1708-1779) recalled that in 1745 Spencer had returned from abroad, recommended by "eminent gentlemen of the Faculty of London, as a most judicious and experienced physician and man-midwife," and claimed that he was "largely engaged." Cadwalader further noted that a Dr. Thompson was practicing midwifery in 1748. This was Adam Thompson, originally from Edinburgh, who advertised his qualifications in physic, surgery, and midwifery in the *Pennsylvania Gazette.* John Redman, trained by John Kearsley and later preceptor to an impressive array of American doctors, including Rush, was an accomplished accoucheur.[4]

In 1762 in the neighboring colony of New Jersey, Dr. Atwood began to practice midwifery exclusively.[5] Atwood also practiced in New York. *Valentine's Manual,* New York City's directory for the 1840s, reflected obvious contempt for the earlier period when women midwives controlled the practice. Before the Revolution, according to Valentine, Atwood was the "first Dr. who had the hardihood to proclaim himself as a midwife: it was deemed a scandal to some delicate ears, and Mrs. Grany Brown, with her fees of two and three dollars, was still deemed choice of all who thought women should be modest."[6]

In 1750 James Lloyd returned to Boston after completing his courses with Smellie and Hunter and his hospital practice with Warner. His early practice was general, but within two years he had begun to concentrate on obstetrics, ultimately confining his work to this field. His superior education and his association with the principal figures in the "new obstetrics" were key elements in Lloyd's emergence as a midwifery specialist. He trained a number of gifted students who, in turn, became accoucheurs. Among these were Isaac Rand (1743-1822), a successful man midwife, and John Jeffries (1745-1819), who studied with MacKensie in London. Jeffries left records of some two thousand of his midwifery cases.[7]

The colonial obstetric experience followed lines of development similar to those in England. Decorum was observed in the colonies, and social norms still dictated that physicians be called only as a last resort to manage abnormal cases. Those few doctors who did include obstetrics in their practices had as yet no opportunities to attend routine deliveries, even among the indigent. In New York, for example, impoverished women were confined to the "Publick Workhouse and House of Correction" built in the 1730s, where they were attended by a midwife hired by the common council and paid out of the city treasury.[8] A few years later the city constructed an infirmary adjacent to the workhouse that served as a "Receptacle and Convenience of Such unhappy poor who are or shall be Visited with any Malignant or Obnoxious disease." This may have been exclusively a pest house. Dr. John Van Buren, who was placed in charge and paid on a per patient basis, does not appear to have acted as accoucheur. Individual payments were made to those who rendered special assistance in cases of abnormal childbirth. In 1762 Dr. John Bard received £7 from the common council as his fee for "Delivering a Woman in the poor House" and attending her during her confinement.[9]

John Bard is an excellent example of the high caliber of doctors the apprentice system could produce. After completing his work with John Kearsley in Philadelphia, Bard moved to New York where he entered into successful practice. With Peter Middleton (d. 1781) he participated in an early anatomical dissection during the course of which the blood vessels were injected and preserved for medical instruction. Occasionally he lectured on anatomy.

Illustrative of his skillful surgery was the laparotomy he performed. In 1759 Bard was called to see a post-partum patient who had been delivered nine weeks earlier. He diagnosed her condition as extrauterine pregnancy and determined that her only hope lay in an almost unprecedented operation to remove the offending fetal mass from the abdomen. With courage exceeded only by that of his patient, for whom anodynes but no anesthesia were available, Bard proceeded with the laparotomy. The woman made a complete recovery.[10]

However comforting it must have been for women to realize that there were a few gifted and experienced practitioners such as Bard and Lloyd who could be summoned to conduct difficult labors, they did not readily abandon their traditional midwives. Hostility directed against the presence of men in the lying-in room persisted. Caspar Wistar, the Philadelphia obstetrician, reviewing the customs from the perspective of the early nineteenth century, commented, "It was only when something very important was to be done that . . . [men] were resorted to—and, very often, when too late."[11] This he attributed to an existing prejudice against male attendants rather than to any necessity. He insisted, in what seems an overstatement, that in his city an ample supply of experienced and able men midwives had been available to attend all childbirths had women wished to call on them. In New York a physician interested in upgrading the practice of the midwives acknowledged the existence of similar prejudice against men. Commented Valentine Seaman, there are some women who "absolutely refuse having a man to attend them in their labours, or at least not till they are convinced of being in a critical or dangerous situation, and oftentimes not until they are beyond the reach of the greatest skill."[12]

Several elements tended to perpetuate the customary employment of midwives in preference to men. Centuries of tradition in England and the jealousies and suspicions of husbands encouraged men to regard their wives as exclusive and absolute possessions. Increasingly as the eighteenth century progressed, the attributes of modesty and delicacy were deemed highly desirable qualities in women. The New York midwife, who in 1771 advertised her assets of "her strict Attendance, great Tenderness, and Delicacy, to her own Sex"[13] was appealing to just these sentiments. Young women were taught from early childhood ideally to cultivate these traits. Illustrative of this emphasis are these guidelines that appeared in an American women's magazine toward the last decade of the century:

> The attempts, so successful in the fashionable world to bring modesty into disrepute, under the name of bashfulness, can never be fully execrated. . . . Oh! my fair countrywomen, be convinced, in departing from the walks of modesty and delicacy you depart from the charms of virtue; instead of being more alluring, you excite compassion and dislike, in proportion to your libertinism. . . . Be convinced, while you retain modesty and delicacy, you will be loved, cherished and esteemed; as you depart from these amiable companions, in the same degree you will depart from the empire of sterling beauty, and satiety will give birth to disgust.[14]

Any successful attempt to supplant the midwives or even to supplement their practice would need to offer inducements potent enough to overcome these tenacious cultural attitudes that increased rather than diminished in the early decades of the following century.

The major element that reversed this traditional pattern was the "new obstetrics" gradually unfolding in England. Objections citing the impropriety of employing men to conduct ordinary labors notwithstanding, the newer ways had begun to take root even before the American Revolution. The initial position of those seeking change seems not to have been that men were preferable to women as midwives, but rather that the trained attendant was preferable to one untrained. A few physicians sought to educate rather than replace the women, but all such efforts were private ventures. At no time did the colonial, state, or national governments make any effort to follow the continental plan of establishing schools where midwives could be instructed.

While it is equally true that no governmental efforts were essayed to sponsor medical education for men either, one important difference must be recognized. Society expected that all men would become self-supporting. The family that could manage to do so, therefore, was willing to secure a son's future by investing in some sort of training. Privately financed education, whether through apprentice programs or formal schooling, was a realistic possibility for upper- and middle-class young men. On the other hand, society defined women as dependent and weak. Women were expected to move from dependence on their fathers to dependence on their husbands. Viewed primarily as wives and mothers, their work was ordinarily thought to be home-centered. In all periods of our history some women have worked outside the home. Still, even in colonial America, before industrialization and urbanization had imposed distinct division between work done inside the home and that performed away from it, woman's employment was regarded as auxiliary to her role as wife and mother. Families with the where-withal to do so were not inclined to invest in a daughter's specialized training, since her future security was predicated on making a satisfactory marriage. Those women who sought employment in midwifery, as in other fields, did so out of financial necessity. Midwives already in practice had little money and even less incentive to invest in upgrading their own skills, especially since they could scarcely have realized the depths of their own limitations, any more than self-made, untrained physicians could have realized theirs.

The implications of this are as obvious as the results are predictable. Although some midwives did receive excellent training through private sources as they became available, the majority received none whatsoever. Criticisms about their ignorance unfortunately hit close to the mark. Dr. Valentine Seaman, who inquired extensively into the means by which women moved into midwifery practice, concluded that most were first *"catched,* as they express it, with a woman in labour." Having managed to receive the child without incident, they considered themselves competent, and thus almost by accident, they were "immediately established in the profession."[15] As men midwives began to introduce instruments into the practice, the midwives were placed at a further disadvantage, since they lacked both the instruments and the knowledge necessary to use them effectively and safely.

Among colonial physicians specializing in midwifery, none deserves a more prominent place than William Shippen, Jr., for it was he who introduced the first systematic series of lectures on obstetrics in America. In 1762, when he returned to Philadelphia fresh from his studies in London and Edinburgh, he was an accomplished accoucheur and anatomist, young, energetic, and determined to upgrade American medicine. Shippen had brought with him a valuable gift for the Pennsylvania Hospital from Dr. John Fothergill. It consisted of a set of eighteen crayon "pretty accurate anatomical drawings, about half as big as . . . life," done by Jan van Rymsdyk, the artist who worked with Hunter on the *Anatomy of the Human Gravid Uterus,* one human skeleton, some anatomical casts, and an injected and preserved human fetus. Fothergill's gift was prompted by a desire to foster medical learning in the Quaker colony. Recognizing the paucity of available "real subjects" for anatomical dissection in Philadelphia, and realizing "that the knowledge of Anatomy is of exceedingly great use to practitioners in Physick and Surgery," Fothergill had encouraged Shippen to initiate a course of anatomical lectures using the preparations and drawings for illustrative purposes.[16]

Shippen did not delay in putting Fothergill's plan into operation. In the fall 1762 he announced a course of anatomical lectures to include surgical operations, bandaging, "an explanation of some of the curious phenomena that arise from an examination of the gravid uterus," and "a few plain general directions" in midwifery.[17] Shippen found the Fothergill drawings particularly useful in illustrating the latter part of his course, for they included representations of preternatural presentations such as breech and arm, the gravid uterus under various conditions, and fetal circulation.[18] The following year he announced a complete course of twenty lectures in midwifery, organized along the lines of Colin MacKensie's in London. Lectures included anatomy, a discussion of natural, difficult, and preternatural cases, the care and treatment of women and children "in the month," and concluded with the "necessary cautions against the dangerous and cruel use of instruments." This last subject clearly reflects the effect of Shippen's association with the ultraconservative William Hunter. Pupils were expected to attend two courses at a total cost of five guineas, and "perpetual pupil" status could be had for the sum of ten guineas. Clinical experience was available, since students were permitted to attend the few poor women "who otherwise might suffer for want of the common necessaries on these occasions" and who were lodged in the small lying-in ward maintained by Shippen near his office in Letitia Court.[19] By emulating the London obstetricians and providing care for the indigent in exchange for clinical teaching opportunities, Shippen introduced Americans to the idea that men might attend normal as well as difficult and preternatural births.

This is not to suggest that Shippen entertained any notions that the midwives would ultimately be replaced. It is not clear whether or not he permitted women to attend his first course in 1762, but he clearly encouraged them to attend his full midwifery course. He promised that women would be "taught privately and assisted at any of their private labours when necessary." When the opening of the course was delayed by insufficient enrollment, Shippen took to the newspaper to announce with a certain sense of urgency his decision to proceed.

Dr. Shippen, Jr., having lately been called to the assistance of a number of women in the country, in difficult labors, most of which was made so by the unskillful old women about them, the poor women having suffered extremely, and their innocent little ones being entirely destroyed, whose lives might have been easily saved by proper management, and being informed of several desperate cases in the different neighborhoods which had proved fatal to the mothers as to their infants, and were attended with the most painful circumstances too dismal to be related, he thought it his duty immediately to begin his intended courses in Midwifery, and has prepared a proper apparatus for that purpose, in order to instruct those women who have virtue enough to own their ignorance and apply for instructions, as well as those young gentlemen now engaged in the study of that useful and necessary branch of surgery, who are taking pains to qualify themselves to practice in different parts of the country with safety and advantage to their fellow citizens.[20]

Regrettably, there is no way to determine the number of women Shippen trained. The tuition of five guineas for attendance at two full courses, while comparing favorably with Smellie's fee of two guineas per course in London twenty years earlier, was nevertheless a large sum of money to women who delivered patients for a few shillings. That some women attended Shippen's courses is known. As late as 1789 midwife Grace Mulligan, who had moved from Philadelphia to Wilmington, advertised that she had been trained and recommended by him; perhaps by the close of the century there were still some Shippen-trained midwives in practice bringing to their patients the benefits derived from attendance at "as good a course as was then available"[21] in the new republic. Before the American Revolution, Shippen's course was a private one, which he did not continue after the war. He then delivered "a short course to his general class"[22] at the Philadelphia Medical School, where he retained the chair in anatomy and surgery to which he was appointed at the school's founding in 1765. In any case, the only women Shippen trained were those who attended his private course, for women were not admitted to the medical school.

William Shippen's teaching was merely an adjunct to the full private midwifery practice he established in Philadelphia. His popularity as an accoucheur was due as much to his sense of decorum as to his outstanding ability. As an innovator in a sensitive field, he was fully aware, as Smellie and Hunter had been before him, of the dangers inherent in appearing too audacious. His personal correspondence reveals his view of the special qualities accoucheurs needed to cultivate if they were "to gain a good opinion . . . [from] the female world." Above all, a grave deportment was requisite. Agreeable conversation in the lying-in room he thought permissible, provided the accoucheur avoided "religiously any jokes about the patient or profession."[23]

Caspar Wistar, a colleague at the University of Pennsylvania Medical School, recalled that Shippen, often a brilliant lecturer, was never better than when he delivered his introductory midwifery lecture devoted to "the subject of address and deportment." Introducing young men to midwifery was always "an affair of great delicacy," requiring good sense and a knowledge of human nature. Shippen's students were "young and . . . unused to reflections of this kind." "In strong colours," continued Wistar, "Shippen portrayed the feelings of delicate women, on such occasions; and from thence inferred the necessity of the physician's avoiding every appearance of officiousness, and of waiting till his interference was really necessary; when, he declared it would ever be gratefully received."[24]

From the journal kept by Elizabeth Drinker, we are able to glimpse the conservative Shippen in practice, for the family frequently employed him as accoucheur. In April 1795 Sally Drinker Downings began a preternatural labor. Her contractions were unproductive, and Shippen prescribed an anodyne after she had been in labor many hours. He was sent for again the following morning, visited the patient, dined with the family, and left. Toward evening he was called once again, and this time questioned unsparingly by Sally Downings, who was suffering to no avail. An analgesic of two opium pills produced little effect. Finally, some thirty hours into labor, Shippen intervened and "by good management . . . brought on a footling labour." Four years later Shippen again attended Sally in a protracted labor that lasted some forty-eight hours. On this occasion he considered, but ultimately rejected, resorting to instruments. Sally's mother found the "Doctor . . . very kind and attentive during the whole afflicting scene," observing that he was in the household "two nights and 2 days and sleep't very little."[25]

Shippen's conservatism was, by the standards of the day, infinitely preferable to the meddlesome midwifery practices in which some of the later accoucheurs would engage. His demeanor was faultless and his ability superior. Educated and cultivated, it is easy to see how he was able to find acceptance among the more affluent and prestigious Philadelphia families, and in so doing, to further the cause of man midwifery in that city. Shippen was not, of course, the only physician to teach and practice midwifery in Philadelphia. In fact, that city took an early lead in midwifery training and retained it for many years. Dr. Thomas Bond (1712-1784), who had been instrumental in the establishment of the Pennsylvania Hospital in 1751, was appointed as a staff physician. In 1766 he inaugurated clinical lectures in midwifery at the hospital, although the institution did not add a lying-in ward until 1807. In 1770 Bond's private pupils were permitted to attend labors at the Philadelphia Alms House, personally supervised by their mentor.[26] In December 1793 William Potts Dewees, who was destined to become one of the nation's leading obstetricians, returned to Philadelphia from Abington, where he had attained "a large share of obstetrical practice" in that country town.[27] Within a short time he announced a "regular and extensive course of obstetrical Lectures,"[28] which he continued to offer for some time. Although he did not yet have the doctor of medicine degree, which he took at the University of Pennsylvania in 1806, Dewees was conversant with obstetrical theory and practice as taught in both the French and British schools. To these he added his careful personal observations taken and recorded from private practice. Available information about the courses taught by Bond and Dewees does not reveal that either teacher solicited or taught women pupils. It is doubtful that they did. Thus, in eighteenth-century Philadelphia there were a number of avenues open to men who wished to add midwifery to their training, but except for Shippen's early course, there were apparently none open to women.

Between 1760 and 1800 in the northern cities, lying-in customs evolved from the almost exclusive employment of midwives for all but exceptional cases to the growing tendency among families of standing to send for a man midwife in the normal as well as the abnormal case. In New York and Boston, as in Philadelphia, traditional assumptions were tested, found wanting, and gradually modified. In the process a bitter struggle resulted that paralled in many ways a similar contest in England. Midwives threatened with loss of their livelihood insisted that only they could preserve the modesty of delicate women, whereas male practitioners sought to add obstetrics to their repertoire both for profit and in the name of progress. Forced into competition with men whose abilities eclipsed their own, the midwives sought to retain their stronghold.

One indication of the developing competition and its effects is found in the growing number of advertisements that appeared in the city newspapers. Before the 1760s a man midwife was almost unheard of in normal cases; he was the interloper who sought to make his availability known. Thus in 1751 Peter Billings advertised himself in the *New York Gazette* as "an experienced physician and man-midwife." Billings's credentials are not known, but one contemporary, William Douglass, thought him a "notorious quack who specialized in quick cures for venereal diseases and sold medicine to prevent the yellow fever and the West Indian dry gripes." In the same period a Parisian surgeon, "Doctor" Guischard, claimed himself "experienced in women's delivery" and promised "with the help of the Lord" to prove himself of service to women "in their extremity."[29] Other surgeons made similar claims. James Smith in 1765 advertised himself as a "surgeon and man-midwife," and a few years later Dr. Aubrey, trained in the Paris hospitals, noted that he specialized in the "obstetric art" in addition to treating toothache.[30] As late as 1782 Mr. Thomas Flloyd, recently arrived from London with a regular and liberal education, offered his services to the public in "Physic, Surgery and Midwifry . . . on the most moderate terms."[31]

The midwives took to the papers as well. In 1769 Mrs. Fisher, who lived near Whitehall, advertised for patients. Two years later, after she had moved to a new address, Mrs. Fisher advised her clientele of the change and added that potential patients interested in determining her ability could "enquire of Dr. Farquhar, and others."[32] Another midwife, Elizabeth Pairidge, newly arrived from London in the late 1760s, informed readers that she was available on the "shortest Notice." Pairidge claimed special authorization to practice in New York by virtue of having been "duly examined by the Faculty" of the city.[33] This last information is curious in view of the fact that midwives were not then subject to licensing examinations but were required merely to take the traditional midwives' oath sworn before city officials. It is possible that as a newcomer in an increasingly competitive field, Pairidge sought the examination as a means of suggesting her superiority. Another recent arrival from England claimed to have studied "under the most celebrated Professors in London," where she had practiced more than twelve years "with Applause and Success." She too claimed to have been examined by "most of the Gentlemen of the Faculty" in the city of New York.[34] Mrs. McLean, formerly Mrs. Glass, did not want her new name and address to cost her patients. Consequently, she advertised her continued availability to both those whom she had previously had "the pleasure of serving, and others who . . . [might] be pleased to oblige her with their commands."[35] That both men and women continued to advertise throughout the decades of the 1770s and 1780s is an indication of the prolonged nature of the competition and the attendant efforts to sway public opinion in favor of employing one sex over the other.

The employment of men midwives for normal deliveries was beginning to find favor in other colonial cities as well. The New Jersey Medical Society established a fee table for physicians in 1766, setting a fee of £1.10.0 for natural deliveries in addition to the fee of £3.0.0 for preternatural and laborious cases.[36] In Philaadelphia, brothers Thomas and Phineas Bond charged "£2 or £3" for a delivery in 1766, but their fee was not broken down into specific charges for normal and abnormal cases. Physicians in New York City set the following rates of individual charges in the 1790s: "Ordinary cases in Midwifery £4.0.0; Extraordinary d°from £5 to £10; Introducing Catheter first time £0.16.0; Every succeeding time £0.8.0."[37]

From an ordinance enacted shortly before the Revolution, it is clear that men had begun to move into midwifery in Albany, New York. The ordinance regulated midwives and was patterned largely after the one first introduced in New York City more than half a century earlier. It contained one significant change; the section prohibiting the male presence with the exception of cases of extreme necessity was omitted. Instead, specific reference was made to men employed in the field in a section that provided that "if any Man or Woman, within the City of Albany, shall, after the Publication hereof, use, or exercise, the office of *Man-midwife,* or *Midwife* . . . before the oath . . . hath been duly administered," the offender would be subject to a fine of forty shillings for each offense.[38]

Keen competition had also developed in Boston. In 1772 midwife Mary Bass announced that she was moving from that city to Salem. She cited as her reason the fact that "men midwives are fairly numerous in Boston."[39] Perhaps one of her rivals was Dr. Spencer, who claimed to have been trained in the hospitals of London and Paris and who advertised for patients in midwifery in addition to those in need of tooth extraction.[40] The success of the Boston doctors in popularizing male attendance at deliveries is clearly suggested by the following advertisement that appeared in the *Boston Evening Post* in 1781:

The physicians of the town of Boston, hereby inform the public, that, in consideration of the great fatigue and inevitable injury to their constitution, in the practice of midwifery, as well as the necessary interruption of other branches of their profession, they shall, for the future, expect that in calls of this kind, the fee be immediately discharged.[41]

By the beginning of the nineteenth century men midwives had gained a substantial measure of acceptance in population centers. General practitioners had managed to replace many midwives, and the special term man-midwife was used less frequently.[42]

With the establishment of the first two medical schools in America, man midwifery received an important boost. In 1765 the medical school of the College of Philadelphia had a faculty of two. John Morgan offered materia medica, chemistry, and the theory and practice of medicine. William Shippen, Jr., taught midwifery as an adjunct to anatomy and surgery. Augmenting the work of these two were the clinical lectures offered by Thomas Bond at the Pennsylvania Hospital. The King's College Medical School in New York, founded in 1767, had a more complete faculty of six professors who taught the requisite courses for the degree Doctor of Physic; unfortunately the absence of a hospital precluded clinical lectures.

From the beginning King's College had a separate chair in midwifery. It is not clear that this was the original intention of the governors of the college. In 1767, however, John Van Brugh Tennent (1737-1770), who had taken the degree of doctor of medicine abroad, wrote to the governors who were then establishing the medical school. Tennent called attention to the fact that no chair had been assigned in midwifery and recommended himself for the position. He claimed to have especially prepared himself in midwifery "with a design sooner or later to give Lectures," which, added Tennent, he would have begun earlier had he not been "discourag'd by observing that those who did attempt any thing of that nature were disappointed."[43] The governors were sufficiently impressed with Tennent to offer him the post.

It is probable that Samuel Bard had wanted the midwifery post at King's. A certain professional rivalry existed between the two men dating back to their student days. Samuel's father, John Bard, was annoyed at Tennent's "very Remarkable boast of . . . having Ingaged all the principal Families" of New York for his practice. Such a "weak and ostentatious" assertion on Tennent's part "Lessend him" in the elder Bard's opinion.[44] Ironically, owing to Tennent's poor health, he did not keep the midwifery post for long. Upon his death in 1770, Samuel Bard, who had been teaching the theory and practice of medicine since the founding of the school, added midwifery to his chair.

Important as the inclusion of midwifery teaching was in the total curricula of the early medical schools, its effect in these formative years must not be overstated. It was far less costly to attend one of the American schools than to finance years of study abroad, yet very few students were graduated in the years before the Revolution. Then too, attendance at such a school was regarded as auxiliary to training with a preceptor. Perhaps the most that can be said is that the inclusion of midwifery by the colleges illustrated that this specialty had advanced to the position where it was considered a legitimate area of practice for physicians.[45]

Unfortunately for the progress of medical education, the effects of the American Revolution were devastating, for doctors were not immune to the politics and the misfortunes of war. King's College's medical school was closed in 1776 when its building was occupied by the British. Not until 1792 was the medical school reopened at what had become Columbia College. Even then it attracted few students; in 1814 it was absorbed by its New York rival, the College of Physicians and Surgeons, but the factionalism within the institution worked against the best interests of medical education. The only other pre-Revolutionary medical school was the College of Philadelphia, which merged with the University of Pennsylvania before the end of the century. It was not until 1810 that midwifery and anatomy were separated at that institution. Even then, the trustees of the university resolved that it was not necessary to attend the professor of midwifery in order to obtain the medical degree. Massachusetts Medical College (Harvard), founded in 1782, did not establish a separate chair in midwifery until 1815, and Dartmouth Medical College, the last of the four medical schools founded in the eighteenth century, combined anatomy, surgery, and midwifery when it opened in 1798.[46] A century after the war obstetrician T. Gaillard Thomas reviewed the period by observing that the United States had shared little in the obstetrical progress achieved abroad because of the Revolution and subsequent postbellum problems. In this period, he noted, America put forth little public or private effort on behalf of any science. The result, he concluded, was that "as an art, practised chiefly by midwives, obstetrics was a vigorous plant, deep rooted and strong; as a science, a delicate shoot, which feebly struggled with adverse circumstances for life; while the very seed of the sister branch of gynaecology may be said to have been unsowed."[47]

There were nevertheless some individual private physicians who continued to demonstrate a keen interest in obstetrics amidst the confusion of the post-war period. William Moore built an extensive and successful midwifery practice in New York City and kept a careful record of the nearly three thousand cases he attended from 1781 to 1823.[48] The work of Valentine Seaman, another New York practitioner, had greater public impact. As a surgeon at the New York Hospital, opened in 1791, Seaman was in a position to experience firsthand the public and private apathy toward medical care. He was convinced that the midwives would continue to find employment among the substantial number of women who still resisted the intrusion of men into the lying-in room. This being the case, Seaman reasoned, in the interest of humanity those women who could not be persuaded to abandon their old habits and submit to the care of physicians still deserved to be properly attended. He had often witnessed the unsound practices of some of the midwives, practices that he attributed to their woefully inadequate background. The New York practitioner advocated emulating the various continental programs designed to provide thorough training for midwives. "Whatever may have been the desire, and whatever may have been done elsewhere, no plan of the kind, so far as I can learn, has heretofore been established in America: consequently," lamented Seaman, "the midwives, with a very few exceptions, are as ignorant of their business as the women they deliver."[50] He acknowledged that some midwives tried to expand their knowledge by reading, but the results of these efforts he pronounced unsatisfactory. The texts available to the women he thought too obscure and technical for them to comprehend readily. Moreover, sound obstetrical practice required that attendants have clinical experience in addition to a theoretical foundation. Succinctly he summarized the midwives' dilemma: "To learn such a handicraft business by reading alone is like shipbuilding without touching timber. Can we expect, but that such workers, in either occupation, must destroy more materials than their good work will ever pay for?"[51]

Seaman soon found an opportunity to act on his ideas. In 1798 private subscriptions had raised sufficient money to permit the establishment of an adjunct to the New York Almshouse. This was "an asylum for the reception of women in a state of pregnancy, who [were] unable to procure the necessary medical assistance and nursing, during the period of their confinement." In December the subscribers met at Tontine Coffee House to discuss the project and appoint a committee to draft a constitution providing for the regulation of the lying-in "hospital."[52] When it opened the following August, Seaman was appointed "physician extraordinary." He saw in the concentration of numerous cases an opportunity to provide midwives with urgently needed training. Seaman proposed to offer a course of lectures in obstetrics to include anatomy and physiology as well as clinical observation at the lying-in ward. *The Medical Repository,* which carried an announcement of the course, was enthusiastic. The editors indicated that it was to be "particularly and exclusively devoted to the education of females" and urged women to take advantage of this valuable opportunity.[53]

Despite the obvious support of the medical community, Seaman's success was limited. Once underway he did not limit the enrollment to women, perhaps because the number of midwives who registered for the course was low. In any case, Seaman later referred to having offered it for "interested physicians and female midwives." "A number" of pupils attended, but the total was disappointing. Unfortunately it is not possible to ascertain the tuition for the course; these charges may have been excessive from the perspective of the limited resources of women then in the labor force. Seaman attributed the low enrollment to other causes. Some women stayed away out of the conviction that they were already sufficiently knowledgeable in their craft, he thought. Others were merely "indolent," while a third group avoided the chance to learn out of "a dread of the retrospect that opening their eyes might present to their senses."[54]

In 1800 Valentine Seaman published the first American midwifery manual. This was a guide for midwives and pregnant women titled *The Midwives Monitor and Mother's Mirror* and consisted of the syllabus of his twenty-six midwifery lectures and the entire contents of the three concluding lectures. This small work met with a favorable reviewer in the *Medical Repository* who found it a useful tool for the midwives. That its usefulness had another dimension was not lost on the reviewer. Modest gravid women, "whose delicacy is too much affected to look to accoucheurs for advice in their own cases, may contemplate themselves before this *Mirror,* without blushing or embarrassment," commented the reviewer approvingly.[55]

An examination of the *Midwives Monitor* clearly reveals the role that Seaman envisioned for the women attendants. His text makes it abundantly clear that they were never to attend any but "natural," that is, normal, cases. To enable them to make intelligent judgments and to send for timely help, he provided them with a useful guide to the correct classification of labors. Natural labors were those where the head presented with no "artificial assistance" necessary and with a duration of up to twenty-four hours. In laborious cases, the head presented, but assistance was required and/or the labor exceeded the normal twenty-four-hour period. Preternatural cases were those where the presentation was other than cephalic, whereas "complicated" labors were those accompanied by "floodings," "convulsions," or other unusual conditions.[56] All but the natural cases Seaman termed "diseases"; as such he considered them absolutely beyond the province of the midwives. In his course Seaman had instructed the women in the techniques utilized by practitioners attending preternatural births and had even permitted them to practice performing version on the "machine." Yet he never expected that women would put this training to practical use. Cautioned the doctor in unmistakable language, this is "a part of the business, well for you *to know,* but not politic for you to practise."[57] To avoid confusion Seaman delineated the duties of the ideal midwife: to bolster her patient's morale during labor, to examine her to determine the degree of dilatation achieved, to support the perineum at the moment of birth, to tie off the umbilical cord, and above all, to refrain from pulling on the cord in an effort to hasten the expulsion of the placenta.[58]

It is regrettable that the absence of evidence makes it impossible to measure the effect of Seaman's work with the midwives. His interest in upgrading their practice suggests that he fully expected the women to remain in the field, albeit limiting their participation to the normal. The same may be said of Samuel Bard, whose interest in fostering the principles of the new obstetrics was long-standing. His interest in the field was encouraged first by his father. Later, his work at Edinburgh and in London with Colin MacKensie fully prepared him to succeed John Van Brugh Tennent as obstetrics lecturer at King's College. After the Revolution, when the medical school was still in disarray, Bard offered a private course in midwifery. Throughout the duration of his long and distinguished career in New York, Bard was "assiduously engaged" in the practice of obstetrics. In the post-war period he experimented with various treatments for uterine hemorrhage, the "floodings" mentioned so frequently in contemporary medical literature. As a result he developed a successful treatment that introduced ice into the vagina. These experiments, however, were said to have given rise to unfavorable rumors about him, "especially among respectable dames and matrons," who may have thought the procedure indecent. Sensitive to the need for quelling these rumors and cultivating the support of influential families, the more especially as a returned Tory determined to reestablish himself, Bard advanced an explanation. In 1788 he published a fifteen-page essay giving the rationale for his use of cold in uterine hemorrhage, but how successful he was in winning acceptance for the treatment is not known.[59]

In 1796, at the age of fifty-five, Samuel Bard turned over his active medical practice to his partner, David Hosack (1769-1835), and retired to his comfortable estate at Hyde Park, along the Hudson. There he busied himself with agricultural pursuits, improving his farm, cultivating his botanical gardens, and experimenting with the breeding and raising of merino sheep. He also retained his interest in medicine. In particular, his contacts with the midwives over the years had convinced him of their need for a sound, precise, yet inexpensive text on obstetrics from which they might learn to correct their erroneous ideas and improve their procedures. Bard realized that the midwives' limited finances and their "deficiency of education" precluded their obtaining information from "systems of midwifery" or "books of science." He began to write a book with the stated purpose of being "useful" rather than "learned." In the resulting *Compendium of the Theory and Practice of Midwifery,* which appeared in 1807, he carefully explained those "facts and observations" that had received "the stamp of time and experience" and avoided offering any "new opinions."[60]

Bard's work, preceded only by Valentine Seaman's slim volume several years earlier, found a ready market. By 1819 it had gone into its fifth edition, and at his death the author left a sixth revision, never published.[61] In the early editions aimed chiefly at reaching the midwives, Bard omitted both descriptions of instruments and directions for their use. Rather he emphasized the importance of noninterference, stressing the desired goal of perpetuating sound procedures by which deliveries were accomplished naturally. In the third edition, however, he reluctantly added a chapter on instruments and their use, carefully stating that the information was provided exclusively for the edification of young male students and practitioners. Bard bowed in the direction of Smellie, widely read in America, and termed him "one of the first and great improvers of the art of midwifery." At once critic and admirer, he charged that Smellie had "certainly . . . not [been] acquainted with all the resources of nature, in their full extent." Bard therefore feared the legacy of Smellie's teaching: "Having greatly improved the instruments of his day . . . [Smellie] described their use with great precision," observed Bard, adding that he was "apprehensive, that many of [Smellie's] readers may thereby be induced to suppose them equally safe in their hands, as they appear to have been in his—and hence be led to a more frequent use of them than modern practice has found necessary or safe." At the close of his own thirty-year practice, Bard had found much less occasion to employ instruments than earlier in his career. Pointedly he commented that "the person, who, in proportion to the extent of his practice, meets with the most frequent occasion for the use of instruments, knows least of the powers of nature; and . . . he who boasts of his skill and success in their application is a very dangerous man."[62]

In 1811 Bard was appointed president of the College of Physicians and Surgeons, into which the medical college at Columbia had been absorbed. A few years later, complying with a request from the Regents of the University of the State of New York, Bard prepared a report comparing contemporary medical instruction in Edinburgh, New York, Philadelphia, Boston, and Baltimore. The section on midwifery indicates his continuing interest and shows how the field had changed during his lifetime. The latter three schools had made midwifery "a distinct and subgraduate course." Considering "its real importance, the universality of the practice among our physicians, or the fatal blunders, which frequently arise from ignorance of its principles," Bard reasoned, the "strictest propriety" mandated that the New York college also offer this branch as a separate course and require it for graduation. Country practitioners in particular, isolated and unable to seek timely professional counsel, were "in every difficult case of midwifery continually called on to decide promptly on measures which may save or sacrifice" mother and child. In no other branch of medicine, he insisted, were these observations more "evidently applicable," and in none other was it "more important that correct information . . . be assured." He further maintained that this specialty could only be "properly taught" when theoretical instruction was augmented with clinical practice. For that reason New York had a special obligation inasmuch as midwifery teaching was limited to the "large and populous City, where only, the poorest women, for the comforts of an Hospital, or for a pecuniary consideration will consent to be attended by Pupils." Admittedly a short and therefore less expensive course than others, it was nevertheless too important to be attached to another professorship, he concluded.[63]

At the time of this report, American urban midwifery practices had reached a crucial juncture. Accoucheurs had successfully moved into the field of normal deliveries. Such proficiency as they acquired was obtained, as Bard indicated, through clinical practice utilizing poor women unable to pay for their accouchements. As the men continued in the field, upper- and middle-class women turned to them, tentatively persuaded that they offered greater safety than the midwives. Yet the physicians realized that the quality of obstetrical care still was questionable. Early in 1822 for example, the Medical Society of the County of New York, only recently organized, appointed a committee to investigate the causes of what it considered to be an "unusual number of still-births." The conclusions reached in the resulting report are revealing not only because they supported the physician over the midwife, a not unexpected position, but also because the tendered solution was replacement rather than education of the latter group. "Considering the general diffusion of correct obstetric information among those who practised as accoucheurs," stated the report, the number of stillbirths was not disproportionate to that found in other cities and countries. Still, concluded the committee members, they were convinced that "the mortality among newly-born children would be materially diminished if the practice of midwifery was more restricted to male attendants," investigation having revealed "that a very large proportion occurred in cases under the charge of midwives."[64]

At the same time, the Medical Society decided to improve the quality of care available to poor parturient women by providing them with "gratuitous professional attendance at and after the period of parturition." The members divided the city into ten districts corresponding to its wards and appointed attending and consulting accoucheurs to serve each. As a safeguard against abusing the "junior members of the profession," among whom obstetrics cases were eagerly sought, women were not to be attended by the society's appointees unless a magistrate had first certified that they were unable to defray the "ordinary expences which must attend . . . lying-in."[65] What is not clear is whether these "ordinary expences" meant those a woman would have incurred through attendance by a midwife or by a doctor. Ordinarily the latter's fee would have been slightly higher, and whether such proffered charity was calculated to undercut the practice of midwives cannot be determined.

By the same token, the absence of statistical data makes it impossible to estimate the number of midwives in the cities who were still in active practice by 1820. Some women continued to employ midwives for reasons that Valentine Seaman had termed "indiscreet and ill-founded prejudice" against male attendants and a sense of "false delicacy."[66] Others chose the midwife for her lower fee. In the cities studied, however, the pattern emerging among trendsetting upper- and middle-class women was that of movement away from the midwives in favor of the accoucheurs. In the professional journals and case histories of the period occasional references to midwives are found. Some of them were highly regarded by physicians. Benjamin Rush's *Commonplace Book* contains, for example, favorable comments about Mrs. Patten, who at age fifty-eight had delivered between "9990 and 10,000 women, inclusive of seven months' children," and had "lost only one."[67] Yet in 1820 Harvard's first obstetrics professor, Walter Channing (1786-1876), in reviewing the field remarked, "Heretofore, where midwifery has been in the hands of women, they have only practised among the poorer and lower classes . . . the richer and better informed preferring to employ physicians." In unequivocal terms he indicated his approval of the new trend in his comment, "It was one of the first and happiest fruits of improved medical education in America, that . . . [women] were excluded from practice; and it was only by the united and persevering exertions of some of the most distinguished individuals our profession has been able to boast, that this was effected."[68]

Such consensus, however, had not always existed among Boston's physicians. John Collins Warren (1778-1856), the eminent surgeon, was an early advocate of specialization. If possible, he would have confined himself to surgery, separating this field from that of general medicine. He also advocated separating midwifery from both.[69] He and his colleague James Jackson (1777-1867) formulated a plan calling for instruction of the midwives. Local opposition was so strong that they abandoned this idea. As a substitute, in 1818 they invited midwife Janet Alexander, who had been trained in Scotland, to emigrate to Boston and take over their cases. Mrs. Alexander achieved a large measure of popularity among the upper-class women of Boston. When she was offered a substantial financial inducement to move to New York, they promptly raised $1,200 in a successful effort to persuade her to remain. She stayed without the support of Warren and Jackson, however, for in the face of condtinued opposition from their medical colleagues, they "agreed to give her up."[70] According to one nineteenth-century historian, Janet Alexander was probably the last midwife who attended "the higher classes in Boston, although," added the author, "many women still found employment among families of moderate means."[71]

The decline of female midwifery and the concomitant growing popularity of employing the general practitioner to act as accoucheur are directly related to the evolution of midwifery from an art to a science that began to develop in England early in the eighteenth century. Tradition, societal definitions of modesty, and the midwives all opposed man midwifery, yet it gained increasing acceptance among many women of influence. It did so in the name of safety and implied progress. Traditional midwives had varied in ability, but almost all had learned their craft empirically. Little more was expected of them than to assist nature, receive the child, and offer post-partum care for mother and infant. Women had little choice but to accept as inevitable and divinely ordained the trauma and risk of childbearing. The pronouncement in Genesis supported this view: "I will greatly multiply thy sorrow and thy conception; in sorrow thou shalt bring forth children."[72]

The resignation with which women faced pregnancy and parturition was captured poignantly by Anne Bradstreet in seventeenth-century Massachusetts when pregnant with one of her eight children:

> How soon, my Dear, death may my steps attend,
> How soon't may be thy lot to lose thy friend,
> We both are ignorant, yet love bids me
> These farewell lines to recommend to thee. . . .[73]

More than a century later, Elizabeth Drinker's private journal echoed this theme:

> They invited this morn.ᵍ at the three meeting houses to the burial of Rebecca Trotter . . .—she has left 7 children, was in the 42 year of her age—probably, had it pleased providence to have spared her, she might never have had another—I have often thought that women who live to get over the time of Child-bareing, if other things are favourable to them, experience more comfort and satisfaction than at any other period of their lives.[74]

Both Bradstreet and Drinker were upper-class women for whom the best available midwifery care could be obtained. Bradstreet's attendants were women, for men had not yet entered the field in seventeenth-century Boston. Drinker's daughters had a choice. It is worth noting that they chose William Shippen and Nicholas Way, both formally educated physicians who represented the new obstetrics at its best.

The continued improvements that comprised the new obstetrics, introduced by physicians trained abroad and perpetuated in both private courses and the new American medical schools, furnished the key to this important transformation. Women midwives were excluded from the new obstetrics because they remained without access to formal training. They were not taught anatomy, the techniques of version, or the use of obstetrical instruments. In the extremely rare instances when a few were given information about these procedures, it was offered with the proscription that they not use it. These limitations were extremely significant in view of the direction midwifery had taken since the early 1700s.

The implications were evident in the assessments offered by nineteenth-century participants. The British feminist physician, Sophia Jex-Blake, offered her opinion that "what really seems to have been the cause of transferring the practice of midwifery from women to men, was the invention of the midwifery forceps."[75] The eminent New York obstetrician, Augustus K. Gardner, concurred. In an introductory lecture titled "Past Inefficiency and Present Natural Incapacity of Females in the Practice of Obstetrics" delivered at mid-century, he reminded his students that the general knowledge of the use of the forceps, the classification of labors, and the understanding of the mechanism of labor revolutionized obstetrical practice, and women midwives had been prevented from participating in this revolution.[76]

As the fashion to employ general practitioners as accoucheurs became more prevalent in New York, Philadelphia, and Boston, the midwives lost their upper- and middle-class clientele. Contemporary opponents and supporters of the midwives agreed on this point. In 1820, alarmed by the implications of the Warren-Jackson proposal to revive female midwifery in Boston, Walter Channing responded with the boast that in Boston, more than in any other city of equal size, "this branch of medical practice has been . . . entirely confined to male practitioners."[77] Three decades later in the same city, Samuel Gregory, who perhaps more than any other person would focus attention on renewed efforts to revive female midwifery, surveyed the past. He asked how it had happened that a branch of medicine so obviously female-oriented had been taken over by the men. "While the various sections of the public have been absorbed, each in their own affairs and interests," he concluded, "the medical profession have very naturally been mindful of theirs, and of course they had no objection, so long as no body else raised any, to letting women remain ignorant, and allowing this whole business, with the honors and emoluments and influence it confers, slide into their hands."[78]

Still, Gregory's assessment was not entirely accurate. It failed to include the well-meaning efforts of physicians such as Shippen, Seaman, Bard, and others to train women for competence in normal deliveries. In their work they had seen the results of incompetence and ignorance, and their efforts on behalf of the midwives suggest agreement with Valentine Seaman's position that if "women cannot be persuaded to submit themselves to the care of male practitioners, it is our duty to instruct females how to give them the necessary aid."[79] As late as 1817 Dr. Thomas Ewell, a strong supporter of perpetuating female midwifery, was instrumental in organizing a society for the purpose of founding and operating a lying-in hospital in Washington, D.C., where women midwives could be trained. Both this effort and his proposal that the federal government establish schools to train women along the lines of the system utilized at La Maternité in Paris failed to garner the support needed for implementation.[80] It was the absence of such facilities and sources of training for women that set the stage for the triumph of man midwifery that would follow.

NOTES

1. *New York Weekly Post-Boy,* July 22, 1745, quoted in Howard W. Haggard, *Devils, Drugs and Doctors,* 4th ed. (New York: Pocket Books, Inc., 1959), p. 75.

2. Irving S. Cutter and Henry R. Viets, *A Short History of Midwifery* 1st ed. (Philadelphia and London: W. B. Saunders, 1964), pp. 69-87.

3. Benjamin Rush, "An Inquiry into the Comparative State of Medicine, in Philadelphia, Between the Years 1760 and 1765, and the Year 1805," in Benjamin Rush, *Medical Inquiries and Observations,* Vol. 4, 2nd ed. (Philadelphia: J. Conrad, 1805), p. 375.

4. George W. Norris, *The Early History of Medicine in Philadelphia* (Philadelphia, 1886), quoted in Cutter and Viets, *Short History,* p. 145; *Pennsylvania Gazette,* November 3, 1748; Caspar Wistar, *Eulogium on Doctor William Shippen . . .* (Philadelphia: Dobson, 1818), pp. 30-31.

5. Francis R. Packard, *History of Medicine in the United States*, Vol. 1 (New York: Hafner, 1963), p. 53.

6. *Valentine's Manual* [*Manual of the Corporation of the City of New-York . . .*], quoted in Herbert Thoms, *Chapters in American Obstetrics* (Springfield, Ill.: Thomas, 1933), p. 13.

7. Cutter and Viets, *Short History,* p. 146; Packard, *History,* Vol. 1, p. 53; Frederick C. Waite, *History of the New England Female Medical College, 1848-1874* (Boston: Boston University School of Medicine, 1950), p. 14.

8. *Minutes of the Common Council of the City of New York, 1675-1776,* Vol. 4 (New York: Dodd, Mead & Co., 1905), pp. 240, 250; Claude E. Heaton, "Medicine in New York during the English Colonial Period, 1664-1775," *Bulletin of the History of Medicine* 17 (January-February 1945):35.

9. *Minutes of the Common Council, 1675-1776,* Vol. 5, pp. 397, 466; Vol. 6, p. 287.

10. At the urging of Cadwallader Colden, a physician and political figure in New York, Bard described the operation in a letter to Dr. John Fothergill in London. Fothergill read it before the Society of Physicians and in 1762 published it in *Medical Observations and Inquiries,* Vol. 2. The success of the laparotomy is appreciated when it is noted that almost one hundred years later, Professor Charles Meigs, the eminent Philadelphia obstetrician, made this observation on "ectopic gestation" in his book on women's diseases: "Such a diagnosis would not lead to any hopeful therapeutics or chirurgical intervention, for nothing is to be done in these melancholy cases beyond the adoption of mere palliative measures. No man would be mad enough, under such a diagnosis, to perform a gastrotomy operation." [Quoted in Lewis C. Scheffey, "The Earlier History and the Transition Period of Obstetrics and Gynecology in Philadelphia," *Annals of Medical History,* 3rd series, 2 (May 1940):221.] See also Samuel Bard to his parents, June 12, 1762, Bardiana Collection, Bard College; Byron Stookey, *A History of Colonial Medical Education in the Province of New York, with its Subsequent Development, 1767-1830* (Springfield, Ill.: Thomas, 1962), pp. 32-33; Cutter and Viets, *Short History,* pp. 152, 209.

11. Wistar, *Eulogium,* p. 30.

12. Valentine Seaman, *The Midwives' Monitor, and Mothers Mirror . . .* (New York: Isaac Collins, 1800), pp. iii-iv.

13. Richard H. Shryock, *The Development of Modern Medicine* (New York: Knopf, 1947), quoted in Herbert Thoms, "William Shippen, Jr., The Great Pioneer of American Obstetrics," *American Journal of Obstetrics and Gynecology* 37 (March 1939):512; *New York Gazette and Weekly Mercury,* June 3, 1771.

14. W., "On Modesty," *The Ladies Magazine and Repository of Entertaining Knowledge* 1 (June 1793):36.

15. Seaman, *Midwives' Monitor,* p. viii.

16. John Fothergill to James Pemberton, London, July 4, 1762, quoted in John Fothergill, *Chain of Friendship: Selected Letters of Dr. John Fothergill of London, 1735-1780,* Introduction and Notes by Betsy C. Corner and Christopher C. Booth (Cambridge, Mass.: The Belknap Press of Harvard University Press, 1971), p. 225. See also pp. 15, 228n.

17. Announcement of William Shippen, Jr.'s Anatomical Lectures, November 11, 1762, quoted in Cutter and Viets, *Short History,* p. 148.

18. R. Hingston Fox, *Dr. John Fothergill and His Friends: Chapters in Eighteenth Century Life* (London: MacMillan Co., Limited, 1919), p. 368.

19. Norris, *Medicine in Philadelphia,* quoted in Cutter and Viets, *Short History,* p. 148.

20. *Pennsylvania Gazette,* January 31, 1765, quoted in Cutter and Viets, *Short History,* p. 149.

21. Richard H. Shryock, *Medicine in America: Historical Essays* (Baltimore: Johns Hopkins Press, 1966), pp. 181-182.

22. Wistar, *Eulogium,* p. 31.

23. Scheffey, "Obstetrics and Gynecology in Philadelphia," 216.

24. Wistar, *Eulogium,* pp. 14-15, 31.

25. Journal of Elizabeth Drinker, quoted in Cecil K. Drinker, *Not So Long Ago: A Chronicle of Medicine and Doctors in Colonial Philadelphia* (New York: Oxford University Press, 1937), pp. 51-52, 59-60.

26. Claude E. Heaton, "Obstetrics in Colonial America," *American Journal of Surgery,* n.s. 45 (September 1939):6-8; Stookey, *Colonial Medical Education,* pp. 64-65.

27. William [Potts] Dewees, *An Essay on the Means of Lessening Pain, and Facilitating Certain Cases of Difficult Parturition* (Philadelphia: John Oswald, 1806), p. 63.

28. *The Medical Repository* 1 (February 1, 1798):385.

29. Quoted in Heaton, "Medicine in New York," p. 35. See also Waite, *History of the New England Female Medical College,* p. 14. The West Indian dry gripes was lead poisoning, commonly the result of drinking rum distilled through lead pipes.

30. *New York Mercury,* April 20, 1765; *Royal American Gazette,* January 15, 1778.

31. *New York Gazette and Weekly Mercury,* November 11, 1782.

32. *New York Weekly Post-Boy,* January 9, 1769; *New York Gazette and Weekly Mercury,* July 8, 1771.

33. *New York Weekly Post-Boy,* July 4, 1768.

34. *New York Gazette and Weekly Mercury,* June 3, 1771.

35. *New York Gazette and Weekly Mercury,* May 4, 1778.

36. Maurice Bear Gordon, *Aesculapius Comes to the Colonies* (Ventnor, N.J.: Ventnor Publishers, Inc., 1949), p. 350.

37. Rates of Medical Charges, New York, 1798. Mss., New-York Historical Society. Whitfield J. Bell, Jr., *John Morgan, Continental Doctor* (Philadelphia: University of Pennsylvania Press, 1965), p. 153.

38. *Laws and Ordinances of the . . . City of Albany* (Albany: Robertson, 1773), p. 61.

39. *The Essex Gazette* (Salem), July 14, 1772, quoted in Francisco Guerra, *American Medical Bibliography* (New York: Lathrop Harper, 1962), p. 498.

40. *The Massachusetts Gazette and Boston Weekly News-Letter,* quoted in Guerra, *Bibliography,* p. 535.

41. *Boston Evening Post,* November 10, 1781, quoted in Heaton, "Obstetrics in Colonial America," p. 608.

42. See Herbert Thoms, *Our Obstetric Heritage* (Hamden, Conn.: The

Shoe String Press, 1960), p. 140; Richard H. Shryock, *Medical Licensing in America, 1650-1965* (Baltimore: Johns Hopkins Press, 1967), p. 103; Waite, *History of the New England Female Medical College,* p. 14; John B. Blake, "Women and Medicine in Ante-Bellum America," *Bulletin of the History of Medicine* 39 (March-April 1965):99-123.

43. John Van Brugh Tennent to the Governors of the College of New York, August 5, 1767, quoted in Stookey, *Colonial Medical Education,* pp. 50-51.

44. John Bard to Samuel Bard, New York, January 17, 1764, Bardiana Collection, Bard College, Annandale-on-Hudson, New York.

45. Stookey, *Colonial Medical Education,* p. 75, lists the following doctor's degrees awarded as follows: 1771-2; 1772-5; 1773-1; 1774-2; 1775-7. For a discussion of early developments see Martin Kaufman, *American Medical Education: The Formative Years, 1765-1910* (Westport, Conn.: Greenwood Press, 1976), Chapter 2.

46. Kaufman, *Medical Education,* pp. 37-38; *Eclectic Repertory* 1 (October 1810):118; Herbert Thoms, "Thomas Chalkey James, A Pioneer in the Teaching of Obstetrics in America," *American Journal of Obstetrics and Gynecology* 29 (February 1935):289-294; *The Medical Repository* 2 (1789-1799): 307; Heaton, "Obstetrics in Colonial America," p. 608.

47. T. Gaillard Thomas, "A Century of American Medicine, 1776-1876; Obstetrics and Gynaecology," *The American Journal of the Medical Sciences* 72 (July 1876):134.

48. Claude E. Heaton, "Obstetrics at the New York Almshouse and at Bellevue Hospital," *Bulletin of the New York Academy of Medicine,* n.s. 16 (January 1940):39.

49. For a sketch of the high caliber of French midwifery training in the period, see Cutter and Viets, *Short History,* especially pp. 92-95.

50. Seaman, *Midwives' Monitor,* p. iv.

51. Ibid., pp. vii-ix.

52. *The Medical Repository* 3 (1800):64-65.

53. *The Medical Repository* 2 (May 2, 1799):437.

54. Seaman, *Midwives' Monitor,* p. xi.

55. *The Medical Repository* 3 (1800):408.

56. Seaman, *Midwives' Monitor,* pp. 80-81.

57. Ibid., pp. 101-102.

58. Ibid., pp. 90-99.

59. Samuel L. Mitchell, *A Discourse on the Life and Character of Samuel Bard . . .* (New York: Fanshaw, 1821), pp. 25-26; Samuel Bard, *An Attempt to Explain and Justify the Use of Cold in Uterine Hemorrhages with a View to Remove the Prejudices which Prevail among the Women of*

this City against the Use of this Safe and Necessary Remedy (New York: Gaine, 1788).

60. Samuel Bard, *A Compendium of the Theory and Practice of Midwifery, Containing Practical Instructions for the Management of Women During Pregnancy in Labour, and in Child-bed;* 5th ed. (New York: Collins, 1819), p. iii.

61. The manuscript for the proposed sixth edition is in the library of the New York Academy of Medicine.

62. Ibid., p. vii.

63. Samuel Bard, Remarks on the Constitution, Government, Discipline and Expenses of Medical Schools; submitted to the Regents of the University of the State of New York, in obedience to their requisition for such information, April 3, 1819, pp. 15-17, New-York Historical Society.

64. *The Medical Repository,* n.s. 8 (1823-1824):224-225.

65. Ibid., p. 225.

66. Seaman, *Midwives' Monitor,* p. iv.

67. Benjamin Rush, *The Autobiography of Benjamin Rush: His "Travels Through Life" together with his Commonplace Book for 1789-1813,* ed. George W. Corner (Princeton, N.J.: For the American Philosophical Society by Princeton University Press, 1948), p. 176.

68. [Walter Channing], *Remarks on the Employment of Females as Practitioners in Midwifery,* By a physician (Boston: Cummings and Hilliard, 1820), pp. 12, 21.

69. Rhoda Truax, *The Doctors Warren of Boston: First Family of Surgery* (Boston: Houghton Mifflin, 1968), p. 95.

70. Edward Warren, *The Life of John Collins Warren* (Boston: n.p., 1860), Vol. 1:pp. 219-220, Vol. 2:pp. 275-276, quoted in Blake, "Women and Medicine," p. 108; Kate Campbell Hurd-Mead, *Medical Women of America* (New York: Froben Press, 1933), pp. 16-17.

71. Ednah D. Cheney, "The Women of Boston," *Memorial History of Boston,* Vol. 4 (Boston: n.p., 1881), quoted in Elisabeth A. Dexter, *Career Women of America, 1776-1840* (Francestown, N.H.: M. Jones, 1950), p. 35.

72. Genesis 3:16.

73. Anne Bradstreet, "Before the Birth of One of her Children," in *The Works of Anne Bradstreet in Prose and Verse,* ed. John H. Ellis (Gloucester, Mass.: Peter Smith, 1962), pp. 393-394.

74. Journal of Elizabeth Drinker, quoted in Drinker, *Not So Long Ago,* p. 48.

75. Sophia Jex-Blake, *Medical Women: A Thesis and a History* (Edinburgh: Oliphant, Anderson & Ferrier, 1886; London: Hamilton Adams and Co., 1886; New York: Source Book Press Reprint, 1970), p. 19.

76. Augustus K. Gardner, *A History of the Art of Midwifery* . . . (New York: Stringer and Townsend, 1852), p. 19.

77. [Channing], *Remarks,* p. 3.

78. Samuel Gregory, *Letter to Ladies in Favor of Female Physicians* (New York: Fowler and Wells, 1850), pp. 25-26.

79. Seaman, *Midwives' Monitor,* p. iv.

80. Thomas Ewell, *Letters to Ladies, Detailing Important Information Concerning Themselves and Infants* (Philadelphia: W. Brown, 1817), pp. vii-viii, 30; Blake, "Women and Medicine," pp. 108-109.

Man Midwifery and the Delicacy of the Sexes

Who wants to know or ought to know that the ladies have abdomens and wombs but us doctors. When I was young, a woman had no legs, even, but only feet, and possibly ankles; now forsooth, they have utero-abdominal supporters, not in fact only, but in the very newspapers. —CHARLES MEIGS, 1848

By the second decade of the nineteenth century, northern urban women of means, convinced that the superior training of doctors equipped with instruments meant safer and shorter parturition, hardly ever employed a midwife.[1] Despite this fact, the doctors' hold on the practice of midwifery was still a tenuous one. The general practitioners who attended upper-class women recognized the rewards accruing to the accomplished accoucheur. Midwifery, in itself, was not especially lucrative, although physicians probably received higher fees for this service than had the midwives. Greater financial rewards could be obtained from a varied practice ranging from vaccinations and minor ailments to the treatment of serious diseases and surgical operations. Midwifery's attraction was that it fed this general practice; the man who acquitted himself well in the lying-in chamber earned the enduring gratitude of patient and husband. As one Boston physician succinctly observed:

Women seldom forget a practitioner who has conducted them tenderly and safely through parturition—they feel a familiarity with him, a confidence and reliance upon him, which are of the most essential mutual advantage in all their subsequent intercourse as physician and patient. It is this which ensures to [doctors] the permanency and security of all their other business.[2]

Obstetrics, reported a committee of the Philadelphia College of Physicians a few years later, had become a highly competitive field precisely because it led "to the highest success in medicine, more certainly than any other department of practice." Even physicians who opposed man midwifery despaired of accomplishing reform, due to the common boast of the doctor "that if he can attend one single case of midwifery in a family, he has ever after secured their patronage."[3]

Consequently, most physicians were eager to add normal midwifery cases, which constituted the majority of deliveries, to the abnormal ones for which they would almost always be called. To accomplish this, they attempted to reinforce the growing acceptance of the idea that the parturient woman's best prospect for eliminating the hazards of childbirth and post-partum complications lay in the employment of the accoucheur. Working in the doctors' favor was the fact that man midwifery was no longer strictly an innovation. Benjamin Rush, reviewing a half century of medical practice in Philadelphia, claimed in 1805 that "death from pregnancy and parturition . . . [was] a rare occurrence" in his city and attributed this directly to the trend that led to midwifery "being exercised by physicians of regular and extensive educations."[4] In 1826 William Potts Dewees (1768-1841), Adjunct Professor of Midwifery at the University of Pennsylvania, prefaced his obstetrics textbook by exhorting medical students to learn the theory of midwifery thoroughly. In general practice "everyone almost" was called upon to attend deliveries. "A change of manners, within a few years," he observed, "has resulted in the almost exclusive employment of the male practitioner," a change chiefly realized "by a conviction, that the well-instructed physician is best calculated to avert danger, and surmount difficulties."[5]

It would have been strange, indeed, had physicians not played their strongest suit. They emphasized the element of safety and stressed the potential for danger that accompanied every normal case. In contrast to the midwives, who lacked opportunities to gain training, the doctors held a virtual monopoly on the use of the forceps, the lever, and other obstetrical instruments. The pregnant woman, vulnerable in her understandable wish for a shorter and safer delivery, permitted the accoucheur to be called because she believed he always offered the best chance for both.

Despite the repeated claims and promises of the profession, evidence suggests that this belief was not always warranted. In the better medical colleges—the University of Pennsylvania, the College of Physicians and Surgeons in New York, and the Massachusetts Medical College (Harvard)—midwifery and the diseases of women and children constituted one separate department. Yet even these schools did not always require completion of this combined course for the medical degree. Although medical students studied anatomy and physiology of the female, they often had little or no clinical experience in obstetrics. In 1832 Dr. Daniel Drake, surveying medical education, noted that the young practitioner would embark on his career with less practical knowledge in obstetrics than in any other branch of medicine. He urged that the student be especially diligent in acquiring theoretical information in midwifery to avoid being "thrown into situations of responsibility most harrowing to his feelings, if not fatal to his patient."[6] Thomas Denman (1733-1815), the celebrated British obstetrician whose works greatly influenced American teaching and practice, rejected unnecessary interference but sanctioned instrumental deliveries. He agreed that ideally "it would be a very desirable thing that every student should have an opportunity of seeing the operation with the *forceps* performed before he goes into practice" but confessed that such experience was not always possible. Denman ventured his opinion that if the medical student were "properly instructed in the principles of the application and use of the forceps, reflects seriously before he determines on performing the operation, and proceeds slowly but not timidly, he can hardly fail to succeed."[7]

Most obstetrics cases were normal ones, however, and the actual services performed by a knowledgeable physician should not have differed appreciably from those that a competent midwife was capable of providing. These were limited to making the patient as comfortable as circumstances permitted, lending encouragement without giving false hope of a rapid delivery, supporting the perineum at the moment of birth to prevent rupture of the tissue, tying off the umbilical cord, and supervising the expulsion of the placenta.[8] That physicians were equipped with obstetrical instruments, however, held a potential for disaster. Doctors tended to resort to mechanical aids in cases where their use was completely unnecessary. Many men poorly trained in midwifery and lacking in experience did not hesitate to use the lever or forceps with appalling disregard for the consequences. Indiscriminate "meddlesome midwifery" persisted, despite the repeated warnings of the authorities that such interference was potentially harmful to mothers and infants.

Samuel Bard, who maintained his interest in obstetrics for over fifty years, prefaced the third edition of his *Compendium of the Theory and Practice of Midwifery* (1815) with a warning. He had, he said, added a chapter on the use of instruments "rather to recommend caution and repress temerity, than to encourage confidence and presumption" on the part of the youthful practitioner. His work extolled the virtues of caution and patience that permitted nature to accomplish its course unimpeded. Bard vividly traced the consequences that followed the physician's hasty resort to instruments:

He will probably fail at first, for want of judgment, to discriminate accurately between one case and another, as well as for want of skill and dexterity in the application of his instruments; and finding himself foiled in the use of the safer lever and forceps, he will become alarmed, confused and apprehensive for his patient's safety, as well as for his own reputation. And now, deeming a speedy delivery essential to both and . . . having taken the case into his own hands . . . he thinks he must not desist before he has accomplished it, he flies to the crotchet, as more easy in its application and more certain in its effect—with this he probably succeeds; and although the poor infant is sacrificed, yet he persuades himself, perhaps honestly believes, this was necessary.[9]

William Dewees' *Compendious System of Midwifery* (1824) also stressed the importance of noninterference.

It is a vulgar prejudice, that great and constant benefit, can be derived from the agency of the accoucheur; especially, during the active state of pain; and this feeling is but too often encouraged by the ignorant, and the designing to the injury of the patient, and to the disgrace of the profession. When all things are doing well, the *active* duties of the accoucheur, are limited indeed—it is but where the contrary obtain, that he can be said to be actively useful.[10]

Dewees was equally critical of those who resorted to the "barbaric practice" of needlessly thrusting a hand into the uterus for the purpose of hastening the discharge of the placenta. Even some of his "obstetric friends" whom he greatly esteemed fell into this error, lamented Dewees.

They grate my ears by boasting how frequently they have carried the hand into the uterus, and with what facility the placenta has been removed: that this operation may be easily effected, I have no doubt; but depend upon it, if you do carry your hand into the uterus on every occasion, to get away the placenta, some women will die at last, and die the victims of your mismanagement.[11]

Another physician, comparing American and French obstetrical training in the *Eclectic Journal of Medicine,* was convinced that the American medical schools placed undue emphasis on abnormal cases. The result was that students gained the mistaken impression that such abnormalities were the rule rather than the exception. Citing the Statistics on Proportion of Labours requiring Instruments kept over a seven-year period at the Dublin Lying-in Hospital, the editor pointed out that in 16,654 deliveries, instrumental assistance had been used only twenty-seven times, or roughly 1:608 childbirths. The physician could do much to contribute to the parturient woman's comfort, safety, and her post-partum recovery, but not, warned the author, "by any instrumental display, or the exhibition of medicine to hasten labour; or by hasty extraction of the placenta."[12]

In 1843 John Metcalf, a Bedford, Massachusetts, physician, reported his midwifery experiences in the *American Journal of the Medical Sciences.* Metcalf had kept a record of more than three hundred cases he had attended over a thirteen-year period. Using the "numerical method of observation" introduced by the French and then gaining popularity among American physicians,[13] he calculated his own ratio of instrument deliveries as 1:300. Experience had taught him that despite the professional attention given to the various delicate manipulations that could be employed, in actual practice the need for them was very rare. The secret of success in obstetrics, he stressed, lay in "letting the patient alone" so long as the physician could reasonably assume that the natural mechanism of parturition could accomplish its end without help.[14]

In 1845 Gunning S. Bedford, who held the chair in Midwifery and the Diseases of Women and Children at the University of New York, warned his students that unrestrained and "unpardonable" use of instruments was still widely prevalent. A young practitioner in discussing operative midwifery with Bedford had mentioned that he brought to his practice great familiarity with instruments. The preceptor with whom he had studied had averaged sixteen embryotomies a year! Bedford was horrified but not surprised, for as he observed to his class, "I have myself witnessed in this city scenes of blood sufficient to satisfy my mind that this is not an exaggerated picture."[15]

Another physician, Augustus K. Gardner, lecturing in New York on operative midwifery in 1851, warned that it was the shortsightedness of the medical profession that threatened obstetrical practice in that city. The average medical student could graduate without ever having attended a delivery. The resulting ignorance led either to meddlesome midwifery on the one hand, or to the equally dangerous doctrine of absolute noninterference on the other. If a doctor encountered only uncomplicated cases at the outset of his career, he was likely to believe that "all the talk of position, presentation, rotation, and such like is all nonsense, or at best theoretical, and he joins the 'expectant' practitioners, trusts to the *vis medicatrix naturae* . . . and by a dull inactivity . . . loses the child, and not unfrequently the mother also, and injures the reputation of the profession."[16]

In 1850 when the *New York Medical Gazette* ran a brief notice describing an improved set of obstetrical forceps recently developed by a Dr. Henry Bond, the editor expressed the hope that improved forceps would not lead to increased use. He observed that there were cases in which the forceps were indispensable but added regretfully "that they are employed very many times when they are wholly uncalled for, is no less certain."[17] With some optimism he predicted that the conservative midwifery currently taught in the schools would make instrument deliveries the exception rather than the rule.

In the first half of the nineteenth century American medical education, on which doctors based their claims to superiority over the midwives, was of variant quality. The period from 1820 to 1860 witnessed a spectacular increase in the number of medical colleges.[18] This proliferation was accompanied by keen competition for students and in turn led to a general lowering of standards both for admission and graduation. The individual colleges, rather than state medical boards, examined the students, and the contemporary professional view was that many who were awarded the doctor of medicine were mediocre, or worse. Dr. George Wood, speaking before the Philadelphia Medical Society in 1824, lamented the inadequate preparation of students on entering medical school:

The pupil, undismayed by his deficiencies, enters with all his mental faculties stiffened by inaction, and paralyzed by neglect. . . . His progress in the attainment of medical knowledge must therefore be exceeding slow, and, at the end of the regular period, unfit as he necessarily must be, he goes forth to encounter diseases and proves, I fear not unfrequently, more an auxiliary than an antagonist.[19]

Still further competition appeared in the form of unorthodox or "irregular" medical sects such as the Thomsonians, Homeopathists, and Eclectics. Under the banner of reform they also established medical schools and produced substantial numbers of graduates with the doctor of medicine.[20] One orthodox or "regular" physician in 1849 blamed the growth of empiricism and general lack of public confidence in the profession on the failure of medical schools to enforce rigorous standards. In many instances, he complained, attendance at lectures was not required, and students matriculated for the degree without relinquishing their regular jobs. The ease with which students passed the examinations and earned the medical degree had overcrowded the profession, he maintained. When they could not find room in the regular profession, he continued, graduates turned to irregular practice, becoming homeopathists, hydropathists, and "consumption doctors." Concluded this critic, "our most powerful and dangerous enemies are to be found within our own ranks."[21]

An indication of the low esteem in which the public held the doctor, as compared with the minister and the lawyer, is suggested in the response of his father when J. Marion Sims (1813-1883) announced his plan to enter medicine. It was a profession for which he had the "utmost contempt," declared the elder Sims.

There is no science in it. There is no honor to be achieved in it; no reputation to be made; and to think that *my* son should be going around from house to house through this country, with a box of pills in one hand and a squirt in the other, to ameliorate human suffering, is a thought I never supposed I should have to contemplate.[22]

Equally disturbing to the regulars was the trend in the state legislatures, given impetus by the spirit of reform individualism in Jacksonian America, to move away from licensing requirements in response to egalitarian demands of white males lower down on the socioeconomic scale. In New York, for instance, the legislature in 1806 had provided for the licensing of doctors under the aegis of the state medical society. By 1844 the movement toward laissez-faire had resulted in the repeal of all New York laws prohibiting unlicensed persons from suing for fees. Those who practiced medicine without a license, moreover, were not liable for criminal prosecution unless convicted of gross ignorance, malpractice, or immoral conduct.[23] In the face of public support for empiricism, members of the Monroe County Medical Society in western New York gave up all hope for improving the profession, as this committee report suggests:

Empiricism is everywhere rife, and was never more arrogant, and the people love to have it so. That restless agrarian spirit that would always be leveling down, has so long kept up a hue-and-cry against calomel and lancet, that the prejudices of the community are excited against it, and their confidence in the medical profession greatly impaired, and no law could be enforced against the empiric and nostrum vender. Every attempt of the kind would only create a deeper sympathy in their favor, and raise a storm of higher indignation against the profession.[24]

Concluded the committee, "This spirit cannot be controlled by arbitrary legislation."

The *Boston Medical and Surgical Journal* summarized a discouraging medical picture with the observation that there was little incentive for the regular physician in an overcrowded profession as long as the public continued to patronize "quacks."[25] The *New York Medical Gazette* voiced less concern about the increased competition than about the lowering of standards. The *Gazette* was highly critical of the state legislature for incorporating irregular colleges, thereby reducing all schools to the same level, and charged that the legislators had contributed to the mortality bills by "throwing open the field of practice in every branch of the healing art, to every presumptuous pretender, or needy adventurer, however ignorant or unprincipled."[26]

Had these deficiencies in medical education been common knowledge, women might have shown greater reluctance in employing male physicians, many of whom had scant midwifery training. As it was, doctors faced a more formidable obstacle to continued dominance in obstetrics in the form of the cultural mores of the period. With the growing urbanization of American life that accompanied nascent industrialism, upper- and middle-class women were confined to a narrow sphere of home and family. There they were expected to cultivate the virtues of "true womanhood"[27] and warned of the dire consequences of immodesty. A society that grew increasingly prudish as the century progressed could not be expected to look with equanimity upon the presence of accoucheurs in the lying-in chamber, regardless of their training.

The doctors themselves were well aware of the conflicting demands of modesty and safety. Even W. Channing, who argued against a proposal to restore midwives in Boston, felt constrained to admit that the honor, virtue, and dignity of women greatly depended on their feelings of delicacy. "There can be no doubt," he observed, "that the attendance of a female must be more grateful to these feelings, and that they must be somewhat wounded at first by the presence of a physician.''[28] He hastened to add, however, that the employment of a doctor did not constitute an indelicacy and had come to be accepted in Boston as a matter of course.

Other physicians were more sensitive to propriety. In 1835 Edward Cutbush, delivering an address before a mixed audience at the opening of the new medical school at Geneva College, commented at length on all branches of medicine except obstetrics. The speaker explained that "delicacy has thrown a veil around this subject which precludes all remarks before this audience.''[29] Cutbush confined himself to lavishing praise on William Shippen, whose "suavity of manner and correct deportment" in the eighteenth century had contributed much to obviating the prejudice against accoucheurs. Neither Shippen's students nor those of the succeeding generations, Cutbush assured his audience, had been guilty of violating strict propriety in the course of their professional obligations.

The eminent Charles D. Meigs, who for many years held the chair in Obstetrics and the Diseases of Women and Children at Jefferson Medical College in Philadelphia, once described to his students the embarrassment with which his own teacher had approached the topic of midwifery. Thomas Chalkley James (1766-1835) was so modest, Meigs recalled approvingly, that as he lectured, the delicate nature of his subject "frequently sent the mantling blood over cheeks and brow to testify that he had the deepest sense of the delicacy of the task assigned to him—that of exposing to hundreds of young men, those trembling secrets of the lying-in chamber, which he had blushed to learn and which he more redly blushed to tell.''[30]

Meigs had overcome his own youthful inclination to regard midwifery as an occupation "fit *only* for old women," as his long and productive career in obstetrics attests. Still, he retained the gentleman's respect for womanhood. In order to be successful, Meigs believed, the accoucheur must fully comprehend those traits that were unique to the female. In 1847 he favored his students with an entire lecture built around these "distinctive characteristics." Woman elevated and civilized mankind; the arts, literature, and science all flourished under her spell; her smile was the propelling force that made man's achievements possible. Naturally prone to be religious, she exerted a salutary effect on society's morals, setting the tone and willingly martyring herself for religion, country, and family. Her head was "almost too small for intellect, but just big enough for love." But of all her attributes, observed this physician, the most charming was her modesty. This modesty stemmed from her "natural" inclination to timidity and dependence and served as one of her strongest attractions as well as one of her most powerful aids. It bound her to home and family, where she transmitted to her children those positive values that elevated mankind. It made her "come out from the world, and be separate from it."[31]

This idealized concept of delicate American woman—modest, docile, submissive, and gentle—found wide acceptance among both men and women of the period. Even when feminist reformers sought greater opportunities for women, many were careful to couch their demands in terms of usefulness within "woman's sphere."[32] Of chief interest here is the incongruity of the situation in which, despite the "innate" modesty and delicacy of her character, the enceinte woman was encouraged to suspend her prejudices and inhibitions—at least temporarily—in order to obtain a safe and rapid delivery at the hands of an accoucheur. The physicians' task in overcoming woman's timidity was made all the more complex by their own recognition of the need to bow to propriety and decorum. One solution, of course, was to provide society with medically trained women attendants. The same cultural attitudes, however, that bound women to their natural "sphere" made it increasingly difficult to accept the notion that "true" women could be competently trained to perform the delicate tasks of the obstetrician and still retain their modesty. Physicians capitalized on this in their determined efforts to keep women out of medical practice.

Anxious to attract obstetrical cases, yet mindful that they were always subject to criticism, the doctors endeavored to strike a balance that would permit them to control the field yet not offend the sensibilities. In 1838 Hugh L. Hodge, Professor of Midwifery at the University of Pennsylvania, put the problem in focus. Deploring the continued presence among women of "prejudice" against the accoucheur, he asserted that medical students must not only totally qualify themselves in obstetrics but must also "diffuse, in every direction a knowledge of the great value of obstetrics, as a practical science." In so doing, they must inculcate the view that parturition was *always* dangerous:

if these facts can be substantiated; if this information can be promulgated; if females can be induced to believe that their sufferings will be diminished, or shortened, and their lives and those of their offspring, be safer in the hands of the profession; there will be no further difficulty in establishing the universal practice of obstetrics. All the prejudices of the most ignorant or nervous female, all the innate and acquired feelings of delicacy so characteristic of the sex, will afford no obstacle to the employment of male practitioners.[33]

While they admitted to the "delicacy of the sexes" and acknowledged what Meigs called "the embarrassments of the practice," some doctors nevertheless belittled objections to the obstetrician by charging that women were cultivating a "false delicacy." The American edition of Hugh Smith's *Letters to Married Ladies* (1829) cautioned women against withholding information from their physicians. Pointing out that a doctor could not prescribe properly without full knowledge of his patient's symptoms, the physician as author warned women against deciding for themselves what they would reveal and what they would not. There was, he assured his readers, no need "for a bold, unblushing declaration of the whole truth; but . . . there should be no desire to conceal" the nature of the case. "True modesty," observed the author, "never interferes, in any respect, with health; it must be nothing less than mock modesty, bearing no alliance to that lovely charm which sheds such lustre over every female grace." He scorned the exhibition of "mere pretence of character" and assured his readers that doctors were not deceived by it.[34]

As doctors expanded their treatment of women to include not only parturition but also that wide range of disorders included in the term "diseases of women," the problems multiplied. Frequently, the woman who could be persuaded to call a doctor to deliver her was loathe to have him treat other "female complaints." If she did consult him, she was reluctant even to describe her symptoms and more often than not would absolutely refuse to submit to a physical examination. The comments of physician Richard Arnold, upon sending his ailing wife to consult with Charles Meigs, reinforce the point. "As the wife of a medical man," wrote Arnold, "she is aware that false delicacy too often injures females, by allowing disease to get beyond the reach of medical art before they speak out. I have told her," he continued, "to answer any questions you should think necessary to ask her."[35]

Drafting its Code of Medical Ethics in 1848, the members of one medical society hoped the chasm between candor and delicacy could be bridged by the physician who was able to make himself a "friend and adviser" to both men and women patients. "Even the female sex," they observed, "should never allow feelings of shame or delicacy" to preclude divulging necessary details to the physician. In ordinary life "delicacy of mind" was highly commendable, but when too strictly observed in medicine, warned the doctors, it often caused the patient to "sink under a painful and loathsome disease, which might have been readily prevented."[36]

Charles Meigs agreed that the woman who was less than candid or who steadfastly refused to permit more than a partial and superficial examination invited grave consequences. Yet physicians, too, must recognize their own responsibilities, he insisted. Many practitioners, observed Meigs, were constrained by their own sense of delicacy from examining women patients thoroughly. To illustrate the point, he cited the case of a woman who had suffered for twenty years from an abnormal uterine condition. Although she had been examined repeatedly over the years, not one of these partial examinations had revealed the actual source of her complaint. As a consequence, she had suffered unnecessarily for years from a condition that could have been remedied if one of the attending physicians had persisted in obtaining the requisite information.

But even Meig's genuine concern about the medically injurious effects of modesty did not prevent his making this astounding observation:

It is perhaps best, upon the whole, that this great degree of modesty should exist, even to the extent of putting a bar to researches. . . . I confess I am proud to say that, in this country . . . there are women who prefer to suffer the extremity of danger and pain, rather than waive those scruples of delicacy which prevent their maladies from being fully explored. I say it is an evidence of the dominion of a fine morality in our society.[37]

Yet it would certainly be erroneous to consider Meig's comment as representative of the views of the entire medical profession. The majority of physicians were inclined to draw a fine distinction between "false" and "genuine" modesty. As Dr. John F. Holston stated in the *New York Medical Gazette,* intelligent women, when not blinded by "modern reform notions," recognized the difficulties involved in training women as obstetrical attendants and wisely agreed that the "bulk" of obstetrical practice should be in the hands of male practitioners.[38] In 1855 John Quackenbush of the Albany Medical College remarked to students that most doctors could expect to be called upon to practice midwifery during their careers. The public, he noted, had learned that childbirth was a risky business and had been persuaded to employ the accoucheur "almost" exclusively. "The natural delicacy of the woman exists *now*; but she permits the knowledge of her danger to override this delicacy of her feelings and the modesty of her nature."[39]

These observations notwithstanding, physicians were vulnerable to the charge of exciting "improper feelings" among their women patients. Professors at the medical colleges were conscious of this fact and repeatedly urged students and colleagues to take every possible precaution to avoid censure. It was essential for a doctor to cultivate a climate of mutual respect with his patient. No true gentleman, asserted one doctor, would commit the error of infringing on the delicacy "which should ever attach itself to the almost sacred office in which he is engaged."[40] Although Caspar Wistar, Midwifery Professor at the University of Pennsylvania, considered it a "self-evident truth" that women should be attended by accomplished male obstetricians, this was not always so apparent to the public. In asking woman to sacrifice some degree of modesty by employing the accoucheur, the doctor incurred a special obligation. He must not betray her trust in him and must strive always to "repay woman's confidence . . . by diligence and . . . [devotion to] duty."[41]

Such prohibitions carried over into the area of clinical teaching as well. Condemning the European practice, Charles Meigs unequivocally denounced "the spectacle . . . of troops of women waiting in succession for a public examination of their genitalia in the presence of large classes of medical practitioners and students of medicine." Modesty and chastity were the foundations of man's love and respect for woman, the cornerstone of "civilization and order" that must be preserved. It would sometimes be the physician's "distressing duty" to "condescend" to conduct vaginal examinations, continued Meigs. Still, "he is but the pander of vice who parades his thousands of uterine cases before the public gaze; and is, himself an unchaste man, who ruthlessly insists upon a vaginal taxis in all cases of women's diseases that, however remotely, may seem to have any . . . connexion with disorder of their reproductive tissue,"[42] pronounced Meigs.

The need to observe strict propriety in the lying-in room made it awkward for physician and patient when it was necessary to conduct a vaginal examination. The young physician was cautioned to examine only when it was essential and warned against unnecessary repetition. Above all, such examinations must always be conducted with decorum and preferably in the presence of a married woman or nurse. William Dewees suggested that even questioning of a delicate nature be accomplished through the intermediary nurse or elderly female friend. This third person should be the one to propose a necessary examination to the patient and to urge it upon her. Permission granted, further precautions were called for. "Before you proceed," advised Dewees, "let your patient be placed with the most scrupulous regard to delicacy, as the slightest exposure is never necessary."[43] Only when all light was excluded from the room could the exclusively tactile examination proceed. Finally, when delivery was imminent, the decorous physician left the room while the nurse positioned the patient. He returned when she was covered entirely except for her head, at which time he delivered the child under the blanket or sheet.

The post-partum mother frequently has difficulty excreting urine. To effect elimination in such cases, a catheter must be passed through the urethra to the bladder. Physicians and patients alike found this procedure unpleasant and offensive. Consequently, doctors could not agree about who was responsible for performing catheterizations. Samuel Bard believed it could be done by a woman attendant, who should introduce the device "under the bedclothes."[44] Thomas Ewell concurred. He emphasized the fact that the passing of the catheter was a simple matter and insisted that it was a "disgrace to the sex" for a man to perform such an "odious" task.[45] William Dewees, who believed that the physician should perform the operation, nevertheless was aware of the potential offense to dignity it involved and carefully advised the young practitioner on correct procedure. Once the patient had been positioned properly at the side of the bed, the doctor lubricated his finger with sweet oil or lard. Then he carefully placed his hand beneath the bedclothes, "so as not to occasion the smallest exposure" of the patient, and inserted the catheter. Relying solely on the sense of touch might seem awkward, but it was considered infinitely preferable to offending etiquette.[46] Charles Meigs favored teaching the patient to insert the catheter herself. "There is," he wrote, "scarcely a more disagreeable operation to be performed than that of catheterism of the female; an operation which, I should think, every gentleman would be glad to commit to other hands than his own."[47] At mid-century Chandler R. Gilman, Professor of Obstetrics at the College of Physicians and Surgeons in New York, stated that he never used the catheter if he could avoid it. When forced to, he normally avoided exposing his patient, although he admitted that in some cases "delicacy must yield to necessity."[48]

The "diseases of women" presented additional challenges to decorum. Gynecology was in its infancy in the early years of the nineteenth century. For the most part doctors treated gynecological disorders medically rather than surgically, prescribing pills and pastes. Digital examination, even when permitted by a reluctant patient, provided doctors with little accurate information and left much to conjecture until the vaginal speculum began to find favor. This instrument, developed in France by Joseph Claude Anthelme Recamier, made possible the inspection of the cervix and uterus, greatly enhancing the possibilities for treating diseased parts effectively. After many years of experimentation and subsequent modification of the speculum to widen the field of vision, Recamier demonstrated its use to colleagues in 1818.[49]

The pervasive climate of modesty in the United States, according to a report in the May 1850 issue of the *New York Journal of Medicine,* hindered acceptance of the speculum, and physicians themselves were reluctant to employ it.[50] In 1844 Fleetwood Churchill, an English physician who modified the speculum, said he considered the instrument highly overrated. He particularly objected to it because its use necessitated exposure of the patient, which digital examination did not, thus making it much more offensive to female delicacy.[51] On the other hand, in the January 1851 issue of the *New York Journal of Medicine* Chandler Gilman charged with negligence those doctors who claimed never to have encountered a patient with a diseased cervix. He insisted that routine use of the speculum led to the discovery of previously undetected cases. Gilman strongly objected to the "anti-progress party" in the profession whose adherents opposed innovation in general and chloroform and the speculum in particular. On June 15, 1851, the *New York Medical Gazette* reported that the recently organized American Medical Association had heatedly debated the "speculum mania."[52] Thus, at mid-century there were many American doctors who still took the position that a competent physician need not resort to visual examination for any reason whatsoever.[53]

The efforts to conform to early Victorian moral precepts created special problems for physicians engaged in obstetrical and gynecological practice. The acute competition for obstetrical cases placed additional strain on medical ethics. In 1823 the Medical Society of the State of New York adopted a System of Medical Ethics. Observed the society, "the life of a physician is, on the whole, a continual struggle against the prejudices and erroneous habits of the mind, and not unfrequently against [public] ingratitude." Doctors must therefore be careful always to conduct themselves as perfect gentlemen, avoiding everything that might lead to censure. Members were reminded of the confidential, even secret, nature of their business. Those outside the profession were apt to misinterpret what they were told about diseases and treatments. Warned the society, "in ordinary practice, common sense, decency, and delicacy should in familiar conversation with females and persons uninstructed in medicine" always exclude details.[54] Often it was easier to state professional and patient obligations than to honor them in a manner acceptable both to medicine and society. Most importantly, the full force of man midwifery criticism had not yet descended on the profession.

NOTES

1. This chapter is a slightly revised version of Jane B. Donegan, "Man-Midwifery and the Delicacy of the Sexes," in *"Remember the Ladies"*: *New Perspectives on Women in American History,* ed. Carol V. R. George (Syracuse, N.Y.: Syracuse University Press, 1975). Reprinted with permission of Syracuse University Press.

2. [Walter Channing], *Remarks on the Employment of Females as Practitioners in Midwifery,* By a physician (Boston: Cummings and Hilliard, 1820), pp. 19-20. In the three cities considered—New York, Philadelphia, and Boston—physicians in New York received the highest midwifery fees. The New York City Fee Bill of 1816 set fees of $25 to $30 for common cases, and $35 to $60 for tedious or difficult ones. In 1817 the Boston Medical Association established fees of $12 for day cases and $15 for night cases, without apparent regard for the nature of the cases. In 1834 the fee table for the College of Physicians in Philadelphia listed $8 to $20 for midwifery. Detailed discussion of fees appears in Henry B. Shafer, *The American Medical Profession, 1783-1850* (New York: Columbia University Press, 1936), pp. 154-160.

3. "Report of the College of Physicians, November 15, 1835," in W. R. Penman, "The Public Practice of Midwifery in Philadelphia," *Transactions of the College of Physicians of Philadelphia* 37 (October 1869):129. The report stated that 170 practitioners had delivered a total of 7,856 infants that year. Had the cases been equally divided among them, they would have averaged roughly forty per doctor. Some, however, had as many as one to two hundred.—W. Beach, *An Improved System of Midwifery adapted to the Reformed Practice of Medicine . . . with Remarks on Physiological and Moral Elevation* (New York: Scribners, 1851), p. 13.

4. Benjamin Rush, "An Inquiry into the Comparative State of Medicine, in Philadelphia, Between the Years 1760 and 1765, and the Year 1805," in Benjamin Rush, *Medical Inquiries and Observations,* Vol. 4, 2nd ed. (Philadelphia: J. Conrad, 1805), pp. 395-396.

5. William Potts Dewees, *A Compendious System of Midwifery, Chiefly designed to facilitate the Inquiries of those who may be pursuing this branch of study,* 1st ed. (Philadelphia: Carey and Lea, 1824), pp. xiv-xv.

6. Daniel Drake, *Practical Essays on Medical Education, and the Medical Profession, in the United States* (Cincinnati: Roff & Young, 1832), pp. 40-41.

7. Thomas Denman, *Aphorisms on the Application and Use of the Forceps and Vectis; on preternatural Labours, on Labours attended with Hemorrhage, and with Convulsions* (Philadelphia: Benjamin Johnson, 1803), p. 25. For his conservative approach, see *An Introduction to the*

Practice of Midwifery, 2 vols. (New York: James Oram, 1802), a work of many editions that was very popular in American medical schools.

8. The use of anesthesia in childbirth was advocated by Walter Channing in his *Treatise on Etherization in Childbirth* (1848). At about the same time, Dr. James Y. Simpson, Professor of Obstetrics at the University of Glasgow, had begun his experiments utilizing chloroform in parturition. American and British obstetricians resisted these innovations, and it was many years before either ether or chloroform won acceptance. In 1851 Dr. Augustus K. Gardner promoted the use of chloroform in "simple and natural as in difficult and instrumental deliveries." He observed that anesthesia was commonly used in Boston, but in New York its use was "exceedingly limited."—Augustus K. Gardner, *A History of the Art of Midwifery: A Lecture Delivered at the College of Physicians and Surgeons, November 11, 1851* . . . (New York: Stringer and Townsend, 1852), p. 24.

Charles D. Meigs, Professor of Midwifery and the Diseases of Women and Children at Jefferson Medical College in Philadelphia, was one of the profession's most adament opponents of anesthesia. He argued that a woman's pain in childbirth was "natural" or "physiological" and therefore "a desirable, salutary, and conservative manifestation of life force" with which doctors ought not interfere.—Howard W. Haggard, *Devils, Drugs and Doctors,* 4th ed. (New York: Pocket Books, Inc., 1959), p. 117. In 1849 Meigs observed that the use of anesthesia had made no real progress in his city, and added, "it is quite . . . true that a lying-in room is, for the most of the time, a scene of cheerfulness and gaiety, instead of one of shrieks and anguish and despair which have been so forcibly portrayed."—Quoted in Lewis C. Scheffey, "The Earlier History and the Transition Period of Obstetrics and Gynecology in Philadelphia," *Annals of Medical History,* 3rd series, 2 (May 1940):221.

9. Samuel Bard, *A Compendium of the Theory and Practice of Midwifery* . . . , 5th ed. (New York: Collins, 1819), pp. iv-vi, 240.

10. Dewees, *Compendious System,* p. 188.

11. William P. Dewees, quoted in A. Curtis, *Lectures on Midwifery and the Forms of Disease Peculiar to Women and Children, Delivered to the Members of the Botanico-Medical College of Ohio,* 2nd ed. (Columbus, Ohio: Jonathan Phillips, 1841), p. 205.

12. "Obstetrics," *Eclectic Journal of Medicine* 1 (November 1836):27-28.

13. Richard H. Shryock, *Medicine and Society in America, 1660-1860* (Ithaca: Cornell University Press, 1962), pp. 126-131, contains a discussion of the influences of the Paris School on American medicine in the second quarter of the nineteenth century, including the adoption of the use of clinical statistics during this period.

14. John G. Metcalf, "Statistics in Midwifery," *American Journal of the Medical Sciences,* n.s. 6 (October 1843):327-330; 334. In one of his cases Metcalf's ultra-conservative definition of "necessary" interference allowed him to stand by and permit a woman with a malformed pelvis to suffer through eighty-four hours of labor before she finally was delivered without mechanical aid! Such reluctance to intervene was extreme even among those within the profession who ranked as the severest critics of meddlesome midwifery.

15. Quoted in [John Stevens], *Man Midwifery Exposed, or the Danger and Immorality of Employing Men in Midwifery Proved; and the Remedy for the Evil Found* (London: William Horsell, 1850), p. 41.

16. Gardner, *History of Midwifery,* p. 30. The poor preparation of medical students in midwifery was still being criticized as late as 1912. J. W. Williams, Professor of Obstetrics at Johns Hopkins, surveyed midwifery teaching in the country's recognized medical schools. Among the responses he received to his questionnaire was one from an obstetrics professor who admitted that prior to assuming his professorship, he had never seen a woman deliver! See J. Whitridge Williams, "Medical Education and the Midwife Problem in the United States," *Journal of the American Medical Association* 58 (January 6, 1912):1-7.

17. *The New York Medical Gazette* 1 (July 20, 1850):45.

18. A partial list of orthodox medical colleges established in the period includes: Jefferson (1824), Geneva (1834), Tulane (1834), Willoughby [Starling] (1834), Cincinnati (1835), Berkshire (1837), Albany (1838), New York University (1838), New York (1850), Miami [Ohio] (1852), and Long Island (1858). Detailed background on these colleges appears in Francis R. Packard, *History of Medicine in the United States,* Vol. 2 (New York: Hafner, 1963), chapter 11. Recent well-documented interpretive studies are Martin Kaufman, *American Medical Education: The Formative Years, 1765-1910* (Westport, Conn.: Greenwood Press, 1976), and Joseph F. Kett, *The Formation of the American Medical Profession: The Role of Institutions, 1780-1860* (New Haven: Yale University Press, 1968).

19. George B. Wood, *An Oration Delivered Before the Philadelphia Medical Society, February 14, 1824* (No place: J. Harding, for the Society, 1824), pp. 9-10.

20. An indication of the wide variety of practitioners in the field in 1836 is seen in the following list appearing in the *Boston Medical and Surgical Journal:* "regular, irregular, Broussaisians, Sangradorian, Morrisonian, Botanic, regular botanic, Thomsonians, reformed Thomsonian, magnetical, electrical, homeopathic, rootist, herbist, florist and quack."— Quoted in Shafer, *American Medical Profession,* p. 202. For a discussion of some of these interesting sects, see chapter 7.

21. I. F. Galloupe, Letter to the Editor, *Boston Medical and Surgical Journal* 41 (November 29, 1849):380-382.

22. J. Marion Sims, *The Story of My Life* (New York: Da Capo Press, 1968: facsimile of first edition, New York: D. Appleton and Co., 1884), pp. 114-115.

23. Kett, *Formation of American Medical Profession,* p. 182. Richard H. Shryock discussed this period in *Medical Licensing in America, 1650-1965* (Baltimore: Johns Hopkins Press, 1967), pp. 3-42. His comment on the effect of the general lack of midwifery regulation is provocative: "It is true that the ancient specialty of midwifery was subject at best to only casual regulation. . . . Hence, midwives (who continued to practice among the poor) lost the status enjoyed by some colonial predecessors." (p. 27) Had the the doctors not been able to reverse this leveling trend in medicine after mid-century, the midwives could have benefitted from a comparative increase in their status.

24. Charles B. Coventry, "History of Medical Licensing in the State of New York," *New York Journal of Medicine,* o.s. 4 (March 1845):160.

25. *Boston Medical and Surgical Journal* 47 (October 1852): 328.

26. *The New York Medical Gazette* 2 (April 1, 1851):74.

27. See Barbara Welter, "The Cult of True Womanhood: 1820-1860," *American Quarterly* 18 (Summer 1966):151-174.

28. [Channing], *Remarks,* p. 16.

29. Edward Cutbush, *A Discourse Delivered at the Opening of the Medical Institution of Geneva College, State of New York, February 10, 1835* (Geneva, N.Y.: Greves, 1835), p. 9.

30. Charles D. Meigs, *Introductory Lecture to a Course on Obstetrics Delivered in Jefferson Medical College, November 4, 1841* (Philadelphia: Merrihew & Thompson, 1841), p. 8.

31. Charles D. Meigs, *Lecture on some of the Distinctive Characteristics of the Female, Delivered Before the Class of the Jefferson Medical College, January 5, 1847* (Philadelphia: Collins, 1847), pp. 6-17. Discussions and analyses of some aspects of medical views of woman during this period are found in Carroll Smith-Rosenberg and Charles Rosenberg, "The Female Animal: Medical and Biological Views of Woman and Her Role in Nineteenth-Century America," *Journal of American History* 60 (September 1973):332-356; Barbara Welter, "Female Complaints," in Barbara Welter, *Dimity Convictions: The American Woman in the Nineteenth Century* (Athens, Ohio: Ohio University Press, 1976); and H. Carleton Marlow and Harrison M. Davis, *The American Search for Woman* (Santa Barbara, Calif.: Clio Books, 1976), chapter 2.

32. William O'Neill shows how this trend became more pronounced later in the century as feminists soft-pedaled earlier radical positions in favor of

more acceptable socially oriented objectives. See William F. O'Neill, "Feminism as a Radical Ideology," in *Dissent: Explorations in the History of American Radicalism,* ed. Alfred F. Young (De Kalb, Ill.: Northern Illinois University Press, 1968), pp. 275-300.

33. Hugh L. Hodge, *Introductory Lecture to the Course on Obstetrics and the Diseases of Women and Children, Delivered in the University of Pennsylvania, November 7, 1838* (Philadelphia: J. G. Auner, 1838), p. 11.

34. Hugh Smith, *Letters to Married Ladies,* 2nd ed. (New York: G. & C. Carvill et al., 1829), pp. vii-viii.

35. Richard D. Arnold to Charles D. Meigs, Savannah, Ga., 1838, in Richard H. Shryock, ed., *The Letters of Richard D. Arnold, 1808-1876* (Duke University Papers of the Trinity College Historical Society), quoted in Shafer, *American Medical Profession,* p. 130.

36. "Code of Medical Ethics," *Transactions of the Medical Association of Southern Central New York, 1848* (Ithaca: Mack, Andrus & Co., 1848), p. 21.

37. Charles D. Meigs, *Females and Their Diseases* (Philadelphia: Lea & Blanchard, 1848), pp. 19, 20-21.

38. John G. F. Holston, "Letter to the Editor," Zanesville, November 10, 1853, *New York Medical Gazette* 5 (May 1854):224.

39. John Van Pelt Quackenbush, *An Address Delivered Before the Students of the Albany Medical College, Introductory to the Course on Obstetrics, November 5, 1855* (Albany, N.Y.; B. Taylor, 1855), p. 7.

40. [Channing], *Remarks,* p. 20.

41. Caspar Wistar, *Eulogium on William Shippen . . . delivered before the College of Physicians of Philadelphia, March, 1809* (Philadelphia: Dobson, 1818), p. 30; Quackenbush, *Address,* p. 8.

42. Charles D. Meigs, quoted in Harvey Graham [I. Harvey Flack], *Eternal Eve* (London: W. Heinemann, 1950), pp. 494-495.

43. Dewees, *Compendious System,* pp. 190-191.

44. Bard, *Compendium,* p. 26.

45. Thomas Ewell, *Letters to Ladies, Detailing Important Information Concerning Themselves and Infants* (Philadelphia: W. Brown, 1817), p. 96.

46. Dewees, *Compendious System,* p. 206.

47. Meigs, *Females and Their Diseases,* p. 572.

48. *Report of the Trial, The People versus Dr. Horatio N. Loomis, for Libel,* reported by Frederick T. Parsons, Stenographer (Buffalo, N.Y.: Jewett, Thomas & Co., 1850), p. 25.

49. James V. Ricci, *The Development of Gynaecological Surgery and Instruments* (Philadelphia: Blakiston, 1949), p. 294.

50. *New York Journal of Medicine and the Collateral Sciences* 4 (May 1850):395.

51. Ricci, *Gynaecological Surgery,* p. 299; Graham, *Eternal Eve,* p. 494. In some sections of the United States in the 1840s, the speculum was virtually unknown. J. Marion Sims, wishing to examine Betsy, a slave woman who had suffered a large fistula during childbirth, bent a pewter spoon handle as an improvised speculum. Inserting it into the vagina, Sims later reported he "saw everything, as no man had ever seen before." Sims, *Life,* p. 234.

52. C. R. Gilman, "The Use and Abuse of the Speculum," *New York Journal of Medicine and the Collateral Sciences,* n.s. 6 (January 1851):12-14; *New York Medical Gazette* 2 (June 15, 1851):133.

53. See *The Medical News and Library* 8 (October 1850):83.

54. *Transactions of the Medical Society of the State of New York, From its Organization in 1807, up to and including 1831,* Vol. 1 (Albany: C. Van Benthuysen & Sons, 1868), p. 232.

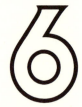

Man Midwifery Exposed

As to myself, I ingenuously own, could my wife's mind be out of the question, I would sooner give her up to the embraces of any one man, once a year, than subject her person to be exposed, touched, and handled, as she who is attended, and delivered of a child, must be, by a male midwife.

—[PHILIP THICKNESSE], *MAN-MIDWIFERY ANALYZED,* 1764

No man should ever be permitted to enter the apartment of a woman in labor, except in consultation and on extraordinary occasions. [Man midwifery] . . . is unnecessary, unnatural, and wrong—it has an immoral tendency.

—WOOSTER BEACH, *AN IMPROVED SYSTEM OF MIDWIFERY,* 1851

One of the demands of nineteenth-century feminists was that women be admitted to the medical profession. Obstetrics and "The Diseases of Women and Children" seemed areas of the practice especially suited to the women's cause.[1] In England as early as 1792, Mary Wollstonecraft, one of the first feminist writers, cast a longing glance in the direction of midwifery. Regretfully acknowledging the trend toward employing men in the field, Wollstonecraft would have reversed the fashion and increased the opportunities for women to participate in medicine. Rejecting the "unnatural distinctions in society" that kept women dependent, she commented:

women might certainly study the art of healing and be physicians as well as nurses. And midwifery decency seems to allot them, although I am afraid the word midwife, in our dictionaries, will soon give place to *accoucheur,* and one proof of the former delicacy of the sex be effaced from the language. . . . How many women . . . waste life away the prey of discontent, who might have practised as physicians, or engaged in other useful occupations?[2]

Yet, it would be erroneous to conclude that the origins of the anti-man midwifery crusade were the same as those of the women's rights movement. Long before the feminists emerged, another group of reformers sought to bar men from the lying-in chamber. These reformers were not motivated by a desire to broaden opportunities for women, but rather by the wish to remove from society the paradox created by conflicting demands of modesty and safety. Their principal goal was to eradicate a practice that, to them, clearly violated the claims of decency and decorum. They were found chiefly in England and the United States, for in neither of these countries were sustained efforts made to develop a midwives' service that would have produced women trained in obstetrics. On the Continent, by sharp contrast, accoucheurs were called in primarily to treat abnormal cases. Well-qualified *sage-femmes* were trained to attend routine deliveries, and in France they also performed simple operative work until late in the nineteenth century.[3] It was not until the last quarter of the nineteenth century that Great Britain moved to establish a midwives' service, and then it was chiefly for the working classes; in the United States, despite efforts in the late nineteenth and early twentieth centuries, the movement made almost no headway.[4]

The criticism of man midwifery erupted with full force in England in the third quarter of the eighteenth century. By then the accoucheur had won a measure of acceptance among upper-class women and the middle-class women who strove to emulate them. The tradition of sending for the surgeon to perform a specialty operation as a desperation measure—and the resulting version, embryotomy, or rare caesarean on an already sacrificed mother—had generated the view of surgeon as an unwelcome intruder too often accompanied by death. Forceps deliveries, especially after instruments and procedures had been refined, worked to produce a revised definition of the male operator. In this he was no longer villain but rather the hero who rescued mothers and infants from almost certain death. Once these operators began to move into the range of normal deliveries by attending and even maintaining indigent women in hospitals so as to gain experience and foster clinical teaching, the first wave of substantial criticism of man midwifery surfaced.

The crusade to reform midwifery by excluding men spanned almost a century. In the end it proved abortive, for the women never regained their monopoly. The effort repays examination, nevertheless, for the light it sheds on the moral values developing in pre- and early Victorian society. The concept of modesty, accompanied by an increasing prudery, provided the basis on which rules for interaction between the sexes were built. Social attitudes were predicated on the male-oriented view of woman that defined her as "innately" passive, docile, easily influenced, and properly dominated by male superiors. Less purely intellectual than man, less rational and logical, she was "intuitively" capable of solving those problems that touched her life directly. Rousseau's pronouncement in *Emile* that women "ought to learn multitudes of things, but only those which it becomes them to know" contained the essence of the prevailing version of ideal woman. These ideas made it increasingly difficult for women to obtain the training requisite to practicing the new obstetrics that depended so heavily on skilled operators conversant with the anatomy and physiology of the female.

Almost a century lay between the 1760s, when English critics battled in vain against the inroads of William Smellie and his "he-practitioners" in London, and 1848, when the Boston Female Medical College in Massachusetts began to train women midwives and physicians. Yet within this time span the central arguments of man midwifery critics remained essentially unchanged. Two elements were fundamental: Man midwifery was offensive and dangerous. As the nineteenth century progressed, the increasing popularity of accoucheurs with middle-class women coincided with the emerging middle-class standards of morality, as well as with a growing awareness of health and safety issues. These trends were reflected in the modifications made by critics in their arguments. Although the rhetoric changed somewhat, the issues remained the same.

As men began to invade the realm of normal midwifery cases, critics of the new obstetrics began the attack. These eighteenth-century reactionaries contended that the institution of man midwifery was immoral. The custom had been introduced from France where, they asserted, "decency . . . [had] long since vanished."[5] In England, "a few women of fashion . . . [had] countenanced it," and because "the middling class of people must be in fashion, and ape the quality; decency . . . [was] kicked down stairs, and modesty put out of countenance."[6] These critics admitted that it was indelicate even to discuss the details associated with the accoucheur's attendance of women, but insisted that society must be alerted to the dangers before the practice became too widely established.

Elizabeth Nihell, an English midwife trained at the Hôtel Dieu, focused her attack on William Smellie and his students, "trained up at the feet of his artificial doll." Nihell suggested that these "he-practitioners" used midwifery chiefly as an entrée to a more general medical practice. They have, she charged, "intrepidly hoisted the standard of a general knowledge of physic, and having originally insinuated themselves into families in the character of man-midwives, have easily maintained their ground in them afterwards on the foot of physicians."[7] The cost to modesty and the safety of women was incalculable, she continued. "What barriers are thrown down— what a door is open to licentiousness, to the admission of this so needless innovation! . . . An army of five hundred pupils, constantly recruiting with the pupils of those pupils, [had been] let loose against the female sex," wreaking havoc and spreading death and destruction.[8]

Critics insisted that only the most depraved individuals would continue to condone a fashion that permitted a man to gaze upon a woman not only when she was in the throes of childbirth and embarrassingly subject to "some other Efforts of Nature" accompanying the occasion, but even months prior to the delivery itself. Proof of the many indelicate offices performed by the "professors of this bawdy profession" was found easily within the treatises of midwifery written by these men. The digital examination, then known by the unfortunate term "touching," enabled the attendant first to ascertain a woman's pregnancy by palpating the soft rounded fetal mass evident in the uterus at ten or twelve weeks. At term, the examination was used to determine both the position of the fetus and the degree of dilatation of the os uteri. Most midwifery treatises gave directions for the procedure and recommended it.[9]

"Touching," explained William Smellie in his *Treatise,* was performed properly "by introducing the fore finger lubricated with pomatum into the *Vagina* . . . and sometimes into the *Rectum*, to discover the stretching of the *Fundus*." It was "impractical" to employ touching to determine pregnancy after the fourth month, advised Smellie, but whenever the procedure was used, the patient for practical reasons was "to submit to the inquiry in a standing posture."[10] These directions, written in the vernacular and including the observation that the *"Fossa Magna* or *Navicularis* [was formed] for the direction of the Penis in coition, or of the Finger in touching, into the *Vagina*" provided evidence enough to one critic of the indecent character of man midwifery and of those who practiced it.[11]

The critic reminded his reader that the examination normally took place in the husband's absence, for he was banished by the attendant and left only to guess at what transpired. Behind the closed door, charged the critic, the virtuous woman was forced to submit to the doctor's embarrassing questions and to permit him to take liberties too indecorous to mention. Who knew what great harm had been committed already as a result of these practices? Human nature was depraved, and virtue, it was pointed out, was not easily preserved, even in the best of circumstances. Accoucheurs posed a special challenge, because "assuming the Character of Matrons . . . [did] not emasculate Men Midwives . . . [and] their Profession therefore does not extinguish those Emotions that a fine Woman naturally excites, especially when heightened by Liberties taken under Colour of that Profession."[12]

Nor could one ignore the effect of touching on the passive and easily led woman. "A woman's passions are very unlike those of men," one critic reminded his readers. Generally, their feelings lay "dormant till stirr'd by the dalliance of a man," he continued:

. . . the design of touching also *may be* to see if any emotions arise in the touched lady's breast, that the Doctor may take advantage of. A man once admitted to such a liberty, knows not himself, and the woman, who through simplicity, (or what she is told, is necessity), consents to it, cannot answer for the consequences that may arise from such transactions.[13]

Tales put forth as notorious truths, were recounted to convince women and their husbands of the accoucheur's degeneracy. Recounted one critic:

one of these modest *gentle-touching* Gentlemen told the Husband, that it was absolutely necessary for his Wife's Recovery, he should refrain from her Bed, and at the same time the Villain was administring [sic] stimulating Medicines to the Lady, in order to gain Admittance there himself; but his Ignorance defeated his wicked Views, for he administer'd the Medicines in so great a Quantity, that it killed the lady.[14]

Interestingly, the sexism of the age caused this critic of man midwifery to take offense not only at the prospect of a husband "robbed of his wife's fidelity" but also at the failure of the man midwife to participate in a plot to shield a husband from the consequences of a similar moral lapse. "A merchant who had a very young and beautiful wife," ran the story, employed "an eminent man-midwife, to cure him of a disorder he had got by going astray, and amusing himself one evening in the environs of Covent-Garden, while his buxom wife imagined he was gone to his country house at Epsom." Having thus contracted a venereal disease, the husband further enlisted the accoucheur's help by requesting that he tell her she must "lie apart from her husband," a prescription made "absolutely necessary" by her gravid condition. The doctor gave the merchant assurances that he would save his credit and keep his secret. Instead of doing so, however, he "informed the wife with the whole truth of the matter; and made such inflammatory observations on the inconstancy of the husband, and the beauty of the wife, that with the advantage of opportunity, her husband's falseness, and large doses of *cantharides,* which he administered, he debauched the woman." Before she died, victim of the accoucheur's medication, the wife confessed all, revealing both the duplicity of the attendant and his immorality.[15]

"Most women," contended another critic, suffered great "agonies" the moment the "mid-men" entered their lying-in chambers; such suffering could be prevented only by supplying parturient women with attendants of their own sex.[16] Elizabeth Nihell insisted that laboring women often found comfort and "mitigation of their complaints" in the gentle soothings of the midwife's hand. Women were "ashamed" to ask for and not "weak" enough to expect such solace "from the delicate fist of a great-horse-godmother of a he-midwife, however softened his figure might be by his pocket night-gown being of flowered calico, or his cap of office tied with pink and silver ribbons," she jeered in the direction of William Smellie and his suggested attire for the accoucheur.[17]

The critics did not stop at railing against men midwives for alleged offenses to morality and their total disregard for both the delicacy of the female and the sanctity of marriage. The accoucheur was dangerous in yet another respect. Unlike the midwives, men were equipped with "Iron Instruments" capable of inflicting great injuries on their patients. The detractors alleged that the doctors themselves were well aware of the lethal potential of their instruments, a fact that explained their motive in resourcefully concealing them from patients and female attendants.[18] Nihell accused the men of maintaining their position by force of "arms . . . those weapons of death!" Vehemently she insisted that instruments were no match for the gentle, "shrewd," and "sensitive" fingers of the female midwife.[19] "Instruments," declared another critic, were "always injurious, often dangerous, and never necessary." Even when they did not inflict harm, the very fact that they had been used on a woman rendered her "less agreeable, and often loathsome to her husband."[20]

As man midwifery became well established among the upper classes toward the close of the century, the doubts and attacks continued. Margaret Stephen, midwife to Queen Charlotte, had fought the use of instruments but finally came to recognize the value of forceps in difficult cases. Still she concluded that the evils of man midwifery far outweighed the good. "Ladies," she observed, had been "induced to dispense with that delicacy which was their greatest ornament, by the insinuations of designing men, who taught them to believe they endangered their own lives, and that of their children, by employing women."[21]

In the 1790s another articulate critic appeared. S. W. Fores, writing under the pseudonym John Blunt, published in book form a series of letters addressed to Alexander Hamilton, the celebrated Edinburgh obstetrician. The title of the work explicitly stated its purpose and defined its character: *Man-Midwifery Dissected; or the Obstetric Family-Instructor. For the use of Married Couples,*

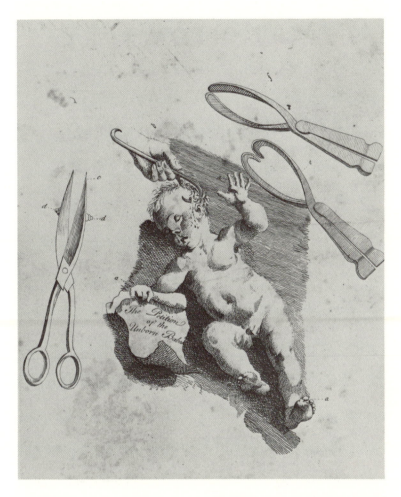

Engraving of a stillborn child mutilated by a man midwife, 1745. Anonymous artist.—From Philip Thicknesse, *Man-Midwifery Analysed,* London, 1765. (Courtesy of the Wellcome Institute for the History of Medicine.)

and Single Adults of both Sexes. Containing A Display of the Management of every Class of Labours by Men and Boy-Midwives; also of their cunning, indecent and cruel Practices . . . Various arguments and Quotations, proving that Man-Midwifery is a personal, a domestic, and a national Evil. . . . The book is of particular interest because it contains a number of arguments and allegations that were resurrected by critics of the new obstetrics in the following century.

The author, who described himself as a former medical student, admitted the value of instruments when judiciously employed. In any instance requiring operative assistance, he insisted that the husband be present to insure against doctors "making too free with women's persons, manually, ocularly, and instrumentally." This was especially important, he argued, in view of the great mischief already done, "owing to the ignorance and impatience of those professors who erroneously imagined, their instruments *must* be used on *all* occasions, whether the labours were natural or difficult." Regrettably, he continued, all too often the decision to use instruments was made not out of consideration for the mother's safety and comfort but rather as a matter of convenience and profit for the operator.[22]

Fores favored training "intelligent" women to be midwives. To facilitate this he proposed the opening of a school in London where young women might study anatomy, physiology, version, and the diseases of women and children. Necessary clinical experience would be obtained through supervised attendance at the deliveries of the poor.[23] He did not recommend that the women learn to use forceps, but he believed them capable of passing the catheter and mastering the technique of simple version. He cautioned that they must not attempt craniotomies or cesarean sections. "Indeed," he wrote, "I think it as presumptuous for a midwife to attempt either, as it is ridiculous for a man, or a boy, to be seen sitting at the tail of a modest woman, who has a natural labour."[24] Unfortunately for the critics of man midwifery, Fores' proposals for training women met with no more success than had those of John Douglas fifty years earlier. It is regrettably impossible to assess the strength of the critics' support among the upper classes of women who had set the fashion for man midwifery and whose patronage allowed it to grow. That they employed men does not necessarily imply that they would not have preferred to employ women, had they been trained.

In the 1760s William Buchan, Fellow of the Royal Society of Edinburgh, had articulated clearly the dilemma of the woman faced with the choice between the services of a skillful male attendant and those of an untrained midwife whose sex made her presence less offensive to female sensibilities. Few women, wrote Buchan in *Domestic Medicine,* went into midwifery practice unless forced into it by reduced circumstances. Consequently, "not one in a hundred of them" had the requisite education and knowledge. Admitting that it was true that nature, when left to its own resources, usually would expel the fetus, he added, "It is equally true, that most women in child bed require to be managed with skill and attention, and that they are often hurt by the superstitious prejudices of ignorant and officious midwives." Buchan believed that the injuries inflicted by women were greater than the public realized. His recommendation was the obvious one, that only "properly qualified" women be allowed to practice. "Were due attention paid to this," he predicted, "it would not only be the means of saving many lives, but would prevent the necessity of employing men in this undelicate and disagreeable branch of medicine, which is, on many accounts, more proper for the other sex."[25]

Buchan was equally outspoken on the credulity of the public that sustained incompetent men midwives. With obvious approval "John Blunt" quoted Buchan's criticism of the faculty:

As matters stand at present, it is easier to cheat a *woman* out of her life than of a shilling, and almost impossible either to detect or punish the offender. Notwithstanding this, people still shut their eyes, and take every thing upon trust that is done by any PRETENDER to *midwifery,* without daring to ask him a reason for any part of his conduct. Implicit faith, everywhere else the object of ridicule, is still sacred here.[26]

Doubtless many of the faculty were well qualified and deserved the public's confidence, continued Buchan; but as every profession had its incompetents, "the safety, as well as the honour of *women*" called for "some check upon the conduct of those to whom they intrust so valuable a treasure."

In 1815 another critic joined the ranks. Dr. R. Kinglake, a practicing physician in Taunton, England, published a paper in the *London Medical and Physical Journal* critical of man midwifery. Kinglake contended that the indiscriminate practice of midwifery by men had created the impression that the doctor could always provide direct assistance. He charged that this faulty view was responsible for a great deal of unwarranted interference by accoucheurs who would not wait for nature to take its course. The remedy he proposed was simple: Limit the practice of men to cases in which the presentation was faulty and those in which hemorrhaging or convulsions signaled grave danger.[27]

Predictably, Kinglake's position was attacked immediately. John Wayte countered that midwifery had passed from women to men out of "necessity" and was surely neither indelicate nor a mere "fashion." The midwives blundered because they were not well versed in anatomy and physiology; having done so they were forced to call in the professional men, "whose attendance assuredly would be solicited at future labours," when new impediments to birth arose. What had once been an occasional occurrence had in time become habitual, continued Wayte, because the midwives were simply not experts. "There is not one woman in a hundred throughout the kingdom," he declared, "who, if able to afford it, will not prefer a male practitioner . . . because they consider themselves more safe."[28] Dr. J. Atkinson agreed. It was midwives and not physicians who were dangerous. They caused women to suffer long, hazardous, and difficult labors simply because they seldom had the requisite knowledge to assess accurately which cases could be left to nature and which required obstetrical art.[29]

In reply to the argument that men must handle all maternity cases to prevent complications, Kinglake protested that it was the doctors themselves who were responsible for the high incidence of childbed disorders. If they were prevented from interfering with normal cases, he predicted, much less would be heard about puerperal fever, uterine "distempers," and "after-pains," not to mention the irreparable damage inflicted on the bodies of poor mutilated infants.[30]

Samuel Merriman responded that quite the opposite was true. More importantly, he cited statistical data to support his contention that as man midwifery had increased, a decline in the number of abortive and stillborn births listed in the bills of mortality had resulted. Merriman claimed that over a twenty-five year period from 1657 to 1681,

there were 273,763 christenings, and 14,397 abortive and still-born children, so that the children dead-born were to those born alive as 1 to 19. But during the last twenty-five years, from 1791-1815, when the practice of midwifery has been more generally conducted by men, the number of christenings is 492,464, and the stillborn children 15,084, which is to those born alive as 1 to 30—diminished more than one third.[31]

Merriman concluded that he was at a loss to explain the diminution of mortality in childbed except by attributing it "to the more careful and judicious management of women in labour and after delivery adopted by accoucheurs."

In the midst of the controversy over meddlesome midwifery, a tragic event in 1817 fanned the flames of the dispute. Princess Charlotte Augusta, only child of the Prince of Wales (George IV), married to Prince Leopold of Saxe-Coburg, and pregnant with the Hanoverian heir, died in childbirth. Although the princess was said to have preferred the attendance of a midwife, Richard Croft (1762-1818) served as her accoucheur. Croft, the son-in-law of Thomas Denman, had inherited much of Denman's practice when the latter died in 1815. Assisted by Matthew Baillie (1761-1823), William Hunter's nephew, and finally by John Sims (1749-1831), Croft had followed a conservative course of noninterference despite the waning strength of his patient. After fifty hours of labor, Princess Charlotte was delivered of a dead male child. Her own death followed several hours later. To some the tragedy suggested malpractice; Croft's suicide in 1818 confirmed the suspicions of many. Supporters of man midwifery criticized Croft's conservative conduct, claiming that he should have interfered and terminated the labor by delivering with the forceps.[32]

An autopsy failed to reveal the cause of death. Reporting the case, the *London Medical Repository* found no reason to criticize Charlotte's accoucheurs. The editors observed that the entire royal family was subject to "spasms of a violent description" and suggested that this hereditary condition, aggravated by the tedious nature of the labor and the consequent "increased excitability" of the patient, was probably responsible for the outcome.[33] As might be expected, the proponents of female midwifery were less charitable. They saw in the death of the young princess dramatic proof of the harm inflicted by obstetricians. Thirty years after the event, they were still citing it as a prime illustration of why men midwives should be barred from practice.[34]

Across the Atlantic some physicians, as noted earlier, initially supported suggestions that women be properly trained to conduct normal cases. Acute competition within the profession had not yet developed, and the busy practitioner sometimes found midwifery burdensome. Valentine Seaman knew that many women preferred the female attendant. Even if that were not the case, he explained, it would be desirable to train midwives, because "the nature of the practice of physic, in this country, is such, that physicians cannot afford to give up so much of their time from their other business, as would be necessarily employed upon such occasions for the small compensation, that the greater proportion of citizens are able . . . to make them."[35] This view was echoed in 1824 by the editor of a Philadelphia medical journal quoting from a British proposal that women be educated as physicians and accoucheurs out of respect for female reserve and delicacy. Remarked the editor, the suggestion might be an especially welcome one to young physicians seeking relief "from some of the immense fatigue attendant on their overwhelming superabundance of business."[36] Once this doctor-patient ratio had altered, however, the physicians' concept of midwifery as a feeder for their general practice caused them to see obstetrics patients in a different light. As man midwifery gained increasing acceptance among the upper classes, American critics soon joined their British cousins in the attack on men midwives.

In 1817 the American physician Thomas Ewell proposed the restoration of all normal cases to the midwives. Although he called for government sponsorship of midwifery schools, after the pattern established by France, Germany, and Denmark, Ewell nevertheless was of the opinion that normal cases required little active assistance beyond "common sense and observation." The "women physicians," that is, accoucheurs, whose popularity he deplored had received their first instruction in obstetrics from books that, according to Ewell, could be readily comprehended by anyone.[37]

Ewell believed midwives capable of conducting digital examinations, provided they were properly cautioned against such abuses as unnecessary repetition and attempted manual dilatation. He was confident, too, that they could learn the procedure of version as applicable to all types of presentation. Despite his confidence, he pointed out that any patient apprehensive about her midwife's skill was justified in calling for a physician to turn the fetus in utero.[38] Stressing the ease with which most deliveries were completed, Ewell contended that in normal cases the "huge fists" of the doctors and their inclination to hurry the process along did infinite harm. To prove the latter point he cited the cautions of conservative authorities such as Thomas Denman and William Buchan.[39]

The dominant theme in Ewell's argument was that the attendance of men at normal births constituted an affront to morality. By encouraging women to submit to "unnecessary" examinations, accoucheurs forced them to sacrifice delicacy, thereby threatening virtue. He charged that the consequent corruption of married women had contributed to the high incidence of adultery in large cities, where man midwifery was most prevalent. "Even among the French so prone to set aside the ceremonies among the sexes," claimed Ewell, "the immorality of such exposures has been noticed." Evidence of this he found in Voltaire's warning to the father of an infant son delivered by an accoucheur: "You are traveling the road to cockoldom [sic]." As British critics had done earlier, he recounted amazing tales of physicians who took unfair advantage of their vulnerable patients:

Time and opportunity to press on a grateful heart, for a favour in regions where magnified favours have been conferred, have been used, and more frequently desired. . . . Many of these modest looking doctors, inflamed with thoughts of the well-shaped bodies of the women they have delivered, handled, hung over for hours, secretly glorying in the privilege, have to their patients, as priests to their penitents, pressed for accommodation, and driven to adultery and madness, where they were thought most innocently occupied.[40]

In one case, Ewell was well assured, "a physician in Charleston, infuriated with the sight of the woman he had just delivered, leaped into her bed before she was restored to a state of nature." It was said that the wife of a prominent congressman was among those seduced by an accoucheur. It was foolish and unnecessary for husbands to be so shortsighted, Ewell pointed out. He approved the conduct of the husband, who upon sending for a doctor to attend his wife warned the accoucheur that he would be "demolished" if he touched or looked at his patient![41]

All women with the least sense of delicacy were humiliated by man midwifery, ran the argument. This sensitivity manifested itself in many forms. It was not uncommon for a woman in the throes of labor to discover that the accoucheur's unwelcome presence so shocked her system that contractions completely vanished! The awful toll of violated delicacy drove others into convulsive states and sometimes totally deranged them. The most virtuous and saintly of women wisely preferred to endure indescribable suffering and torment in childbed rather than stain their honor by resorting to the man midwife, Ewell summarized.[42]

The theme of modesty versus temptation was elaborated in England and the United States over the next forty years. The very foundations on which "civilized" society rested were threatened by a practice at once "disgusting, degrading, and injurious." One need not look far to see the effects. Doctors took advantage of "the unbounded familiarity of approach necessary in the duties of midwifery . . . for the gratification of the most prurient lusts."[43] Unfortunately, temptation could never be totally eliminated, admitted the critics. Yet, as one British author remarked in the book he addressed to the Society for the Suppression of Vice, "there are many men, and many women, who have virtue enough to protect them if let alone; if assailed, or thrown into temptation, they fail."[44]

No less an authority than Sir Anthony Carlisle, Fellow of the Royal Society, surgeon to the king and to the Westminster Hospital, had given his opinion of the practice. If man midwifery were not abolished, claimed Sir Anthony, the pretensions to female modesty and the respect for the decorums of society eventually would disappear from the female character.[45] William Cobbett, the popular British journalist, lamented the increasing prostitution and growing numbers of children born out of wedlock in *Advice to Young Men and Women*. These things made it "impossible for men in general to respect the female sex, to the degree that they formerly did." And to what did he attribute these signs of decaying morality? Clearly they were fed by the presence of "man-operators" in the lying-in chamber and the equally obnoxious practice that allowed physicians, with impunity, to exhibit before an audience of men the dead body of a virtuous female.[46]

By taking over obstetric practice, the medical profession had profaned the sanctity of the female character and of conjugal vows. God had decreed that every man should have his own wife free from "pollution," declared William Hosmer, who warned that any tampering on the part of the medical faculty destroyed the marriage compact.[47] A "privileged class of physicians," by failing to keep its ministrations within proper limits, had contributed to the ruination of society and in so doing had "rendered itself one of the severest scourges that ever afflicted mankind."[48]

Critics insisted that physicians were notoriously wicked. Had not one of the great health reformers himself, "Dr." [Sylvester] Graham, repeated one physician's remark that young doctors actually boasted of having committed adultery with women even as their husbands were at home?[49] Nurses testified that many doctors took advantage of sick, weak women by taking their leave of them with an affectionate kiss. This act alone was a dangerous symbol of corruption. Another nurse reported overheard conversations among young doctors:

When speaking of attending the young wives on the first occasion . . . [they] called it 'halter-breaking them' . . . rejoicing in their occupation. 'There,' they would say to each other, as they looked out into the street, 'There goes one that I halter-broke a few weeks ago—and there, yonder, comes another that I will break in soon.'[50]

All too often husbands and wives did not realize until after their marriage that a medical imposition would violate their vows. The wife became ill and the husband called the physician. "Before there . . . [could be] opportunity to resist or time to reflect, all . . . [was] swept away in the tide of fashionable depravity."[51] "Shameless old hags," who had permitted doctors to handle them until all sense of modesty was lost, perpetuated the evil by convincing younger women that their only choice lay between death and the physician.[52]

Obstetrics textbooks were rife with observations taken by critics as evidence of the doctors' corrupt and indecent work. Smellie's casebook proved that he had permitted students to examine an exposed patient as he demonstrated to them the manner in which to apply forceps. In passages such as "I had the patient laid supine across the bed, and her legs supported by two of my pupils," Smellie had seemingly indicted himself.[53] Credulous women were led to the faulty belief that if they submitted to the indignity of an examination per vaginam, the doctor could relieve or eliminate the pains of childbirth.[54] Anyone who doubted the veracity of the allegations of farce and deception practiced by many physicians needed only to be referred to telling passages such as the following from the *London Practice of Midwifery:*

A patient, after the waters are discharged, requires a little management. It is not just to stay with her at the time; and yet it is necessary, if we leave her, to leave her in confidence. Therefore we may give her the idea of making provision for whatever may happen in our absence: We may pass our finger up the vagina or opening to the womb, and make a moderate degree of pressure, for just a few seconds, on any part of it, so that she may just feel it; after which we may say to her, "there ma'am, I have done something that will be of great use to your labor." This she trusts to; and if, when she send for us, we get there in time, it is well: if later than we should be, we easily satisfy her. . . . "Yes! you know I told you I did something which would be of great use to your labor." If the placenta is not yet come away— "Oh, I am quite in time for the after-birth, and that, you know, is of the greatest consequence in labor!" And if the whole has come away—"We are glad the after-birth is all come away in consequence of what we did before we last left, and the labor terminated just as we intended it should."[55]

Demanded the critics, what motives other than lust or greed could induce physicians to pass the catheter or make "frequent examinations with the finger or the speculum" when the "highest" authorities in medicine believed these examinations to be unnecessary and harmful?[56] Female virtue could not hope to survive in the hands of the physician whose "licentious character" made him quick to "seize upon any advantages . . . which his profession . . . [threw] in his way."[57] Wives and husbands must be alerted to the immoral tendencies in present society that would not be tolerated even in "heathen" lands. Insisted one critic:

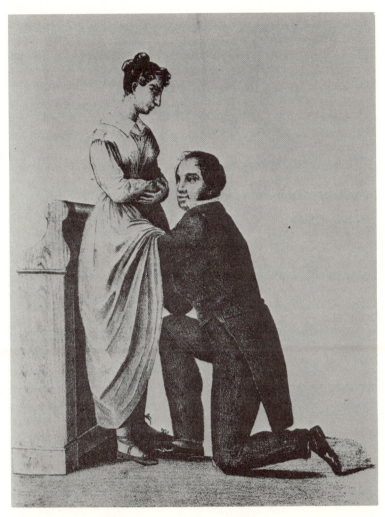

These plates, taken from an American edition of a French midwifery text, illustrate recommended procedures for "touching," the digital examination to determine pregnancy. Critics of man midwifery regarded plates such as these indecent.—From Jacques Pierre Maygrier, *Midwifery Illustrated,* New York, 1834; facsimile edition, Medical Heritage Press, 1969. (Courtesy of the State University of New York Upstate Medical Center.)

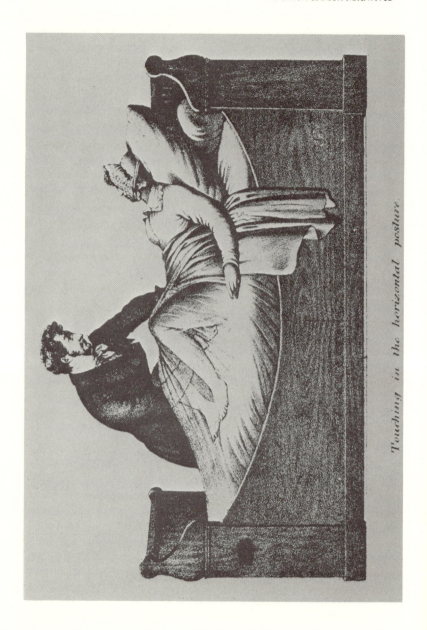

Touching in the horizontal posture.

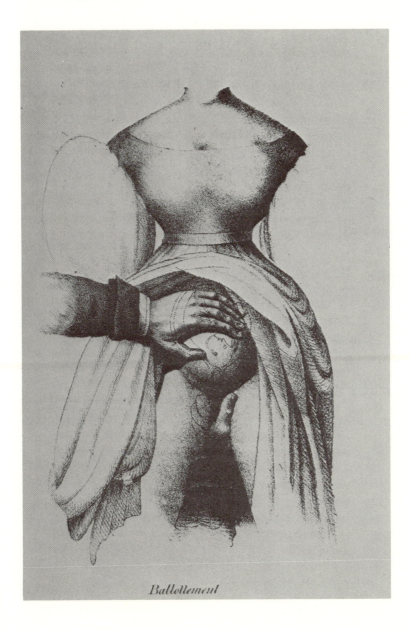

Ballottement

The manner in which women are obliged to submit themselves—sometimes months before the time of accouchment—to the shocking liberties which male-midwives may and often do take with them, under the *pretence* of performing professional duties, but really to test their willingness to sacrifice their virtue to lust, must be brought to public attention.[58]

The "good" men and women deeply interested in "the establishment and preservation of chaste and delicate customs in society" realized that "the tone of public virtue" depended chiefly upon the influence of woman. All members of society should be interested in so vital a reform, for "female friends and relatives will necessarily partake of the prevailing character of the times," and pernicious habits uncorrected would be the legacy transmitted to succeeding generations.[59] Now that the veil of secrecy with which physicians had surrounded their nefarious deeds was being lifted, claimed another critic, public indignation was on the rise. Within a short time, only the "most abandoned women" would suffer the indignities produced by the male presence in the birth chamber.[60]

That many women had accepted man midwifery was seen by critics as one of the greatest hurdles to be overcome. Unless these women became convinced of the evil engendered by the practice, they would perpetuate it indefinitely. A Methodist minister affirmed that the woman who submitted herself to the medical attentions of a man was no better than the physician himself. "Any woman who would willingly submit to have a Doctor to deliver her of a child, would let that same Doctor afterwards get her with child, if he chose to do so," was the terse assessment.[61] Observed another critic, "It would be ten times less disgraceful for women to employ men to attend them at the water closet, and quite as excusable," as to have men employed as accoucheurs.[62] Unfortunately women generally preferred to be attended by physicians, remarked Dr. Kinglake. The very fact that so many ladies had allowed themselves to be cajoled into believing there was nothing immoral in the practice of man midwifery proved to him the "incorrectness" of appealing to them on the subject.[63] The women of primitive societies were sensitive enough to seek privacy and seclusion during parturition; no less should be expected of "civilized" women.[64] Time and again these critics alluded to the unenviable plight of the genuinely pure and modest women. Unable to bring themselves to surrender their modesty for the sake of fashion, they suffered silently rather than conform.[65]

Physicians had insinuated their way into normal cases by claiming superiority over the midwives. Critics maintained that repeated allegations of incompetency among midwives had terrorized the public into believing that when wives employed women, they deliberately courted danger and death. The truth, insisted critics, was that the doctors' claims were "erroneous." If women learned the truth and understood that physicians were not guarantors of safety, their sense of propriety would lead them back to the midwives.[66] Not all reformers were optimistic about the possibility of change. Women had placed great confidence in man midwifery, and it might be too late to overturn the practice.[67] Then too, those who had surrendered themselves to the dictates of this "depraved" fashion perpetuated the notion that it was "indelicate" to employ women.[68]

Although the medical profession sometimes claimed that the doctors who practiced obstetrics tended to specialize, expecting "little employment in any other branch,"[69] critics disputed the point. The truth, they asserted, was that the best physicians gave up midwifery as soon as they were well established. Once secure, they agreed only to attend their favorites in childbed. The result was that their other women patients found it necessary to resort to other accoucheurs, thus exposing themselves to still more men.[70] These replacements often were young and inexperienced, even "quacks." Men with sound training and genuine medical knowledge, it was said, considered it beneath their dignity to practice obstetrics. Preferring to devote their energies to branches more in keeping with their mental capacities, they abandoned midwifery as soon as they were able to do so.[71]

The reactionary critics called upon all sincere and virtuous physicians to assist the reformation directly by training women to replace accoucheurs. They appealed to influential, established doctors to set the proper example by refusing to lend themselves to a business that licensed "hundreds of libidinous fiends in human shapes . . . under the cloak of the medical profession, to plunder thousands of women of the dearest pearl of their human, domestic, social life."

It was incumbent upon all responsible people to halt the activities of poseurs whose "mal-practice and immoral conduct, from generation to generation plunge[d] husbands, wives, parents, children and friends, into irretrievable wretchedness and disgrace."[72]

As to safety, continued the critics, candid physicians admitted that prudent women were capable of managing all normal cases. They cited with approval the view of one doctor whose personal experience combined with the reports of surgeons led him to conclude that "not . . . one case in three thousand" called for "uncommon assistance."[73] Estimates varied, but all critics of man midwifery were agreed that the abnormal case occurred rarely. One British reformer pointed out that William Dewees, the eminent obstetrics author and teacher of Philadelphia, had admitted this was so. If the ladies in the United States were once made aware of the truth, remarked this critic, Dewees and his colleagues would soon be out of business. Unfortunately, he concluded, "American obstetricians are determined to make the people believe that it is necessary for them to examine and finger over every case, for fear that it should be difficult, when not one in a thousand ever needs their assistance."[74]

However, the "indecent and immoral" practice of man midwifery continued to be urged upon the public. Among the grave consequences, warned the critics, was the rash and untimely interference by accoucheurs. Sir Anthony Carlisle, openly critical of his colleagues, had insisted that they realized how demeaning it was for them to occupy the lying-in room. In their efforts to compensate for this, they taught students "to assume directorial offices, and to be curiously or officially medling, under various pretenses." Carlisle attributed the alleged increase in maternal and infant mortality directly to such malpractice.[75] Botanic practitioner A. Curtis, citing the works of the regular obstetricians under the heading of "Butchery," used their own words to emphasize the dangers. Dewees had stated his belief that "the frequent mention of difficult, dangerous and rare operations" often led practitioners to the "*unnecessary* use of instruments, not always so much from the *necessity* of the case, as the *éclat* which attends them, however unsuccessful." William Smellie, continued Curtis, had warned that "the work of nature is too often spoiled by officious hands." More terrifying still was the warning of Dr. Blundell, who had written in *Obstetricy:*

I strenuously dissuade you from making familiar companions of your instruments because they are not wanted. . . . The very fact that an accoucheur, on all occasions, puts the lever into his pocket when he goes to attend a labor, proves that he is an officious, a meddlesome, and therefore, to my mind, a bad accoucheur. Some men seem to have a sort of instinctive impulse to put the lever or forceps into the vagina. "Lead yourselves not into temptation"; if you put your instruments into your pocket, they are very apt to slip out of your pocket into the uterus. Patience and good nature, are two useful obstetric instruments which may be fearlessly carried to every labor.[76]

There was some basis for the allegations of critics that accoucheurs were guilty of meddlesome midwifery. The repeated warnings of responsible authorities on both sides of the Atlantic for more than a century are indicative of the continuing problem. In 1754 William Smellie had cautioned young practitioners "to beware of being too hasty in offering assistance," counseling them to let nature "effectuate the delivery" when possible.[77] In his *Aphorisms,* Thomas Denman emphatically stated, "It has long been established as a general rule, that no instruments are to be used in the practice of midwifery; the cases in which they are used are therefore to be considered merely as exceptions to this rule."[78] William Dewees was "persuaded" that infants fell victim to "the crotchet . . . wantonly employed . . . where a little address in the use of the forceps, or even a little more patience, would have preserved the child from a premature death."[79]

In his *Compendium,* Samuel Bard stressed the adaptability of the pelvis and the flexibility of the fetal head that afforded wide latitude for normal delivery, even when considerable disproportion existed between the two.[80] James Ewell explained to the "sensible woman" in labor the importance of giving "her mind to patience," so as not to tempt a "designing and unskilful" attendant into employing unnecessary interference.[81]

In 1872 the eminent obstetrician J. H. Aveling, writing on the need to improve midwifery training, claimed that the nineteenth century had seen more abuse of patients and a greater resort to unnecessary instrument deliveries than had the two preceding centuries, when male obstetricians had been more inclined to depend upon nature, "that perfect operatrix."[82] As late as 1884 Thomas

Manley told his colleagues in the New York State Medical Association that because of the relatively small fees the general practitioners were able to command for their obstetrics cases, they were inclined to resort to instrument deliveries and other artificial aids to "terminate labor hastily."[83]

Whatever the truth of the matter may have been, the charges leveled against the profession by reformers sometimes bordered on the absurd. Critics seized upon Dewees's remark that "every accoucheur . . . [at some time] witnessed a temporary suspension of pain on his first appearance in the sick chamber" as evidence that the presence of a man so shocked the parturient woman that it suspended her labor indefinitely![84] As a result of the delay, ran the argument, physicians anxious to return to the duties of their general practice became impatient. To promote delivery they found it necessary to resort to "ergot, to stupefying chloroform, the crushing forceps, or the murderous perforator."[85] Haste produced other abuses. Critics asserted that doctors attempted to hurry along the expulsion of the placenta and in so doing provoked hemorrhaging or inversion of the uterus by their perilous practice of introducing the hand and "sweeping the womb." Conversely, to give themselves time to attend other patients during a protracted labor, maintained the critics, physicians deliberately delayed a woman's labor by drawing blood from her.[86]

Some charged that behind the physicians' insistence upon attending routine cases lay their recognition of the value of obstetrics as a feeder for building a large medical practice and concluded that in order to increase their incomes, they deliberately kept the public in medical ignorance.[87] The low esteem in which critics generally held doctors is apparent in the remark of William Hosmer, that to the physician "medicine is only a livelihood," the doctor having no interest in it other than the financial advantages that might accrue.[88] A physician who had gone over to the reforming Eclectics appealed directly to the pecuniary interests of his colleagues. Were they to return midwifery to the women, he pointed out, doctors would be able to devote themselves exclusively to the more profitable cases within the general practice. At the same time, they would rid themselves of the onerous chore of staying up throughout the night to attend cases of protracted labor.[89]

In advocating the revival of female midwifery the reformers prior to mid-century thought largely in terms of routine cases. They still expected that physicians would attend the abnormal cases that called for their special skills. On such occasions the male presence was not always thought to exceed the bounds of propriety. When a woman was in serious danger, wrote critic Ewell, she was not the object of lust but rather the "subject of commiseration; and the solicitude to remove her danger and agonies" must surely be the only thought in the mind of the accoucheur."[90] Medical students must therefore continue to study obstetrics, just as they did surgery, for those infrequent occasions when they would be called upon to render the particular assistance of which only they were deemed capable.[91]

In spite of the critics, the years following the emergence of the new obstetrics saw a steady increase in the number of general practitioners acting as accoucheurs among the upper classes. Opponents had long advocated the training of midwives as a solution to the apparent dilemma posed by demands for modesty and safety. It is a measure of the critics' definition of woman as inferior that they tended not to demand that women be trained to use the surgical instruments that had given the men primacy, but rather to insist that these instruments were dangerous and unnecessary. The few private efforts to train women for normal deliveries—for example, courses given by Smellie, Shippen, and Seaman—failed to produce any large pool of women practitioners and were not duplicated. Proposals such as those of S. W. Fores and Thomas Ewell calling for the establishment of state-sponsored midwifery schools along the European pattern met with even less success. Throughout the 1830s and 1840s the reactionary reformers continued to emphasize the need to train women, but even the increasing prudishness of the age was not enough to persuade women to abandon the general practitioners, who were at once their perceived guarantee of safer parturition and greatest source of embarrassment.

Man midwifery was not yet so firmly established as to be invulnerable. Physicians realized the need to constantly reinforce their own arguments, especially in view of growing competition within the profession and a recognition of the role midwifery could play in assuring the success of a doctor's practice. If man midwifery were to be overturned, it would take more than sporadic, poorly organized attacks by reactionaries reiterating threadbare arguments. Given leadership and organization, the reforming impulses of the period that worked against elitism and promoted a newer and more positive definition of women's abilities would soon merge with the reactionary goals to produce society's most serious challenge to man midwifery.

NOTES

1. The relation between the women's rights movement and the entrance of women into modern medicine has been noted by historians. See, for example, William Frederick Norwood, *Medical Education in the United States Before the Civil War* (Philadelphia: University of Pennsylvania Press, 1944), pp. 407-408; John B. Blake, "Women and Medicine in Ante-Bellum America," *Bulletin of the History of Medicine* 39 (March-April 1965):104-105; Frederick C. Waite, "Dr. Martha A. (Hayden) Sawin, The First Woman Graduate in Medicine to Practice in Boston," *New England Journal of Medicine* 205 (November 26, 1931): 1053; Richard H. Shryock, "Women in American Medicine," *Medicine in America: Historical Essays* (Baltimore: Johns Hopkins Press, 1966), pp. 178-179.

Recent publications reflecting modern feminism include: Gerda Lerner, "The Lady and the Mill Girl: Changes in the Status of Women in the Age of Jackson," *American Studies Journal* 10 (Spring 1969) reprinted in Jean E. Friedman and William G. Shade, *Our American Sisters: Women in American Life and Thought,* 2nd ed. (Boston: Allyn and Bacon, 1976); Barbara Ehrenreich and Deidre English, *Witches, Midwives and Nurses: A History of Women Healers* (Old Westbury, N.Y.: The Feminist Press, 1973); Barbara L. Kaiser and Irwin H. Kaiser, "The Challenge of the Women's Movement to American Gynecology," *American Journal of Obstetrics and Gynecology* 120 (November 1, 1974):652-665.

2. Mary Wollstonecraft, *A Vindication of the Rights of Woman* (London, 1792), ed. Carol H. Poston (New York: W. W. Norton & Company, Inc., 1975), pp. 148-149.

3. J. M. Munro Kerr, R. W. Johnstone, and Miles H. Phillips, *Historical Review of British Obstetrics and Gynaecology* (Edinburgh & London: E. & S. Livingstone, 1954), pp. 4-5. A recent history of English midwifery is Jean Donnison, *Midwives and Medical Men: A History of Inter-Professional Rivalries and Women's Rights* (New York: Schocken Books, 1977); see especially pages 39-41 for her comparison of English and

Continental midwives. In 1845 the *Southern Medical and Surgical Journal* reported the new regulations governing the instruction of midwives in Paris. Literate women of good moral character and at least eighteen years of age were admitted to the government-sponsored clinical lying-in hospital (La Maternité). There they took a twelve-month course that included two full courses of lectures on the theory and practice of midwifery. See *Boston Medical and Surgical Journal* 32 (July 9, 1845):467.

4. In both countries midwives continued to practice among the lower classes, and humanitarian considerations ultimately led to efforts to provide training. On late nineteenth-century British reform, see J. H. Aveling, *English Midwives: Their History and Their Prospects* (London: Churchill, 1872), especially his preface and pages 158-160; J. T. Mitchell, "On the Necessity of Adopting Laws by which the Wives of the Labouring Classes and the Poor Shall Have Secured to them In their Labours the Attendance of Qualified Accoucheurs, Female as Well as Male," *Transactions of the Obstetrical Society of London for the Year 1873,* Vol. 15 (London: Longmans, Green & Co., 1874), pp. 3-9; and Donnison, *Midwives.* In the United States midwives found patients, especially among the wives of the workers, whose ranks were swelled by an immigrant population from southern and eastern Europe long accustomed to female midwifery. In 1884 health officers in Boston, Brooklyn, and Philadelphia indicated that over one half of the working-class confinements were attended by midwives, the majority of them ignorant and untrained. See Thomas H. Manley, "Women as Midwives," *Transactions of the New York State Medical Association for the Year 1884* (New York: Appleton, 1885), p. 371. In 1911 only fifteen of forty-eight states had enacted regulatory legislation, and in two of these the law permitted unrestricted practice. See Thomas Darlington, "The Present Status of the Midwife," *American Journal of Obstetrics and Diseases of Women and Children* 63 (April 1911): 871. An excellent study of attitudes toward midwifery in the early twentieth century is Frances E. Kobrin, "The American Midwife Controversy: A Crisis of Professionalization," *Bulletin of the History of Medicine* 40 (July-August 1966): 350-353. A recent, well-documented account of the later period is Judy Barrett Litoff, *American Midwives: 1860 to the Present* (Westport, Conn.: Greenwood Press, 1978).

5. [Philip Thicknesse], *A Letter to a Young Lady* (London: R. Davis et al., 1764), p. 3.

6. [Philip Thicknesse], *Man-Midwifery Analysed: and the Tendency of That Practice Detected and Exposed* . . . (London: R. Davis, 1764), p. 4.

7. Elizabeth Nihell, *A Treatise on the Art of Midwifery. Setting Forth Various abuses therein, especially as to the practice with instruments: the*

Whole serving to put all Rational Inquirers in a fair way of very safely forming their own Judgment upon the Question; which it is best to employ, In cases of Pregnancy and Lying-in, a Man-Midwife or, a Midwife (London: Morley, 1760), p. 123.

8. Elizabeth Nihell, *Art of Midwifery,* quoted in [John Stevens], *An Important Address to Wives and Mothers on the Dangers and Immorality of Man-Midwifery,* By a Medical Practitioner (London: O. Hodgson, 1830), p. 18.

9. See, for example, Edmund Chapman, *Treatise on the Improvement of Midwifery* . . . 3rd ed. (London: L. Davis and C. Reymers, 1759), p. 136; John Memis, *The Midwife's Pocket-Companion* . . . (London: Edward and Charles Dilly, 1765), pp. 24-25. Eventually doctors substituted the phrase "taking a pain" for the term "touching," presumably to avoid the indelicate inference the original term suggested.

10. William Smellie, *A Treatise on the Theory and Practice of Midwifery,* 3rd ed. (London: D. Wilson and T. Durham, 1756), pp. 184-185.

11. [Thicknesse], *Man-Midwifery,* pp. 6-7.

12. [Thicknesse], *Letter to a Young Lady,* p. 4.

13. [Thicknesse], *Man-Midwifery,* p. 7.

14. [Thicknesse], *Letter to a Young Lady,* p. 7.

15. [Thicknesse], *Man-Midwifery,* pp. 13-14.

16. John Douglas, *A Short Account of the State of Midwifery in London* (London, 1736), quoted in Sophia Jex-Blake, *Medical Women: A Thesis and a History* (Edinburgh: Oliphant, Anderson & Ferrier, 1886; London: Hamilton, Adams and Co., 1886; New York: Source Book Press Reprint, 1970), p. 23.

17. Nihell, *Art of Midwifery,* quoted in Philip J. Klukoff, "Smollett's Defence of Dr. Smellie in 'The Critical Review,' " *Medical History* 14 (January 1970):39.

18. [Thicknesse], *Letter to a Young Lady,* p. 15.

19. Harold Speert, "Midwifery in Retrospect," in *The Midwife in the United States: Report of a Macy Conference* (New York: Josiah Macy, Jr. Foundation, 1968), p. 174; Klukoff, "Smollett's Defence," p. 37.

20. [Thicknesse], *Man-Midwifery,* pp. 10, 18.

21. Margaret Stephen, *Domestic Midwife; or the best means of Preventing Danger in Childbirth considered* . . . (London: n. p., 1795), quoted in Aveling, *English Midwives,* p. 128.

22. S. W. Fores, *Man-Midwifery Dissected* . . . (London: S. W. Fores, 1793), pp. 143, viii, 57.

23. Ibid., pp. 182-186.

24. Ibid., pp. 65, 61.

25. William Buchan, *Domestic Medicine: or a Treatise on the Prevention and Cure of diseases by Regimen and Simple Medicines* (Fairhaven, Vt.: James Lyon, 1798), p. 353.

26. Fores, *Man-Midwifery Dissected,* pp. xxiii-xxiv.

27. R. Kinglake, "On Obstetric Practice," *London Medical and Physical Journal* 34 (October 1815):290-292.

28. John Wayte, "On the Necessity of Accoucheurs," *London Medical and Physical Journal* 34 (December 1815):450-452.

29. J. Atkinson, "Remarks on Dr. Kinglake's Observations on the Obstetric Practice," *London Medical and Physical Journal* 35 (January 1816):7.

30. R. Kinglake, "In Reply to Messrs. Wayte and Atkinson, on Obstetric Practice," *London Medical and Physical Journal* 35 (March 1816):178.

31. Quoted in Aveling, *English Midwives,* pp. 157-158. For more on the controversy, see Joseph Adams, "On Midwives and Accoucheurs," *London Medical and Physical Journal* 35 (February 1816):84-88; Samuel Merriman, "On the Art of Midwifery as exercised by Medical Practitioners in Reply to Dr. Kinglake," *London Medical and Physical Journal* 35 (April 1816):282-291; John Wayte, "Remarks on Dr. Kinglake's Opinions Concerning the Obstetric Art," *London Medical and Physical Journal* 35 (May 1816):359-363.

32. Irving S. Cutter and Henry R. Viets, *A Short History of Midwifery,* 1st ed. (Philadelphia and London: W. B. Saunders, 1964), p. 187; Harvey Graham [I. Harvey Flack], *Eternal Eve* (London: W. Heinemann, 1950), pp. 536-539.

33. "Case of Her Royal Highness, the late Princess CHARLOTTE of Wales," *London Medical Repository* 8 (December 1, 1817):537. A century and one half after Princess Charlotte's death, three British physicians studying the prevalence of porphyria among members of the royal houses of Stuart and Hanover shed new light on the case. Porphyria, which is hereditary, presents a combination of seemingly unrelated symptoms, including abdominal colic, vomiting, constipation or diarrhea, spasms localized in the chest, muscular weakness, and cerebral symptoms ranging from convulsions, coma, insomnia, and headache. George III apparently suffered from repeated attacks of porphyria, which would explain his erratic behavior at times. Princess Charlotte's previous medical history included frequent attacks of headache, abdominal pain, depression, insomnia, loss of appetite, and rapid pulse, the combination of which suggests that she inherited the illness. If so, her death in 1817 may have resulted from a "fulminating attack of porphyria" which set in a few hours after her dead son was delivered. See Ida Macalpine et al., "Porphyria in the Royal Houses of Stuart, Hanover, and Prussia. A Follow-up Study of

George III's Illness,'' *British Medical Journal* 1 (January 6, 1968):14; and Ida Macalpine and Richard Hunter, *George III and the Mad-business* (New York: Pantheon Books, 1970).

34. See, for example, [John Stevens], *Man Midwifery Exposed, or the Danger and Immorality of Employing Men in Midwifery Proved; and the Remedy for the Evil Found* (London: W. Horsell, 1850), p. 7.

35. Valentine Seaman, *The Midwives Monitor, and Mothers Mirror . . .* (New York: Isaac Collins, 1800), p. v.

36. "Female Doctors," *Aesculapian Register* 1 (August 12, 1824):79.

37. Thomas Ewell, *Letters to Ladies, Detailing Important Information Concerning Themselves and Infants* (Philadelphia: W. Brown, 1817), p. 29.

38. Ibid., pp. 153, 163, 174-186.

39. Ibid., p. 144. See Thomas Denman's *Aphorisms on the Application and Use of the Forceps and Vectis . . .*, 1st American ed. (Philadelphia: Benjamin Johnson, 1803), p. 49 for an example of conservative counsel.

40. Ewell, *Letters to Ladies,* pp. 25-26. This assertion that the immediately post-partum woman was capable of exciting man's uncontrolled passion is reminiscent of the view expressed in [Thicknesse], *Man-Midwifery,* pp. 16-17: ". . . a fine woman . . . can appear in no situation, except in the act of death, but such as may stir the most unconquerable of passions."

41. Quoted in William Hosmer, *The Young Lady's Book; or Principles of Female Education* (Auburn & Buffalo, N.Y.: Miller, Orton & Mulligan, 1855), pp. 199-201.

42. Ewell, *Letters to Ladies,* p. 27.

43. Letter to the Editor, *The Examiner,* June 17, 1827, quoted in M. Adams, *Man-Midwifery Exposed! Or What it is, and What it Ought to Be: Proving the practice to be injurious and disgraceful to Society; the frequent cause of jealousy and disgust; and of serious mischief to delicate and modest females: With Broad Hints to New Married People, and Young Men & Women* (London: S. W. Fores, 1830), p. 50.

44. [Stevens], *Man-Midwifery Exposed,* p. 15.

45. Ibid., p. 1.

46. William Cobbett, *Advice to Young Men and Women,* quoted in ibid., pp. 45-46.

47. Hosmer, *Young Lady's Book,* pp. 187-189.

48. William Hosmer, *Appeal to Husbands and Wives in Favor of Female Physicians* (New York: G. Gregory, 1853), p. 8.

49. [Stevens], *Man-Midwifery Exposed,* p. 14.

50. Ibid.

51. Hosmer, *Appeal,* p. 16.

52. Hosmer, *Lady's Book,* p. 202.

53. [Stevens], *Man-Midwifery Exposed,* p. 16.

54. Adams, *Man-Midwifery Exposed!,* pp. 20, 23, 80.

55. *The London Practice of Midwifery,* quoted in W[ooster] Beach, *An Improved System of Midwifery adapted to the Reformed Practice of Medicine . . . with Remarks on Physiological and Moral Elevation* (New York: Scribner, 1851), p. 19. *The London Practice of Midwifery* was a pirated edition of the lectures of the celebrated London practitioner Joseph Clarke. See Charles D. Meigs, *Females and Their Diseases* (Philadelphia: Lea & Blanchard, 1848), p. 27.

56. *An Appeal to the Medical Society of Rhode Island, In Behalf of Woman to be Restored to her Natural Rights as "Midwife," and elevated by education to be the Physician of her own sex* (Printed for the author, 1851), p. 6.

57. Hosmer, *Young Lady's Book,* p. 204.

58. James Boyle, quoted in Beach, *Improved System,* p. 17.

59. George Gregory, *Medical Morals, Illustrated with Plates and Extracts from Medical Works; Designed to Show the Pernicious Social and Moral Influence of the Present System of Medical Practice . . .* (New York: Published by the author, 1853), p. 5.

60. *Appeal to the Medical Society of Rhode Island,* pp. 6-7.

61. *Belmont Medical Society Transactions for 1850-51* (Bridgeport, Ohio: n.p., 1851), pp. 57-58, quoted in James H. Young, *The Toadstool Millionaires: A Social History of Patent Medicines in America Before Federal Regulation* (Princeton: Princeton University Press, 1961), p. 53.

62. Adams, *Man-Midwifery Exposed!,* p. 83.

63. Kinglake, "Reply to Wayte and Atkinson," p. 177.

64. [Stevens], *Man-Midwifery Exposed,* p. 29.

65. See, for example, Adams, *Man-Midwifery Exposed!,* p. 51, *Appeal to the Medical Society of Rhode Island,* p. 6; Hosmer, *Appeal,* p. 8; Beach, *Improved System,* p. 18.

66. [John Stevens], *An Important Address to Wives and Mothers on the Dangers and Immorality of Man-Midwifery, By a Medical Practitioner* (London: O. Hodgson, 1830),. p. 29.

67. Beach, *Improved System,* p. 13.

68. Adams, *Man-Midwifery Exposed!,* p. 85.

69. "Early Practitioners of Midwifery in England," *London Medical and Physical Journal* 27 (February 1812):117.

70. Ewell, *Letters to Ladies,* p. 29.

71. Samuel Gregory, *Letter to Ladies in Favor of Female Physicians* (New York: Fowler and Wells, 1850), p. 36.

72. James Boyle, quoted in Beach, *Improved System,* p. 18.

73. Quoted in [Stevens], *Man-Midwifery Exposed,* pp. 42-43.

74. [Stevens], *Man-Midwifery Exposed,* p. 34. See also Adams, *Man-*

Midwifery Exposed!, pp. 54-55.

75. Sir Anthony Carlisle, "Address to His Majesty's Judges, Coroners, and Justices of the Peace," *The Times,* May 1, 1827, quoted in Adams, *Man-Midwifery Exposed!*, pp. 37-39.

76. A. Curtis, *Lectures on Midwifery and the Forms of Disease Peculiar to Women and Children, Delivered to the Members of the Botanico-Medical College of Ohio,* 2nd ed. (Columbus, Ohio: Jonathan Phillips, 1841), pp. 200, 198-C; 201.

77. William Smellie, *A Collection of Cases and Observations in Midwifery to Illustrate His Former Treatise, or First Volume on that Subject* (London: D. Wilson and T. Durham, 1754), p. iv.

78. Denman, *Aphorisms,* p. 13.

79. William Potts Dewees, *A Compendious System of Midwifery, Chiefly designed to facilitate the Inquiries of those who may be pursuing this branch of study,* 1st ed. (Philadelphia: Carey and Lea, 1824), pp. 556-557.

80. Samuel Bard, *A Compendium of the Theory and Practice of Midwifery . . .* (New York: Collins, 1819), pp. 18-19.

81. James Ewell, *The Medical Companion* (Philadelphia: Anderson & Meehan, 1816), pp. 431-432.

82. Aveling, *Midwives,* p. 176. Even more damaging accusations fell from the pens of the reformers. See Beach, *Improved System,* p. 13; Ewell, *Letters to Ladies,* pp. 147-148; [Stevens], *Address,* pp. 9-10; Fores, *Man-Midwifery Dissected,* p. 32.

83. Manley, "Women as Midwives," p. 372. Dr. Manley advocated training women to attend normal labors.

84. [Stevens], *Man-Midwifery Exposed,* p. 28. See also ibid., p. 44; Gregory, *Letter to Ladies,* p. 24; Fores, *Man-Midwifery Dissected,* p. 33.

85. *Appeal to the Medical Society of Rhode Island,* p. 5. John Stearns is credited with introducing ergot to American obstetrics in 1807. It was administered to excite uterine contractions, and its use, as in the case of anesthesia, was highly controversial for many years. See August K. Gardner, *A History of the Art of Midwifery . . .* (New York: Stringer and Townsend, 1852), p. 23.

86. [Thicknesse], *Man-Midwifery,* p. 23; [Stevens], *Address,* pp. 17-18, p. 25, cf. Fores, *Man-Midwifery Dissected,* pp. 106-107.

87. Adams, *Man-Midwifery Exposed!*, pp. 63-64; W. Beach, quoted in [Stevens], *Man-Midwifery Exposed,* p. 25; James Boyle, quoted in Beach, *Improved System,* p. 17; Fores, *Man-Midwifery Dissected,* p. 197.

88. Hosmer, *Appeal,* p. 3.

89. Beach, *Improved System,* p. 19.

90. Ewell, *Letters to Ladies,* p. 31.

91. Gregory, *Letter to Ladies,* p. 25.

7

Midwives and "Female Doctresses"

The question of propriety and delicacy had better not be raised—
it will thin the ranks of the male practitioners when it comes up.
Women will decide whether they must forever remain only sufferers
and subjects of medical indelicacy, if they are once wakened up to
the discussion.

—DR. WILLIAM ELDER, *THE NORTHERN CHRISTIAN ADVOCATE,* 1849

At mid-century the opponents of man midwifery were still unable
to build a base of popular support. Neither the press nor the medical
journals took serious notice of their tirades. Publicity for their
cause turned inward, relying chiefly upon the pamphlets and books
that they wrote and circulated among themselves. Although anti-
man midwifery critics had occasionally counted some physicians
among their champions, the majority of orthodox doctors favored
perpetuating the system that preserved the role of the accoucheur.
Many eminent practitioners recognized the abuses meddlesome
midwifery produced and abhorred the resulting mutilation of
women and infants. The remedy they favored was improving obstetrics training for men physicians rather than returning the field
to women. Lost to reactionaries, then, were these potential allies.[1]

In advocating changes the reformers looked to the past. In defending their proposal to train women as midwives, they did not envision a medical revolution that would draw women into the competitive arena of general medical practice monopolized by men. Their primary goal was to purify society, thereby sharpening the distinctions that separated the sexes and assigned specific role expectations. Late in the 1840s Samuel Gregory appeared with the leadership potential requisite to further the cause of the reactionary critics. Gregory was not a feminist, nor did he sanction women occupying positions of leadership. Yet in the course of his activities he raised the expectations of a number of women chafing at the confines of their narrowly defined sphere. Unwittingly he helped move reactionary criticism closer to the broader radical reform currents then sweeping through American society.

Samuel Gregory took a Bachelor of Arts from Yale College in 1840 and a Master of Arts five years later. In his senior year he had attended a course in anatomy and physiology, which may have sparked his interest in medicine. He never formally studied for the degree of medicine, although in 1853 the Eclectic Penn Medical College awarded him an honorary medical degree. Shortly after leaving Yale, he toured the lecture circuit in New England, lecturing at various times on English grammar, phrenology, and mesmerism. In 1844 his first published pamphlet dealt with *Facts and Important Information for Young Men on the Self-Indulgence of the Sexual Appetite.* The work went into many editions and sold over forty-two thousand copies.[2]

Sometime before the mid-forties Gregory was struck by the curious fact that midwifery, "a feminine occupation, as the name implies . . . [was] exclusively in the hands of males."[3] In 1845 his first work on the subject, *Licentiousness, its Cause and Effects,* appeared. The pamphlet discussed unfavorable aspects of man midwifery, and in it Gregory set forth the need for both a supply of women midwives and for "a class of female physicians, qualified at least to attend to the peculiar complaints of their own sex." Frederick Waite credited Gregory with being the first to propose in print the establishment of an institution in which women could receive medical training beyond that of basic midwifery.[4]

Gregory's opposition to male accoucheurs was founded on the earlier views of reactionary critics. Little in his published works suggests originality beyond his insistence that women be given training in general medicine. Unlike earlier critics, however, he succeeded in carrying the cause into the lecture hall. Public activity such as this was bound to make him a controversial figure and to focus attention upon the plan for what detractors termed his "midwives' Manufactory."

Since Gregory was young, unmarried, and not formally trained in medicine, opponents considered his interest in the details of childbirth abnormal. They were inclined to write him off as merely another itinerant reformer out to line his pockets at the expense of a gullible public. Why Gregory chose to concentrate on this particular reform is not clear. The stringent limits imposed by Victorian morality sometimes created ambivalent attitudes toward sex in many young people, yet available evidence does not support his critics' charge that Gregory's attitudes were prurient. In comparison with other contemporary tracts attacking man midwifery, his rhetoric was, in fact, temperate.

Gregory's pamphlets and articles were repetitive, and an examination of one gives a good summary of his views. In *Letter to Ladies in Favor of Female Physicians* he argued society's need for midwives. Decorous women opposed to employing men to attend them would, in the absence of available trained midwives, be forced to patronize those who were ignorant and untrained.[5] He contended that gestating women were especially sensitive and nervous and that the "artificial state of society" in the nineteenth century had made modern women considerably more delicate than their ancestors. During the crisis of confinement they neither needed nor wanted the "strong arm of a protector," preferring the sympathy and compassion of other women who could appreciate their travail.[6]

Setting aside objections based on sex, Gregory observed that in the course of general practice most Boston physicians encountered very few obstetrics cases. Their own experience thus limited, when confronted with preternatural cases they were compelled to seek assistance from men "more exclusively engaged" in midwifery.

He proposed the education of women as the logical solution to the multiple problems posed by necessity and decorum. The training of midwives he saw as a first step in the right direction. It would be better still to find some means, through public or private financing, of providing women with three or more years of concentrated medical study that would encompass all branches. Given such opportunities, women soon would acquire the requisite skills, judgment, and temerity obstetric practice admittedly demanded.[7] Once set on this course, he argued, society could find its way back to the "true refinement and modesty" of an earlier age. Genuine refinement, such as that displayed in colonial society, did not consist of rendering pregnancy and parturition unmentionable conditions nor of driving gravid women into seclusion for months prior to their deliveries. Rather it was obtained by the simple expedient of never permitting "male intruders within the sacred precincts of the lying-in room."[8]

In 1847 Gregory began to deliver public lectures, first exclusively to men and later to women, on the need to provide medical education for women. These lectures created a stir in Boston. The official journal of the Boston Medical Society viewed his activities with a jaundiced eye. New England already was "wholly overstocked with anti-isms of every possible shade and texture," the advocates of which made a lucrative business from their itinerant lecturing to the "great irresponsible public." The *Boston Medical and Surgical Journal* accused Gregory of being more objectionable than most, pandering to a corrupt curiosity and using the lecture platform to utter opinions that under any other circumstances would only be termed "abominable." He had no medical qualifications, and his only sources of information were books and the "leaky vessels" with whom he conversed. Continued the editor, his frequent references to the Eclectic physician Wooster Beach were sufficient alone to discredit him. The journal disclaimed any opposition to qualified midwives or to efforts designed to improve midwifery. It did oppose Gregory and his "altogether unchaste" allusions, which, insisted the editor, were "calculated to beget a prurience of thought at once at variance with propriety, and at war with the first principles of virtue."[9] The tirade concluded with the hope that community leaders would discourage further lectures of this kind.

Undaunted, Gregory replied to the editor, claiming overwhelming popular support for his crusade and citing a great deal of favorable comment from clergymen who had attended his lectures.[10] The editor remained unconvinced. In March he charged that Gregory was merely another "wind-mill reformer," ostensibly attacking man midwifery from a sense of duty but actually using the cause for personal gain.[11]

Encouraged by his supporters, Gregory went forward with plans to establish the Boston Female Medical College. By recruiting twelve women he formed the Female Medical Education Society later termed the "first class of females ever assembled in America for the purpose of qualifying themselves to enter the medical profession."[12] On November 1, 1848, the first three-month course of instruction in midwifery began, followed by a second course in April 1849. Gregory later claimed that twenty women in all, instructed by a single professor, had attended more than three hundred cases of labor during the course of these first two sessions.[13]

Late in November 1848 Gregory organized the American Medical Education Society for the purpose of raising funds. The society's constitution stated its aim to "educate Midwives, Nurses, and (so far as the wants of the public require) Female Physicians."[14] In April 1850 the Massachusetts legislature incorporated the society under the name of the FEMALE Medical Education Society. Lifetime memberships were available for twenty dollars, annual memberships for one dollar. One of the paradoxes of the age—and an indication of Gregory's conservatism—was that initially women were excluded from membership in the society. They were encouraged to contribute financial support and were permitted access to the school's rooms. At a later date women were permitted to join the society but were denied any management role.[15] In 1850 Gregory claimed a membership in excess of eight hundred, including fifty clergymen representing various denominations. Among the members listed were Horace Mann, Charles Francis Adams, and Nathanial Silsbee, Jr., mayor of Salem. Harriet Beecher Stowe and William Lloyd Garrison were among those who made financial contributions to the society.[16]

A printed report issued in 1851 of the Boston Female Medical School set forth the prospective courses of study for midwives, nurses, and physicians. The emphasis laid upon the training for midwives is evident:

Candidates for Diplomas as Practitioners in Midwifery, must be at least twenty years of age, and must present testimonials of good moral character; they must have studied at least one year, including the Lecture terms; must have attended two full courses of Lectures, one of which must have been in this institution: and must pass a satisfactory examination before the Board of Examiners, in Anatomy and Physiology, in Obstetrics and the diseases peculiar to Women.[17]

Courses of lectures and instruction for nurses were given "in reference to their important and responsible vocation of attending the sick." Those women seeking to become candidates for "full Medical Diplomas" and desiring status as "Female Physicians" were required to pursue "a course of Education equivalent to that required in other medical institutions; and at least two terms of their instruction" were to be taken at the Boston Female Medical School.

In its first two years of operation the college had no permanent location. Students met by invitation at the homes of various classmates. Between fall 1848 and spring 1851 six semi-annual courses leading to the midwifery certificate were given. An historian of the college has estimated that attendance at each of the six sessions ranged from twelve to twenty-eight women. Initially the college did not award the degree of medicine but merely gave its graduates certificates of proficiency. After 1853 these certificates were no longer awarded and the school began to award the degree. In the early years probably most of the women who attended planned to work as midwives or nurses. Two members of the first class, Martha Hayden Sawin and Lucinda Capen Hall, later earned medical degrees, Sawin from the Female Medical College of Pennsylvania (1851) and Hall from Worcester Medical College (1852).[18]

In his enthusiasm for the new cults of mesmerism and phrenology, his admiration for Eclectic medicine, and his assault upon the "regulars" for perpetuating man midwifery, Samuel Gregory was representative of the unorthodox forces sweeping through American medicine in the Age of Reform. When he took up the cause of female midwifery, he was able to build the base of popular support that had eluded earlier reactionaries. The original campaign to restore obstetrics to the midwives had been peripheral to the emerging feminist movement. By opening the Boston Female Medical College and providing women with the opportunity to obtain the medical training they needed to give them credibility, Samuel Gregory unintentionally altered the direction of the crusade against man midwifery. Within a few years the college shifted its emphasis from training midwives to preparing women as physicians. This shift moved the anti-man midwifery crusade closer to the goals of the larger and ultimately more significant women's rights movement, despite the fact that Gregory did not sympathize with the radicals. Gregory had expected that the school's graduates would limit their practice to obstetrics and the diseases of women and children. He boasted that they were not "upstarts" or "old maids" but "true women" with no wish to "encroach upon physicians, in the treatment of the other sex."[19] Such protestations could not alter the fact that by preparing women to enter the medical profession on any terms, Gregory's school appeared to be endorsing the assertions of radical feminists.

As the question of whether or not women should be trained as midwives gave way to the more formidable issue of whether or not women should, or even could, be thoroughly educated as physicians, bitter controversy ensued. Foreshadowing these events were the comments of a student at the Boston Female Medical College in 1849. Just as man midwifery had gained acceptance as honorable employment for men:

so too the time will come when it will no longer be regarded as disgraceful for a woman to administer to the necessities of her own sex. Already the light of physiological knowledge is beginning to dawn upon many who have been groping in darkness, and a spirit has been aroused which will not be allayed until such knowledge is diffused throughout the land.[20]

At approximately the time that Sameul Gregory and the Female Medical Education Society were formulating their plans, two women, strangers to each other and drawn from entirely different backgrounds, were independently attempting to acquire an education in medicine. For over a decade Harriot Kezia Hunt had been practicing medicine without a license among the women of Boston. In the fall 1847 at the age of forty-two, she applied to Harvard Medical College for permission to attend the lectures. In a terse reply to her letter she was informed that the president and fellows of the university found it "inexpedient" to consider her application.[21]

The death of Hunt's father and subsequent mismanagement of his estate had made it incumbent upon Harriot to find some means of supporting her mother and sister Sarah. Her interest in medicine stemmed originally from Sarah's illness. Early in the 1830s the sisters consulted a number of orthodox physicians, but Sarah's condition did not improve. In desperation they visited an unlicensed sectarian doctor, Elizabeth Mott, who with her husband Richard had established a practice in Boston. The Hunts were "open to all sorts of opposition for even thinking of such a thing as employing 'a quack'," Harriot later explained. "But we were weary and tired out with 'regulars'; and it did not occur to us that to die under regular practice, and with medical etiquette, was better than any other way."[22]

Sarah's health improved dramatically, and the sisters, attributing this to the effect of Mott's irregular therapeutics, soon established a similar medical practice of their own. From the outset they avoided home visits and obstetrics cases, aware that if they engaged in either of these the "doctors would say, as we were women, that we were insinuating ourselves into families, and weakening confidence in the faculty." At the time, most women knew very little about even the fundamental "laws of hygiene." The Hunts made a point of instructing patients about their bodies and stressing prevention of illness through sound health practices. Thus they invited the criticism of those orthodox physicians who were of the opinion that "it is not fitting for women to know about themselves; it makes them nervous!"[23]

After Sarah's marriage, Harriot continued the practice alone. It was in the hope of acquiring some formal medical knowledge that she attempted to attend the lectures at Harvard.

Concurrent with Hunt's activities, an Englishwoman who had emigrated to the United States as a young girl was attempting to gain access to an orthodox medical education. Elizabeth Blackwell, obliged to support her mother and a family of younger siblings, was first a teacher—one of the few acceptable occupations for middle-class women at the time. Her interest in medicine as a career stemmed from the remark of a friend. Victim of a painful disease, "the delicate nature of which made the methods of treatment a constant suffering to her,"[24] this woman commented that her misery would have been far less had she been able to consult a woman physician.

Blackwell studied medicine privately with liberal preceptors in Asheville, North Carolina, Charleston, and Philadelphia. Determined to obtain orthodox credentials, she applied for admission to medical colleges in Philadelphia and New York but met with no success. In the fall 1847 she received word quite unexpectedly that the students at Geneva Medical College, located in the Finger Lakes region of central New York, had voted unanimously to admit her. She learned later that the students at first thought themselves victims of a hoax perpetrated by a rival medical school; apparently they did not expect that a Miss Blackwell actually would appear at the college.[25] In 1849 Blackwell graduated at the head of her class to become the first woman to earn the M.D. in the United States.

It was not entirely fortuitous that in the 1840s Samuel Gregory, Harriot Hunt, and Elizabeth Blackwell shared the conviction that a body of trained women physicians would benefit American society. In the second quarter of the nineteenth century, several elements were conducive to just such sentiments. Pervasive modesty played its part by creating the "shrinking delicacy," whether genuine or ·affected, that made it uncomfortable at best for women to consult male physicians. Men, too, often were troubled by what Charles Meigs termed "the Embarrassments of the Practice." The criticism that women preferred to suffer silently for years rather than subject themselves to the mortification of even a superficial physical examination is met with frequently in the literature. In his treatise on obstetrics Meigs had offered the opinion that "no woman can be placed in a sanitary condition, compelling her to appeal to the aid of the accoucheur, without some sense of mortified delicacy."[26]

Most physicians, however, believed that these embarrassments could be minimized by the sensitive doctor and that women must of necessity endure the residue. As one physician stated, men had inherited the practice of obstetrics "naturally and legitimately" because of their exclusive competence at coping with cases of difficult parturition. The fact that women had skillful, trained accoucheurs available to attend them, he insisted, "counterbalance[d] the inconveniences incident to the existing sytem," the more so because of the frequency with which complicated childbirths "multiplied and [were] aggravated . . . by the artificial habits of society."[27]

Yet, responsibility for safeguarding society's health was not the exclusive province of the physician. To women fell the task of child rearing. Successful performance of this function required that they supervise the general family health and its morals, religion, and

education. Unfortunately these women, for the most part deprived
of the knowledge of rudimentary principles of hygiene and physiology, were poorly prepared to protect the family health.

Urban middle-class women especially were notorious for their
own poor health. Physicians attributed this to the notion that
woman's physical system was more easily affected than man's by
external elements such as "climate, the state of society and manners."
That "luxury and indulgence" took their toll upon the uterus was
not disputed.[28] As early as the middle of the eighteenth century,
William Smellie had explained the death of a patient in childbirth
by observing that her earlier pregnancies had been uneventful and
her constitution healthy before she moved into London. "One
would be apt to imagine," theorized Smellie, "that this fatal
catastrophe happened from her constitution's altering and becoming more delicate by a city life."[29] In the years that followed,
medical authorities insisted that the urban life-style of the leisure
class created "the feeble females of civilized countries." Women,
confined to "domestic affairs," but with servants to labor for
them, spent their days indulging in irregular and excessive amuse-
ments, complained Dr. John Vaughan. The "lady of fashion" so
far removed from the "mere child of nature" paid a heavy price by
aggravating her "sexual complaints . . . especially those incidental
to pregnancy."[30]

The physical distress that women experienced was not caused by
engaging in activities that physicians deemed frivolous. Women
uninstructed in their own anatomy and uninformed about their
physiology unwittingly injured themselves by confining their bodies
in tightly laced corsets to attain the desired fashionable figure with
its unnaturally slender seventeen- or eighteen-inch waist. Mothers
dressed daughters in corsets at an early age. It was argued that if
tight lacing were begun when a girl was young enough, it was not
harmful. "The supple and growing frame of a young girl is not like
the hard and unyielding works of a watch," reasoned one advocate
of the fashion. If the watch case were compressed, the inner work-
ings would be broken; if initially, however, a young girl's organs
were prevented by tight lacing from developing as they normally
would, ran the assurance, they would harmlessly "accommodate
themselves to any other [form or direction] with perfect ease."[31] In

truth, of course, once a girl was thus encased, the muscles of her torso could serve little purpose and became incapable of supporting her frame without continued artificial assistance. The familiar fainting spells then considered proof of delicacy and breeding were merely one result of this abuse. As leisure-class women were held to be constitutionally weak as well as helpless and dependent, such proof was eagerly sought, regardless of the physical price. It was the welcome visible sign of "an ethereal, spiritual nature, a moral sensitiveness and purity superior to man's."[32]

Knowledgeable physicians recognized the destructive effects of fashionable dress. In 1845 Dr. Joel Wing, delivering his presidential address before the New York State Medical Society, told assembled colleagues that women were afflicted with spinal irritations twice as often as men. Among the predisposing causes he cited were the peculiar female constitution, woman's nervous temperament, and the effects of wearing corset cords and stays that compressed the walls of the chest and impeded the action of lungs and heart.[33] Addressing the Medical Association of Southern Central New York in 1854, that organization's president urged parents to learn more about anatomy and physiology. If thus informed they would understand the ill effects of tight lacing. He maintained that the direct tendency to ill health produced

by an arbitrary and high-pressure system of applying wearing apparel, will be so apparent to you, and the inevitable consequences so well understood, that you would never permit such a system of practice to wrest from you that daughter, to add another to the already numerous catalogue of self-immolated victims, upon the altar of so inhuman a custom as has prevailed in the application of female costume.[34]

Foreign observers commented on the lack of stamina and the general tendency toward malaise exhibited by American women.[35] In 1851 an Eclectic physician attributed the difficulties encountered by "fashionable women" during pregnancy, parturition, and postpartum to the artificial habits fostered by city life, including poor diet, tight lacing, and lack of exercise.[36] Sarah Josepha Hale, editor of the popular and influential *Godey's Magazine,* warned that the "constitutional ill health in the mothers is fast making us a nation of invalids."[37] Margaretta Gleason, one of the first women to earn a doctor's degree, complained that the fashionable education of ladies taught that weakness and dependence were virtues. As long as a lady's charms were thought to lie in "delicate weakness and imbecility," she warned, there was little or no hope of American women developing sorely needed self-reliance.[38] In a similar vein, a Quaker physician speaking at the Female Medical College of Philadelphia in 1851 had harsh words for the "weakness and imbecility" of those women who lacked high aspirations, followed the dictates of fashion, and wasted youth and health in the pursuit of pleasure at the expense of knowledge.[39]

Another unfortunate consequence of the sorry combination of ignorance and excessive modesty was that women were led to seek help from a variety of unreliable sources. The lucrative patent medicine industry flourished on women's patronage in part because its nostrums promised cures without embarrassment.[40] Dr. S. P. Townsend, proprietor of New York's Temple of Health at 82 Nassau Street, dispensed an extract of "Sarsaparilla" that he advertised as especially prepared for use in female complaints. This "most extraordinary Medicine in the World" safely and effectively purified the system and relieved the sufferings attending parturition, claimed Townsend extravagantly. Among other virtues he attributed to this catholic remedy was its ability to provide quick cures for "incipient consumption, barrenness, Prolapsus Uteri, or Falling of the Womb, Costiveness, Piles, Leucorrhoea, or Whites [and] obstructed or difficult Menstruation."[41] Medical manuals were written with an eye toward the "ladies." One dollar would purchase *The Married Woman's Private Medical Companion,* containing "important secrets" for women of all ages. Within its pages a lady could discover in the privacy of her own home "the causes, symptoms, and the most efficient remedies, and the most certain modes of cure in every complaint."[42]

There was also an understandable tendency among women to seek out those who would not ask discomfiting questions. Dr. and Mrs. Drake established themselves in New York as successors to the latter's mother, Elizabeth Mott, the widely known "Female Physician" who in the 1830s had exerted such an influence on Harriot Hunt. The Drakes treated patients botanically with various flowers, roots, herbs, barks, gums, balsams, vegetables, and oils. Mrs. Drake confined her practice to women and children. She assured women "laboring under any of the various complaints so peculiar to their sex, that they . . . [could] consult her with the utmost confidence of gaining relief." For those too retiring to consult Mrs. Drake in person, she offered diagnoses and prescribed medications by mail.[43]

Joseph Kett has observed that much of the phenomenal success enjoyed by sectarian medicine may be attributed to its ability to attract support from women. Thomsonianism, an early, influential medical sect, illustrates the point. In 1813 Samuel Thomson received a federal patent on his system of treating ailments with a wide variety of botanical remedies. For twenty dollars individuals could purchase from Thomson the right to form "friendly botanic societies" in which his system would be practiced.

Just as orthodox physicians understood that their key to success lay in winning the confidence of women, so too did Thomsonians make special efforts to obtain female support. Women found several aspects of botanical medicine appealing. The system aimed at eliminating the services of regular doctors by making a physician of each Thomsonian. The method was learned easily and practitioners required no formal medical training. The woman who adopted it could practice within the bosom of her family without incurring the embarrassments attending outside practice. Thomsonianism had a crusading flavor. In the interest of democracy its adherents advocated a number of social and political reforms. Among reforms sought was the elimination of monopolies. Thomsonians considered medical licensing a form of monopoly, and they were primarily responsible for the reduction and elimination of licensing requirements in the ante-bellum period. Thomsonians also advocated female midwifery. In 1834 John Thomson, son of the founder, expressed the view that the capacity of women to practice medicine exceeded that of men. "Although men should reserve to themselves the exlusive right to mend broken limbs and fractured skulls, and to prescribe in all cases for their sex," commented Thomson, "they should certainly give up to women the office of attending upon women."[44]

By 1840 Thomsonianism had gone into decline, but other reformed systems such as neo-Thomsonianism, homeopathy, and eclecticism survived. These arose as a reaction against the "heroic" practice of the regular or "allopathic" physicians. Orthodox medicine relied essentially upon bleeding, purging, or sweating the patient to recovery by eliminating the particular irritation thought to be causing fever or disease. Venesection on a grand scale had been popularized by Benjamin Rush, who taught that it was "a very hard Matter to bleed a Patient to Death provided the Blood be not drawn from a Vital Part."[45] The process consisted of opening a vein with a lancet and drawing as much as four-fifths of the patient's blood in extreme cases.

As early as 1803 Rush had argued that women need not suffer in childbirth. Since he defined parturition as a "disease" that took the form of a "clonic" spasm, it followed that "remedies for difficult and painful parturition should be the same as for all other convulsive and spasmodic diseases." He advocated drawing thirty ounces of blood at the onset of labor to lessen pain and shorten its duration. This procedure was thought to be particularly effective when accompanied by purging and preceded by a regimen of proper diet. Rush insisted that the results had proved so satisfactory that in Philadelphia bleeding had been "generally adopted by the practitioners of midwifery, of both sexes."[46] Certainly "copious bloodletting" gained popularity among the accoucheurs. Peter Miller, lamenting the fact that physicians were rarely consulted about prenatal care, found that help was consequently limited to drawing twenty to forty ounces of blood when labor began. Although he admitted to lack of experience in gauging the effects of "nauseating doses of emetics," he reasoned that these might prove helpful, as suggested by the "common observation of the old women 'that a sick labour is an easy one.' "[47]

Citing clinical cases from his own practice in an essay on difficult participation, William Potts Dewees explained how the loss of blood "caused the necessary relaxation of the os uteri in tedious and painful cases [arising] from rigidity." Dewees recommended venesection also to ward off puerperal fever, milk abcess, and edema. In a later edition he gave unqualified approval to copious blood-letting to produce nausea, vomiting, and finally syncope with its consequent relaxation of the entire system. Dewees even depicted the conservative William Shippen as having converted to heroic medicine with his comment that he could have spared many of his patients pain and misery had he "used the lancet more freely."[48]

The regulars did not limit venesection to parturition, of course. To many it was the viable treatment for almost every disease. They augmented it with local bleeding achieved by cupping and scarification, as well as by the application of leeches. Purging and sweating were accomplished by administering massive doses of medication, much of it harsh and even dangerous. Among the cathartics regularly prescribed were tamarind, magnesia, jalap and calomel, or mercurous chloride. Tartar, antimony, zinc sulphate, and ipecac were common emetics.

The understandable rebellion of patients and of some orthodox physicians against heroic medical practices led to the development of various medical sects. One of these was homeopathy, introduced into America in the 1820s by those who had adopted the doctrines of the German physician, Samuel Hahnemann. To Hahnemann two principles were fundamental. The first, summarized in the phrase *similia similibus curantur* (like cures like), was that diseases could be cured by giving patients those drugs that produced in healthy people the symptoms exhibited by the diseases themselves. Hahnemann's second doctrine was the law of infinitesimals, which held that the smaller the dose, the more effective its action.[49] By mid-century homeopathy had attracted a large following, including some who came over from the regulars. Practitioners assured perpetuation of their system by establishing their own medical colleges and journals.

The eclectic or Reformed System of Medical Practice, founded by Dr. Wooster Beach of New England, represented another major sect of the period. By the 1840s it had absorbed earlier botanical groups and for several decades it enjoyed enormous popularity. As its name implies, the principle feature of eclecticism was the acceptance of some "redeeming traits" along with a rejection of the "defects" in all other systems. Practitioners selected those medical principles that were "good and useful," discarding anything considered "deleterious."[50] One convert explained the "peculiar characteristics" of the system by noting that Eclectics looked upon "*Mercury, Antimony, Arsenic* and *Lancet* . . . as very uncertain in their effects and liable to produce serious injury; and aim[ed] to substitute for these agents more *certain* and efficient remedies, unattended by injurious results.''[51] Beach and his followers emphasized the value of medications derived from indigenous plants. They substituted vegetable emetics for the harsher drugs of orthodox practitioners and denounced blood-letting as dangerous and useless. They also prescribed opium and digitalis, both condemned by Thomsonians as "vegetable poisons." Taking a cue from the homeopaths, eclectics were sparing in their use of all drugs, recommending minute doses only.

Eclectics also established professional journals, hospitals, and medical schools. In the 1850s they welcomed the attendance of women students. That they courted women is evident from Beach's *Improved System of Midwifery,* in which he alluded frequently to the desirability of female midwives. Eclecticism was especially popular in New England, central and western New York, and southern and central Ohio. Among the medical reformers in these regions, the movement for the education of women physicians found its greatest strength in the 1850s. Unlike Samuel Thomson, who had no formal medical training, Wooster Beach held the doctor of medicine. In the 1820s he operated the unchartered Reformed Medical College in New York City, along with a hospital known as the United States Infirmary.[52] In 1852 Beach returned to Boston, where he "planted his eclectic banner" and officially opened the Reformed Medical College. The editor of New England's only orthodox medical journal gave his opinion that the Reformed Medical College was run by dishonest adventurers. He voiced strong disapproval of a college that admitted women with men, granted diplomas without conducting formal examinations, and advertised that students would have the opportunity of "learning the healing art without the useless and dangerous practice of dissection."[53]

Grahamism was another product of the Age of Reform that women found attractive. Sylvester Graham, founder of the movement, had suffered from ill health during much of his youth. He entered Amherst College at the age of twenty-nine but was expelled on charges of criminal assault and suffered a breakdown. Upon his recovery he began to preach to Presbyterian congregations, often on the advantages of temperance. He taught himself some anatomy and physiology, and in 1830 he was invited by the Pennsylvania Temperance Society to deliver a series of lectures. Thus launched upon the lecture circuit, he spoke on a variety of topics, including temperance, chastity, courtship and marriage, the treatment for cholera, and diet reform.[54] In the 1830s he began his campaign to improve American habits of diet and hygiene. Imbued with the same sort of missionary zeal that characterized the crusades for botanic medicine, temperance, and abolition, Grahamism was genuinely scientific in the sense that it was founded on principles of physiology and hygiene as then understood.[55]

In 1837 Graham and William Alcott established the American Physiological Society to disseminate information to men and women. Human physiology was too delicate a subject for mixed discussion, and in the thirties and forties a number of ladies' physiological reform societies were organized under Graham's influence. Lectures were delivered on anatomy, physiology, diet, and hygiene by Paulina Wright Davis, Mary Gove (later, Nichols), Harriot K. Hunt, Lydia Folger Fowler, and Martha A. Sawin. Harriot Hunt, who helped with the formation of the Ladies' Physiological Society in Charlestown, explained the idea behind the movement.

If women could be induced to meet together for the purpose of obtaining a knowledge of physical laws, it would enable them to dispense in great measure with physicians, put them on their own responsibilities, and be a blessing to themsleves and their children.[56]

The free and open discussion of the diseases peculiar to women especially might enable them to halve their medical bills.

That women were anxious to obtain information about their own bodies, there can be little doubt. Hunt claimed that membership in the Charlestown organization climbed from about a dozen women to more than fifty within the first year.[57] George Combe, the Scottish phrenologist touring the United States in the late thirties, wrote that his daughter had attended one of Mary Gove's lectures on the injurious effects of tight lacing and poor ventilation. Three hundred women were present. An impressive audience of two thousand turned out to hear her free lecture on tight corsets.[58] Although these audiences were segregated, women were shocked by discussions of anatomy and physiology. During the lectures of Paulina Wright Davis, they frequently had to resort to smelling salts.[59]

Davis had retired from public lecturing by the time the movement for women physicians was underway, but she wrote to lend her support. During the four years she had lectured to hundreds of women, she became convinced that the "shrinking delicacy of their feelings" prevented many women from confiding to any man the real nature of their sufferings.[60] All of the other women lecturers cited above not only continued their interest in the health movement but practiced medicine as physicians. Harriot Hunt, of course, continued her practice in Boston and at the same time increased her feminist activities. Throughout her life she continued to promote the cause of women in medicine, encouraging others to enter the field.[61]

Mary Gove Nichols, rebelling against orthodox medicine, became an avid proponent of hydropathy, or the use of water in the treatment of disease. Ultimately she considered it her duty to enlist women in the cause. As she put it, medical practice "was the last atonement I had to make in the world of duty, and the opening up of a way for me, and for many of my sisters, to come into a world of attraction—that new heaven and new earth wherein dwelleth righteousness." Freed from her disastrous first marriage when Hiram Gove divorced her, she later married a writer, Thomas Low Nichols. Together they enthusiastically taught the water-cure system along with radical views on free love and marriage reform to women and men students enrolled in their various hydropathic institutes.[62]

Lydia Folger Fowler, married to Lorenzo Fowler, a well-known phrenologist, accompanied him on his lecture tours. In 1847 she began to lecture women on anatomy, physiology, and hygiene. Before she entered Central Medical College in Syracuse and became the second woman in the United States to earn the medical degree, Fowler already was widely known as a lecturer in her own right. As Dr. Fowler, she taught at eclectic, physiopathic, and hydropathic medical schools and practiced medicine in New York City.[63]

Martha A. Sawin also studied medicine formally in the 1850s. Later, she established herself in Boston, the first woman graduate physician to practice in that city.[64] Sawin criticized doctors for their failure to furnish women with instruction in physiology and "true scientific knowledge" and complained that the five hundred members of the Ladies' Physiological Institute of Boston had received almost no cooperation from the medical profession. Not all women were interested in medical careers, but many did want and need "General rules of physiology, which physicians *can* give without *injury* to themselves, and with incalculable benefit to Society," she insisted. Those physicians who were genuinely interested in winning public approval could best demonstrate the fact by agreeing to lecture to the membership. Long-range benefits would accrue to the doctors, she observed, for women once in possession of accurate medical information would be in a better position to discriminate between genuine physicians and quacks.[65] Ten years later Elizabeth Blackwell argued the need for a connection between the medical profession and "the every-day life of women" too little affected by medical science. Women physicians, she thought, with their knowledge of the domestic life could bridge this gap by lecturing on physiology and hygiene. This she termed "the first work" for women in the profession.[66]

Sawin and Blackwell were not alone in voicing concern about society's generally uninformed state regarding the laws of health. In 1849 James Gordon Bennett, who had once published the *New York Lancet,* renewed his appeal for medical reform. Public education in medicine, claimed the influential publisher of the *New York Herald,* would provide a remedy for the gross ignorance displayed by physicians practicing among all classes. "Why should not the masses of the people be taught the elements of medical science?" asked Bennett. The basic principles of medicine, he insisted, "should form a part of the system of education in our public schools and in all our seminaries for the instruction of youth of both sexes."[67] Samuel Gregory argued that all women could profit from acquiring a general knowledge of the mechanics of parturition. If they were better informed, the terror and anxiety surrounding childbirth would be greatly allayed, and in emergencies, women would be able to cope until professional help arrived.[68] In an enlightened country, commented another reformer, "all business has a scientific character." Unless women were educated, they could not hope to perform competently any of the duties in which a knowledge of science was essential.[69]

To the uninformed, cults and medical sects with exaggerated and spurious curative claims had great appeal. Orthodox physicians denounced all irregular sects and criticized women especially for patronizing empirics. Dr. Augustus K. Gardner was among those who charged that charlatans grew rich by deceiving women patients, permitting them "to run any risk, and to suffer any calamity which their temerity and ignorance might cause."[70] Quackery, wrote another physician, "in ninety-nine cases out of a hundred," owed its popularity to the women. He further asserted that the most zealous advocates of the new systems of medicine were those who had "an abiding faith in mesmerism" and a proclivity to support extremist religious sects.[71]

Thomas Ewell, ardent champion of female midwifery, was another regular physician who condemned the propensity of modest women to resort to quacks. Medicine, he insisted, was a "rational science"; only trained physicians knew the laws to which the human frame was subject and the proper principles to be applied in the treatment of disease. Ewell cautioned women, for the "respectability" of the profession and for their own good, to avoid empirics and seek out "the man of sound mind who reads the books of the profession, instead of the pliant, finical 'lady's doctor.' "[72]

Yet as P. W. Leland explained to the members of his medical society in 1852, empiricism was the legitimate offspring of the reforming spirit then gripping America. "That spirit comes to us," he noted, "in the voice of a free, thinking, restless multitude, in the fresh exercise of its own great prerogative, untrammeled and eager to question." If the current crop of empirics could be vanquished, he continued, another group, perhaps of a worse sort, would soon appear to replace them. "Even now, looming up in the distance," he warned, "is seen approaching, Madam in boots and *bloomer,* ready to meet you at the portals of life, in order that affected modesty may save her blushes for some less worthy and less holy exposure!"[73]

In a similar resort to the all too familiar weapon of ridicule, another practitioner advised his colleagues to "yield the point in these degenerate days of 'women's rights,' for female doctresses are multiplying, and sick *men,* especially bachelors, are giving preference to the Bloomers and the petticoats. So you gentlemen of the press may as well exercise a 'masterly inactivity' on that subject, for you are doomed to be supplanted by the ladies now crowding into the profession.''[74]

By the late 1840s the various reform crusades in which women were active participants had reached the stage where supporters for the concept of female medical education could be found. For feminists actively enlarging woman's role in American society, campaigns for health reform and the education of women physicians were appealing. The latter not only provided an important and sorely needed service to sisters too modest to confide in men but demonstrated that given the opportunities, women were capable of mastering formal medical studies and displaying the stamina necessary to practice medicine as an occupation.[75]

Not unexpectedly, resistance to women physicians was strong, for society does not readily tolerate challenges to its institutions. Advocates of women's rights, whether they promoted broader education, property rights, job opportunities, suffrage, or less ambitious goals, discovered that whenever they moved into the public spotlight, they invited suspicion and ridicule. The paraphrasing comments of the editor of the *American Medical Gazette* were fairly typical: "When we see or hear a woman lecturing on the rostrum on any subject, we do not expect her to do it well but our marvel is that she can unsex herself by doing it at all."[76]

Public sentiment was mixed. To the degree that women doctors represented the personification of the ideals of higher education and professional work for women, they commanded the support of many but by no means all reformers. Horace Greeley, who termed the domination of obstetrics and gynecology by men "monstrous," predicted that "fifty years hence, it will be difficult to gain credit for the assertion that American women acquiesced through the former half of the nineteenth century, in the complete monopoly of the medical profession by men, even including midwifery, and the diseases peculiar to women."[77] Although sympathetic to feminism, Greeley did not advocate total economic equality. In a letter to Paulina Wright Davis he expressed the view that friends of the movement should set a good example by resolving "never to pay a capable, efficient woman less than two thirds the wages paid to a vigorous, effective man employed in the same corresponding vocation."[78] Abolitionist Gerrit Smith regretted the ridicule heaped upon women for their professional aspirations. He claimed that whether or not they were suited to these positions remained to be determined; in the interim, just as blacks ought to be given a fair field, the same opportunities were owed to women.[79] The first women's medical college in Philadelphia owed much of its early success to the sympathetic support of the Quaker community. In Boston patrons of the Female Medical Education Society included some of the city's richest and most respected citizens, despite Samuel Gregory's propensity for alienating potential friends of the cause.[80]

In 1852 the *Boston Medical and Surgical Journal* reported that several women physicians were enjoying increasingly thriving practices, a fact that "very much surprise[d] the gentlemen." Many had predicted that once the "novelty" wore off, sensible people would drop the women and return to the "legitimate source of medical assistance." These estimates, along with similar ones forecasting the decline of homeopathy, had proved erroneous, volunteered the editor, because of backlash resulting from the profession's intense vocal opposition. More than anything else this, complained the editor, was responsible for the likelihood that "prosperity now awaits" the women.[81] Two years later he reported the public still sympathetic, with financial support flowing in "as it always does upon favorite objects of a public nature in this country."[82]

The profession's lack of enthusiasm for proposals to educate women as doctors was mingled initially with curiosity. The *Boston Medical and Surgical Journal* first objected vehemently to Gregory's school, but after 1853, when members of the Boston Medical Society had begun to teach there, this position was modified. In 1854, for example, when the institution awarded its first medical degrees, the commencement address was delivered by Boston's mayor, Dr. Jerome Van Crowinshield Smith, former editor of the *Journal*. Six years earlier Smith had been in the forefront of the opposition.[83] When the Boston journal reported Harriot K. Hunt's first attempt to gain admission to the Massachusetts Medical College [Harvard], it asked, "Why should not well-educated females be admitted? This is a suitable point to be discussed on some convenient occasion."[84] That same issue revealed that "a young lady [Elizabeth Blackwell] made her appearance in the lecture rooms" of one of the medical colleges. Her presence at Geneva was even reported to have had a salutary effect upon the behavior of the notoriously rowdy medical students of that period.[85]

In spite of the successful example of Blackwell, the profession withheld approval. Blackwell's admission, explained one dean of Geneva Medical College, had been "an *experiment,* not intended as a *precedent.*"[86] The extent of orthodox opposition may be gauged in part by the fact that in the decade of the 1850s only three women, Nancy Talbot Clark, Emily Blackwell, and Marie Zakrzewska, succeeded in following the elder Blackwell's lead by securing admission to regular medical colleges and earning the medical degree there.[87]

The reluctance of the regular colleges to accept women students was unfortunate, for it forced women to accept alternative medical education that was less than satisfactory. Degrees from the sectarian schools were suspect in the eyes of the regulars in any case, and women who held them were doubly branded by those who blocked the path to orthodox medicine. On the other hand, supporters of the concept of women physicians were enthusiastic about Blackwell's achievement. The editor of the *Northern Christian Advocate,* noting the embarrassments to which Blackwell had been subjected while attending a male school, reported approvingly the formation of the Boston Female Medical College. Here was a "laudable enterprise" worthy of Christian philanthropy.

There are hundreds of females in the country who could in no other way be so useful to the world as by qualifying themselves for medical practice among their own sex. . . . All who know any thing of the matter, know full well that the modern practice of medicine too nearly overlooks the distinction of sex, and that there is no remedy for this evil but the medical education of females. Nature suggests it, reason approves it, and religion demands it.[88]

In response to the argument that the qualified obstetrician must have a thorough knowledge of all branches of medicine, proponents of medical training for women shifted their emphasis on mere midwifery to that of providing a complete course of study culminating in the degree of medicine. Gregory and the trustees of the Boston Female Medical College had announced at the outset their intention to offer a full course, but opposition from the profession hampered efforts to obtain the requisite teachers. At first the entire faculty consisted of two regular physicians: Enoch Carter Rolfe, who lectured on obstetrics and the diseases of women and children, and William Mason Cornell, who taught physiology and hygiene.[89] In February 1852 the school came closer to realizing its goal by completing arrangements, not uncommon in the period, for sharing faculty with another institution. The choice of the Female Medical College of Philadelphia, founded in 1850, was unsatisfactory. The arrangement was cumbersome, but more importantly, the Philadelphia faculty included several eclectics, whose presence tainted the Boston school with the suspicion of irregularity. By 1854 Gregory had severed his ties with Philadelphia and added three members of the Massachusetts Medical Society to the faculty. The school ceased to issue midwifery certificates and concentrated on offering a complete course leading to the medical degree. In 1856 a new charter specifically authorized the school to confer the degree and to change the name to the New England Female Medical College. Three years later Gregory added clinical practice, inducing Marie Zakrzewska to leave the Blackwells' New York Infirmary to supervise the clinical department and offer instruction at the college's newly acquired hospital. Between 1854 and 1873, when the New England Female Medical College merged with the new, homeopathic Boston University Medical School, ninety-eight women earned the doctor of medicine degree.

Throughout its history the New England Female Medical College experienced fiscal problems and crises in leadership. Although dedicated to the school, Samuel Gregory was hampered by his lack of medical education, limited vision, and distrust of feminism and its supporters. Yet, for all its defects, his college did offer young women the opportunity to acquire formal medical training at a time when few alternatives existed.[90]

The second college established exclusively for the education of women physicians was the Female Medical College of Philadelphia. As in Boston, opposition from the regular medical community was a serious problem. Badly in need of faculty, the trustees hired three eclectic physicians, thereby incurring still more opposition from the regulars. During its brief "irregular" period from 1850 to 1852, the college granted degrees to seventeen women.[91] In 1853 the eclectics withdrew from the school, whereupon the Female Medical College of Philadelphia embarked upon a course of orthodox instruction from which it did not stray. Under the successive leadership of dedicated and capable educators like Ann Preston, the first woman dean, Rachel Bodley, Clara Marshall, and Martha Tracy, the renamed Women's Medical College of Philadelphia survived fiscal problems and professional hostility.[92]

However, it was the sectarian medical schools that in the decade of the fifties were destined to play the most significant role in the education of women physicians. Just before mid-century, two small eclectic institutions merged to form Central Medical College in Syracuse, New York. The trustees of the New York State Eclectic Association, which founded the school, had not planned originally to enroll women. When several women requested admission, the founders reached what proved to be an historic decision. The same openness that allowed the eclectics to choose the "good" from all systems permitted them to extend their reforming impulses to social questions. Thus in 1849 the trustees adopted a resolution approving the course of action at nearby Geneva and opened Central Medical College to women on a coeducational basis. William Hosmer, the reforming editor of the *Northern Christian Advocate* in neighboring Auburn, hailed the decision: "This is a step worthy of men, and entitles those concerned in it to the lasting gratitude of their country."[93]

Eclectics discussed female medical education repeatedly over the next few years. The resolution they adopted at the semiannual meeting of the New York State Eclectic Medical Society in June 1851 shows their unequivocal dedication to the cause:

Whereas the progress of all reforms in society absolutely demands that no factitious distinction shall be made in the enjoyment of scientific privileges, and in assuming the responsibilities which devolve in consequence thereof: and whereas this principle applies especially to the subject of *Female Education,*

Resolved, That we regard the extension of the privileges of medical education to women as demanded by justice, the necessities of the age, and by the progressive genius of Reform; *nor do we countenance that immodest fastidiousness which would keep them in ignorance and consequent degredation.*[94]

In a commencement address Stephen H. Potter, Dean of the College, reviewed the decision to accept women and reminded his audience of the historic precedent that had been set. With obvious pride Potter observed:

This college was the first medical school in America to open its doors to both sexes and give each *equal* advantages without partiality or hesitation. It is not possible that an act so obviously right in itself, and a step so much in advance of the spirit of the age, will fail to enjoy a conspicuous page in the history of the surprising improvements of the nineteenth century.[95]

Five women attended the first session: Lydia Folger Fowler, well-known lecturer on physiology and hygiene, Rachel Brooks Gleason, Mrs. Montgomery, Miss Taylor, and Fidelia Warren. Fowler and Gleason continued their studies in Rochester, where the school soon transferred. Fowler graduated in June 1850, becoming the second woman in the United States to earn the medical degree. In February 1851 Sarah Read Adamson (later, Dolley) and Rachel Brooks Gleason were awarded the medical degree.[96]

From its inception until its final closing, internal dissension plagued Central Medical College. Several body-snatching incidents, in which students and faculty allegedly participated, strained relations with the local Syracuse citizenry and added to college problems. In January 1850 the *Syracuse Standard* reported the arrest of several instructors and students, following the discovery of a desecrated grave in nearby Navarino. A search of the college rooms yielded three bodies. Among those arrested and charged with stealing corpses for the purpose of dissection was the physician who attended one of the victims prior to his death.[97]

Following the first session in Syracuse in the fall 1849, half of the faculty was dismissed and the remainder of the college moved to Rochester. A college announcement appearing in February cited several advantages of the new location: the larger and more hospitable Rochester population, the use of suitable college buildings, and an available botanical garden. In Rochester the college continued its coeducational policy, but male and female students did not attend all the lectures together. Lydia Folger Fowler, "Principal," and Rachel Brooks Gleason, "Associate," were placed in charge of a new Female Department. There they were to teach "such portions of Anatomy and Midwifery as propriety dictates."[98] The following fall a new announcement claimed that a number of ladies had attended previous terms. When several women indicated an interest in attending the next session, the Board of Trustees retained the Female Department. "Mrs. L. N. Fowler, M.D., who from her spirit of investigations, and scientific and medical acquirements . . . [had] obtained a wide spread and merited popularity," once again was placed in charge of the department, assisted by Mrs. Gleason.[99]

In January 1851 the dismissed Syracuse faction, including Dr. Stephen Hollister Potter, organized a rival eclectic institution, Syracuse Medical College. A college announcement advertised that women would be "admitted to the lectures on the same terms, and enjoy equal advantages with those of the other sex." Emphasizing that the principle of coeducation had been "thoroughly and satisfactorily tested," with the result that "not a doubt remains of the propriety and practicability of educating ladies and gentlemen together," the notice indicated that at least four women planned to enroll for the next session.[100]

Successive reports indicate continued interest among women, although it is not possible to determine whether the fifteen to twenty ladies who would have comprised "the largest number ever collected for Medical Lectures" did in fact materialize for the winter session in 1852.[101] It is known that in March 1851 Margaretta Gleason and perhaps one other woman graduated, and evidence suggests that many others attended sessions. When the school acquired a new five-story building, a separate "ladies dissecting room" was included. Clinical facilities were not available in the town. Interestingly, the eclectic *American Medical and Surgical Journal* reported in May 1851 that two women graduates, Sarah Reed Adamson (later, Dolley) and Margaretta Gleason, had made arrangements to attend the Pennsylvania Hospital (Blockley). Boasted the journal, "They have the honor of being the first female students regularly admitted at any hospital in the Union, but we are sure they will not be the last." Gleason and Adamson studied and practiced obstetrics, gynecology, and pediatrics there unsalaried.[102]

In 1852 Syracuse Medical College absorbed the Rochester school, and the merged institution continued to operate until 1855. The two schools had granted a total of seventy-one degrees by that date. Of these at least eight, and possibly nine, were awarded to women. In his commencement remarks in 1855, Dean Potter proudly stated that beginning with the first session in 1849, "each session had enjoyed the harmonizing and refining influence of women in these halls, and between 40 to 50 others have here been qualified to go forth to benefit and elevate their long neglected and oppressed sex."[103] These "others" presumably did not take the degree, but following the then current practice, probably enrolled as "matriculants" or "hearers" and attended partial courses.

Thus the obscure and short-lived Syracuse Medical College, established by the reforming elements that threatened orthodox medicine, inaugurated its successful policy of coeducational medical training. Eclectic enthusiasm for the medical education of women was not limited to central New York. In the winter 1853 two eclectic physicians, Abraham Liverzey and Joseph Longshore, withdrew under pressure from their teaching positions at the Female Medical College of Philadelphia. Immediately they organized Penn Medical College, chartered in February. Penn was the first totally eclectic institution in Philadelphia, then recognized as the medical capital of the United States. Apparently no women attended the first session, but in the fall 1853 the college opened a separate Ladies' Institute. Dr. Hannah Longshore, graduate of the Female Medical College of Philadelphia, was in charge of anatomical demonstrations. Twenty-one women attended the fall session, but only rarely did they attend classes with men. Just as Central Medical College inaugurated coeducation in medicine, Penn Medical College introduced the principle of coordinate medical education. Until April 1861 one-third of those who took degrees from Penn were women. Through 1864 approximately seventy women graduated from Penn Medical College, more than from any rival institution.[104]

As expected, the medical establishment looked askance at institutions that admitted women students and taught irregular systems. Orthodox journals fell back on ridicule and misrepresentation. The

New York Medical Gazette, erroneously reporting a merger of Penn
Medical College and the Female Medical College of Philadelphia,
editorialized: "We see it suggested that the graduates of this concern, of both sexes, should bear the characteristic title of A. S. S.,
which will have the merit of truth, if it be not poetical. As they will
be the first fruits of this hybrid amalgamation, they will probably
be mulish, and the race soon die out."[105] In September the editor
corrected his mistake about the merger. Abraham Livezey, Dean of
Penn and editor of the *Anti-Lancet,* explained to him the origins of
the eclectic school whose founders were critical of the "illiberal
doctrines and dogmatical dictations" of the Female College.[106]
Explanations such as these, of course, did nothing to stop the attacks.

Hannah Longshore, then on the Penn faculty, charged the
Gazette with opposing in principle the idea of medical education
for women. This drew a sharp reply. The *Gazette* claimed to favor
"medical education of females" and welcomed to the profession
qualified women such as Elizabeth Blackwell. If either female
medical schools or female physicians were worthy of confidence,
they would find it. Continued the editor, the *Gazette* did object to
women "being imposed upon by the medley of ignorance, conceit,
presumption and temerity of such men and women as either of the
Faculties proferring to lead 'silly women' astray, by a mongrel of
so called Chronothermal, Eclectic, Botanic, Physopathic, Homeopathic and Hydropathic quackeries which they falsely dignify with
the title 'Medical Education'." In his opinion the doctors at Penn
Medical College were not properly educated themselves, and "a
medical education worth having" could not be obtained from any
of them. This applied as well to "the 'school' of Dr. Thomas L.
Nichols, and his wife Mary Gove Nichols, at Port Chester [a hydropathic institute that accepted women students]. . . . Both profess
to make doctors, while the teachers in both are ever betraying themselves to be dunces." If Doctor Livezey and his colleagues "were
not the veriest blockheads," he concluded, "they would have perceived, that however desirable Female Physicians are, *they* are not
the men to teach a science which they have yet to learn."[107]

The editor's assessment of the quality of education available in
the sectarian schools may or may not have been justified, but it was
patently unfair to condemn women who attended unorthodox

institutions. Irregular colleges were "reform minded" and willingly accepted women in the belief that women physicians were valuable additions to the community. Wooster Beach's Reformed Medical College in Massachusetts taught "Females as well as males," and in 1855 the National Eclectic Association formally approved coeducation.[108] Sectarian schools encouraged and admitted women, whereas orthodox schools, almost without exception, did neither. Some women who sought training as physicians might have preferred to study orthodox medicine. Their inability to gain admission to regular men's colleges left only the alternatives of sexually segregated schools and those of the irregulars. Regardless of their choice there would be criticism.

It is difficult to determine the soundness of the medical education available to women as compared with that offered men in antebellum America. There is evidence that the instructional quality of the two women's colleges improved after shaky starts. Once the eclectics were dismissed from the Female Medical College of Philadelphia, trustees attempted to upgrade the program by adopting a five-month course of instruction, the longest then offered by any medical school in the country.[109] Harriot Hunt had a poor opinion of the New England Medical College, claiming that its standards had "never been such, as to induce the highest minds to graduate there. The cultivated—thoughtful—go to Philadelphia, if they prefer a Female College, and to Ohio [Cleveland] if a general one."[110]

The journal for the Massachusetts Medical Society, still not enthusiastic about medical education for women, was by 1854 less antagonistic than previously. The seventh session had opened with "a respectable number of students," apparently somewhat younger than in earlier classes. The editor added that "intelligent females, who will take a thorough course of study in this College (and we understand it encourages no other), will be prepared for usefulness in the community, by the practice of their profession."[111] The *New York Medical Gazette* was also more charitable, characterizing Dr. William M. Cornell's introductory lecture as "able and instructive."[112]

In 1855 the directors had brought the school's requirements into line with those of its contemporaries by insisting that students present three years of study with a preceptor and complete a medical thesis for graduation.[113] Even so, Marie Zakrzewska was critical of Gregory's school after she had joined the faculty, complaining of poorly prepared students and refusing to certify several degree candidates at the end of her first year. She finally concluded that "no physician in Boston" would acknowledge her as long as she maintained her connection with the institution.[114] Yet the school was more advanced than many others by making hospital practice available although not required.

Mary Putnam Jacobi continued her education in France after taking the medical degree from the Women's Medical College of Philadelphia. Surveying the history of women in medicine at the close of the century, Jacobi claimed that those associated with the New England Female Medical College had been engaged in "an essentially dishonest affair" because of their ignorance of what constituted legitimate medical education. She further maintained that similar naïveté characterized "all efforts for the isolated medical education of women" between 1850 and 1870.[115]

Elizabeth Blackwell held that separate women's colleges were a mistake, regardless of quality. She believed that among the many advantages accruing to women who could attend regular men's schools was the important association with male doctors and students.[116] Despite this opinion, however, the continued overt discrimination of the men's colleges led her in 1865 to add a woman's college to the New York Infirmary. Blackwell realized that many women were unaware of the limitations of their education until they had left medical school and attempted to practice. "Many of them," she observed, "having spent all their money, abandon the profession; a few gain a little practical knowledge, and struggle into a second-rate position."[117] A similar assessment was offered by an anonymous British author arguing in favor of standardized courses of study and examinations for both sexes. In America, maintained this writer, the women's colleges had been organized hurriedly by people who were ignorant of what should constitute genuine medical education.

Half-measures . . . gained a considerable amount of popular sympathy and support; the schools . . . obtained . . . State recognition, and students have steadily flowed into them; but the meagre curriculum and the low standard of examination—a standard so low that it is said to be difficult for a student *not* to get the M.D. at some of the female schools—sufficiently explain the inferior professional position taken by most of their graduates.[118]

He concluded by insisting that women who wished a thorough medical education "still have to seek it in one of the men's colleges."

Despite the limitations of sexually segregated medical schools and sectarian institutions, their role was obviously crucial. The demands of man midwifery critics and the goals of feminists had both moved closer to realization in the fifties. Had the matter been left to the regular medical profession, the education of women physicians would have been postponed many years. As it turned out, the profession, although capable of hampering the movement, was unable to prevent it. Public distrust of the allopaths' elitism, feminist demands, and the lingering charges of violated decency combined to create a more serious challenge than the profession had yet encountered.

NOTES

1. A portion of this chapter originally appeared in Jane B. Donegan, "Early Medical Coeducation in Central New York," Onondaga County Medical Society *Bulletin* 7 (July 1976):18-22. Reprinted with permission of the editor.

2. Frederick C. Waite, *History of the New England Female Medical College, 1848-1874* (Boston: Boston University School of Medicine, 1950), pp. 11-13.

3. Samuel Gregory, *Letter to Ladies in Favor of Female Physicians* (New York: Fowler and Wells, 1850), p. 5.

4. Waite, *History of the New England Female Medical College,* p. 17.

5. Gregory, *Letter to Ladies,* p. 7.

6. Ibid., pp. 17, 27.

7. Ibid., pp. 20-22.

8. Ibid., p. 39.

9. *Boston Medical and Surgical Journal* (hereinafter referred to as *B.M.S.J.*) 37 (September 29, 1847):184-185.

10. Samuel Gregory, "Letter to the Editor," February 28, 1848, in Ibid., p. 121.

11. *B.M.S.J.* 38 (March 8, 1848):122-123. Seven years later Helen Gassett similarly assessed Gregory's activities. From 1849 to 1851 Gassett had

been employed by Gregory's American Medical Education Society as an agent entrusted with soliciting contributions. In 1851, accused by the society of fraud, she was dismissed. Gassett sued for libel. When her lawsuit foundered, she published a polemic condemning Gregory and his associates, implying that they had made improper use of the funds raised. She claimed that Gregory, as a bachelor without a medical background, was unfit and incompetent to lecture on midwifery. Gassett further accused him of violating propriety in his lectures, especially by exhibiting to his male audiences plates depicting the specifics of man midwifery practices. See Helen M. Gassett, *Categorical Account of the Female Medical College to the People of the New England States* (Boston: Printed for the author, 1855), pp. 92, 110-11.

12. *Fourth Annual Report of the Female Medical Education Society and the New England Female Medical College* (Boston: n.p., 1853), quoted in Frederick C. Waite, "American Sectarian Medical Colleges Before the Civil War," *Bulletin of the History of Medicine* 19 (February 1946):160. Elsewhere Waite noted that the popular press was slightly more enthusiastic about the project than was the medical profession in Boston. See Waite, *History of the New England Female Medical College*, p. 19.

13. Gregory, *Letter to Ladies*, p. 7.

14. "Constitution of the American Medical Education Society," reprinted in ibid., inner cover.

15. Mary Roth Walsh, *"Doctors Wanted, No Women Need Apply": Sexual Barriers in the Medical Profession, 1835-1975* (New Haven and London: Yale University Press, 1977), pp. 50-51, 56-57, 63. Walsh demonstrates convincingly that Samuel Gregory consistently prevented women from participating in the formulation of policy decisions. By limiting women to the roles of student and/or financial supporter, Gregory was never able to capitalize upon the support from Boston feminists that could have ensured the school's success.

16. Waite, *History of the New England Female Medical College*, pp. 112-113, 36-37.

17. Quoted in Agnes C. Vietor, ed., *A Woman's Quest: The Life of Marie E. Zakrzewska, M.D.* (New York and London: D. Appleton and Company, 1924; New York: Arno Press, 1972), pp. 248-249. Most of this book consists of an autobiographical account by Marie Zakrzewska published in 1860 by Caroline H. Dall as *A Practical Illustration of 'Woman's Right to Labor'; or A Letter from Marie E. Zakrzewska, M.D., late of Berlin, Prussia.*

18. Waite, *History of the New England Female Medical College*, pp. 24, 30; Vietor, *Woman's Quest*, p. 249.

19. Quoted in Walsh, *"Doctors Wanted,"* p. 56.

20. "Letter to the Editor on the Practice of Midwifery by Females, written by a member of the class of the Boston Female Medical College," *B.M.S.J.* 41 (August 22, 1849):61.

21. Harriot K. Hunt to O. W. Holmes, Boston, December 12, 1847, and James Walker to Harriot K. Hunt, Boston, January 5, 1848, quoted in Harriot K. Hunt, *Glances and Glimpses; or Fifty Years Social, Including Twenty Years Professional Life* (Boston: John P. Jewett & Co., 1856), pp. 217-218.

22. Ibid., p. 110.

23. Ibid., pp. 135, 151-152.

24. Elizabeth Blackwell, *Pioneer Work for Women* London: J. M. Dent & Sons Ltd.; New York: E. P. Dutton, 1915), p. 21.

25. Ibid., pp. 53-59.

26. Quoted in George Gregory, *Medical Morals* . . . (New York: Published by the author, 1853), p. 7.

27. "Clerical Encouragement of Empiricism," *B.M.S.J.* 41 (August 8, 1849):10-11.

28. See, for example, John R. B. Rodgers, "Annual Address to the New York State Medical Society, 1815," *Transactions of the Medical Society of the State of New York, from its organization in 1807 up to and including 1831,* Vol. 1 (Albany: Van Benthuysen & Sons, 1868), pp. 89-90. An elaboration of the theme of feminine fragility and the middle-class cult of invalidism appears in Barbara Ehrenreich and Deirdre English, *Complaints and Disorders: The Sexual Politics of Sickness* (Old Westbury, N.Y.: The Feminist Press, 1973), pp. 17-32. Medical theories regarding the effect of education on the uterus of the adolescent are examined in Vern L. Bullough and Martha Vought, "Women, Menstruation and Nineteenth-Century Medicine," *Bulletin of the History of Medicine* 47 (January-February 1973):66-82.

29. William Smellie, *A Collection of Preternatural Cases and Observations in Midwifery,* 2nd ed. (London: D. Wilson and T. Durham, 1766), pp. 410-411.

30. John Vaughan, "An Inquiry into the Utility of Occasional Blood-Letting in the Pregnant State of Disease . . ." *Medical Repository* 6 (1803):31-33.

31. Amy Louise Reed, "Female Delicacy in the Sixties," *Century* 90 (October 1915):858.

32. Ibid., p. 859.

33. Joel A. Wing, "On Spinal Irritation," *Transactions of the Medical Society of the State of New York,* Vol. 6 (Albany: Munsell and Tanner, 1844-1846), pp. 79-80.

34. "Presidential Address, June, 1854," *Transactions of the Medical Association of Southern Central New York* (Auburn, N.Y.: W. J. Moses, 1854), pp. 11-12. Another example of the warnings issued is "Additional Letter on Corsets," by the American editor, in Hugh Smith, *Letters to Married Ladies,* 2nd ed. (New York: G. & C. Carvill et al., 1829), pp. 200-206.

35. Elisabeth A. Dexter, *Career Women of America, 1776-1840* (Francestown, N.H.: M. Jones, 1950), pp. 42-43.

36. W[ooster] Beach, *An Improved System of Midwifery Adapted to the Reformed Practice of Medicine . . .* (New York: Scribner, 1851), p. 97.

37. Sarah J. Hale, "An Appeal to American Christians on Behalf of the Ladies' Medical Missionary Society," *Godey's Magazine and Lady's Book* 64 (March 1852):187.

38. Margaretta Gleason, "Medical Education of Women," *American Medical and Surgical Journal* 1 (May 1851):190.

39. Quoted in "M. F. S." to J. V. C. Smith, September 5, 1851, in *B.M.S.J.* 45 (September 17, 1851):139.

40. The patent-medicine business in the nineteenth century is detailed in James H. Young, *The Toadstool Millionaires . . .* (Princeton: Princeton University Press, 1961).

41. *New York Herald,* January 21, 1850.

42. *New York Daily Times,* September 7, 1853.

43. *New York Daily Times,* September 22, 1851.

44. *Thomsonian Botanic Watchman* 1 (December 1, 1834):182, quoted in Joseph F. Kett, *The Formation of the American Medical Profession: The Role of Institutions, 1780-1860* (New Haven and London: Yale University Press, 1968), p. 119. In chapter 4 Kett presents an analysis of various aspects of the Thomsonian system, upon which I have relied heavily. Although he was a botanic physician, Elisha Smith expressed disapproval of "pretended friends of the rights of mothers" who advocated replacing accoucheurs. Claimed Smith, the physician who supported this idea was motivated by his own unwillingness and incompetence to "perform the arduous and responsible duties of a faithful accoucheur and would rather see the female, in all weathers and under all circumstances, leave her family and domestic duties to discharge" those duties that were properly those of doctors. See Elisha Smith, *The Botanic Physician, Being a Compendium of the Practice of Medicine, upon Botanic Principles* (New York: Daniel Adee, 1844), pp. 126-127.

45. Quoted in Martin Kaufman, *Homeopathy in America . . .* (Baltimore and London: The Johns Hopkins Press, 1971), p. 2. In chapter 1 Kaufman gives a useful survey of the heroic practice and its rationale.

46. Benjamin Rush, "On the Means of lessening the Pains and Danger of Child-Bearing, and of Preventing its Consequent Diseases," *Medical Repository* 6 (1803):27-28; Benjamin Rush, "A Defence of Blood-Letting as a Remedy for Certain Diseases," *Medical Inquiries and Observations,* Vol. 4, 2nd ed. (Philadelphia: J. Conrad & Co., 1805), pp. 289, 354. When contractions were weak and the labor prolonged, Rush prescribed opium. In view of the mid-century controversy that developed over the use of anesthesia in childbirth, it is interesting to note that Rush had thought it desirable to locate a "medicine so powerful" that it "might succeed in destroying pain altogether" without impairing the labor. See Benjamin Rush, "On the Means of lessening the Pains and Danger of Child-Bearing . . . ," *Medical Repository* 6 (1803): 30. An overview of Rush's ideas is found in M. Pierce Rucker, "Benjamin Rush, Obstetrician," *Annals of Medical History,* 3rd series, 3 (November 1941): 487-500.

47. Peter Miller, *An Essay on the Means of Lessening the Pains of Parturition* (Philadelphia: Maxwell, 1804), pp. 28-29, 35.

48. William [Potts] Dewees, *An Essay on the Means of Lessening Pain, and Facilitating Certain Cases of Difficult Parturition* (Philadelphia: John Oswald, 1806), pp. 65-66; 95; 2nd ed. (Philadelphia: Thomas Dobson, 1818), p. 129.

49. Kaufman, *Homeopathy,* pp. 23-27.

50. "Annual Announcement of the Eclectic Medical College of Pennsylvania, Session of 1851-52," *American Medical and Surgical Journal* (hereinafter referred to as *A.M.S.J.*) 1 (June 1851):113.

51. B. S. Heath, "What is the Eclectic Medical System of Practice?" *A.M.S.J.* 1 (February 1851):34.

52. Francis R. Packard, *History of Medicine in the United States,* Vol. 2 (New York: Hafner, 1963), p. 1230. Kett, *Medical Profession,* p. 105.

53. *B.M.S.J.* 47 (December 22, 1852):450.

54. Mildred V. Naylor, "Sylvester Graham, 1794-1851," *Annals of Medical History,* 3rd series, 4 (May 1942):236-237.

55. Richard H. Shryock, "Sylvester Graham and the Popular Health Movement," in Richard Shryock, *Medicine in America: Historical Essays* (Baltimore: Johns Hopkins Press, 1966), p. 116.

56. Hunt, *Glances,* pp. 170, 177-179.

57. Ibid., p. 177.

58. George Combe, *Notes on the United States of North America, 1838-39-40* (Philadelphia: n.p., 1841), in Dexter, *Career Women,* p. 44; John B. Blake, "Mary Gove Nichols, Prophetess of Health," *Proceedings of the American Philosophical Society* 106, no. 3 (June 1962), p. 221.

59. Shryock, "Sylvester Graham," p. 117.

60. Paulina Wright Davis to J. V. C. Smith, Providence, January 1850, *B.M.S.J.* 41 (January 6, 1850):521.

61. See Hunt, *Glances,* p. 280; Vietor, *Woman's Quest,* p. 134; Walsh, *"Doctors Wanted,"* p. 33.

62. Blake, "Mary Gove Nichols," pp. 225-229.

63. Frederick C. Waite, "Dr. Lydia (Folger) Fowler, The Second Woman to Receive the Degree of Doctor of Medicine in the United States," *Annals of Medical History,* n.s. 4 (May 1932):294-295.

64. Frederick C. Waite, "Dr. Martha A. (Hayden) Sawin, The First Woman Graduate in Medicine to Practice in Boston," *New England Journal of Medicine* 205 (November 26, 1931): 1053-1055.

65. M. A. Sawin to J. V. C. Smith, Malden, September 20, 1849, *B.M.S.J.* 41 (October 10, 1849):201-202. Mary Gove found physicians helpful as she prepared to lecture to the Boston Physiological Society, in the fall 1838. See Blake, "Mary Gove Nichols," p. 220.

66. Elizabeth Blackwell, *Medicine as a Profession for Women* (New York: Trustees of the New York Infirmary for Women, 1859), pp. 9-10.

67. *New York Herald,* August 12, 1849.

68. Gregory, *Letter to Ladies,* p. 20.

69. William Hosmer, *The Young Lady's Book; or Principles of Female Education* (Auburn & Buffalo, N.Y.: Miller, Orton & Mulligan, 1855), pp. 86-87.

70. Augustus K. Gardner, *A History of the Art of Midwifery: A Lecture Delivered at the College of Physicians and Surgeons, November 11, 1851, Introductory to a Course of Private Instruction on Operative Midwifery . . .* (New York: Stringer and Townsend, 1852), p. 31.

71. "Lady Abettors of Quackery," *B.M.S.J.* 36 (March 10, 1847):128.

72. Thomas Ewell, *Letter to Ladies, Detailing Important Information Concerning Themselves and Infants* (Philadelphia: W. Brown, 1817), p. 32.

73. P. W. Leland, "Empiricism and Its Causes," *B.M.S.J.* 47 (November 3, 1852): 285, 294.

74. "Letter to the Editor," *New York Medical Gazette* 4 (May 1853):232.

75. A number of historians have called attention to the relationship between feminism and health reform. See, for example, John B. Blake, "Women and Medicine in Ante-Bellum America," *Bulletin of the History of Medicine* 39 (March-April 1965):104; Shryock, "Sylvester Graham," p. 117; Walsh, *"Doctors Wanted,"* p. 44.

76. *American Medical Gazette* 10 (August 1859):624.

77. *New York Tribune,* 1853, quoted in Mary Putnam Jacobi, "Woman in Medicine," in Annie Nathan Meyer, ed., *Woman's Work in America* (New York: Holt, 1891), p. 139.

78. *Proceedings of the Woman's Rights Convention, Held at Syracuse, September 8th, 9th, and 10th,* 1852 (Syracuse: J. E. Masters, 1852), p. 10.

79. Ibid., pp. 28-29.

80. *B.M.S.J.* 43 (August 28, 1850):84; Walsh, *"Doctors Wanted,"* pp. 63-64; Vietor, *Woman's Quest,* pp. 256, 272.

81. *B.M.S.J.* 46 (June 23, 1852):425.

82. *B.M.S.J.* 51 (October 25, 1854):263.

83. Waite, *History of the New England Female Medical College,* pp. 34-35.

84. *B.M.S.J.* 37 (December 14, 1847):405.

85. Ibid.

86. A. E. Wager, "Women as Physicians," *The Galaxy* 6 (December 1868):781.

87. Nancy Talbot Clark earned her degree in 1852 at Cleveland Medical College, the medical department of Western Reserve College. See Frederick C. Waite, "Dr. Nancy E. (Talbot) Clark, The Second Woman Graduate in Medicine to Practice in Boston," *New England Medical Journal* 205 (December 17, 1931):1195. Emily Blackwell, who was refused admission at Geneva, finally succeeded in enrolling at Rush Medical College in Chicago in 1852. There she completed the first year's course of lectures. When the Illinois State Medical Society censured the Rush faculty for admitting a woman, Blackwell was refused permission to continue. She, too, enrolled at Cleveland and graduated with distinction in 1854. See Wager, "Women as Physicians," pp. 282-283. Zakrzewska, a Polish-Prussian immigrant befriended by the Blackwells, was an accomplished midwife who under the tutelage of the Professor of Obstetrics at the University of Berlin had become chief of the midwifery school there before emigrating to the United States. In 1856 she, too, graduated from Cleveland. She was so outstanding a student that the faculty paid her an unusual tribute by voting to return the entire $120 she had paid in lecture fees. See Wager, "Women as Physicians," pp. 783-786; Vietor, *Woman's Quest,* pp. 46-50.

88. *Northern Christian Advocate,* May 16, 1849.

89. Waite, *History of the New England Female Medical College,* pp. 18-19.

90. Ibid., pp. 30-36, 82, 87; Vietor, *Woman's Quest,* chapter 13; Walsh, *"Doctors Wanted,"* pp. 35, 82-83.

91. Frederick C. Waite, "Medical Education of Women at Penn Medical University," *Medical Review of Reviews* 39 (June 1933):246; Waite, "Sectarian Colleges," p. 159.

92. Kate Campbell Hurd-Mead, *Medical Women of America* (New York: Froben Press, 1933), p. 55; Gerda Lerner, *The Female Experience: An American Documentary* (Indianapolis: The Bobbs-Merrill Company, Inc., 1977), pp. 408-415.

93. *Northern Christian Advocate,* October 24, 1849.

94. "Resolutions of the New York State Eclectic Medical Society Meeting, Syracuse, New York, June 16, 1851," *A.M.S.J.* 1 (July 1851):132-133.

95. S. H. Potter, "Commencement Remarks, February 22, 1855," *A.M.S.J.* (April 1855):152.

96. Waite, "Dr. Lydia (Folger) Fowler," p. 292.

97. *Syracuse Daily Standard,* January 14, 1850.

98. "Announcement, Central Medical College (Rochester)," *Northern Christian Advocate,* February 13, 1850. Editor Hosmer cited the body-snatching incidents as a contributing factor in the move.

99. *Northern Christian Advocate,* September 11, 1850.

100. *A.M.S.J.* 1 (January 1851):20.

101. *A.M.S.J.* 1 (June 1851):120-120a; 1 (October 1851):204-207.

102. *A.M.S.J.* 1 (October 1851):207; 1 (May 1851):100. Adamson's uncle was Hiram Corson, M.D., a Philadelphia Quaker and pioneer promoter of women physicians. He used his influence to obtain the admissions to Blockley. See Hurd-Mead, *Medical Women,* p. 43. Margaretta Gleason's husband was a physician in Philadelphia. See Waite, "Dr. Lydia (Folger) Fowler," p. 292.

103. Waite, "Dr. Lydia (Folger) Fowler," pp. 291-293; Waite, "Sectarian Colleges," pp. 157-158; Potter, "Commencement Remarks," p. 152. Waite used medical college announcements, catalogs, and journals as sources, but found the files scattered and incomplete. Many students, perhaps half of the total enrolled, were "matriculants" or "hearers," who attended partial courses. In some cases students enrolled but never attended courses. Both the New England Female Medical College and the Women's Medical College of Philadelphia also permitted students to attend lectures, even if they did not plan to work toward the doctor of medicine degree.

104. Waite, "Medical Education of Women," pp. 256-260; Waite, "Sectarian Colleges," p. 161.

105. *New York Medical Gazette* 4 (July 1853):332.

106. *Anti-Lancet* 1, quoted in *New York Medical Gazette* 4 (September, 1853):410-411.

107. *New York Medical Gazette* 4 (September 1853):411-412.

108. *B.M.S.J.* 47 (December 22, 1852):450; Waite, "Sectarian Colleges," p. 158.

109. James R. Chadwick, "The Study and Practice of Medicine by Women," *International Review* 7 (October 1879):460.

110. Hunt, *Glances,* pp. 271-272.

111. *B.M.S.J.* 51 (November 22, 1854):347.

112. *New York Medical Gazette* 5 (September 1854): 39. In his preceding

introductory lecture, Cornell had stated that the lecturers associated with the school would permit the graduation of only those who had attended the full course. He indicated a willingness to permit the counselors of the Massachusetts Medical Society to serve as an examining committee. See *B.M.S.J.* 49 (December 21, 1853):419.

113. Waite, *History of the New England Female Medical College,* p. 30.

114. Vietor, *Woman's Quest,* pp. 272-273, 277.

115. Jacobi, "Woman in Medicine," p. 146.

116. Blackwell, *Pioneer Work,* p. 192.

117. Quoted in Jacobi, "Woman in Medicine," p. 163.

118. "Women Physicians," *Macmillan's Magazine* 18 (September 1868): 370.

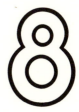

Resistance and Change

We have no sympathy with the hue and cry about 'woman's rights,' 'woman's degradation' and the like. . . . If the Almighty did not intend that woman should occupy a subordinate place, why . . . wasn't Adam given to Eve, instead of Eve to Adam?

—OHIO MEDICAL AND SURGICAL JOURNAL, 1849

Too much has already been said and written about woman's sphere. . . . The widening of woman's sphere is to improve her lot. Let us do it, and if the world scoff, let it scoff . . . So the first female physician meets many difficulties, but to the next the path will be made easy.

—LUCY STONE, NATIONAL WOMAN'S CONVENTION, 1855

Early in the 1850s the Philadelphia physician Dr. Hannah Longshore called upon a druggist for a prescription that she had ordered for a patient. The druggist not only refused to fill the prescription but reproved her by advising that she go home and darn her husband's stockings.[1] Sexist incidents such as this were all too common in the experience of those with the audacity to challenge established male-defined convictions of what constituted woman's role. Medical women trod "a new, true, elevating path"[2] leading away from the narrowly circumscribed "woman's sphere" of home and family into a larger world of action, ideas, and competition. In their search for autonomy they invited criticism and abuse. For the pioneers of the fifties their position was often an anomalous one in which, as Elizabeth Blackwell remarked, they stood "alone in medicine—so often opposed or ignored by the profession, not acknowledged by society, and separated from the usual pursuits and interests of women."[3]

Yet medical women were not totally without allies, for some reformers were anxious to enlarge women's opportunities. The early feminists who asserted sexual equality as a natural right insisted upon a redefinition that pushed women beyond the "circumscribed limits which corrupt customs and a perverted application of the Scriptures" had marked out for them. Participants at the Rochester Convention, held in the aftermath of the historic Seneca Falls Convention of 1848, saw in the "persevering and independent course" of Elizabeth Blackwell "a harbinger of the day when woman" would stand forth "redeemed and disenthralled," able to "perform those important duties which . . . [were] truly within her sphere."[4] Not all of the women who sought access to medical knowledge were motivated by the same reasons. Nevertheless, by demanding not only the right to learn medicine but the right to practice it professionally as well, they were tangible examples of feminist principles translated into action.

Mindful of the value of sisterhood, proponents of the women's movement stressed unity and the need to continue their support of women doctors. In 1852 the Syracuse Woman's Rights Convention urged all sympathizers to employ "the woman physician, phrenologist, [and] artist, rather than a man." A similar meeting the following year at the Broadway Tabernacle in New York City reiterated the right of "each human being" to be the "sole judge of his or her sphere, entitled to choose a profession without interference from others." The group urged supporters to help in reshaping public opinion so that it would no longer be considered "indecorous for women to engage in any occupation which they deem[ed] fitted to their habits and talents."[5]

The women who entered medicine in this period had little choice but to limit themselves to the two branches in which they were most likely to gain acceptance: obstetrics and the treatment of the diseases of women and children.[6] Although reactionary opponents of man midwifery had little sympathy for radical feminism, they were unwitting allies in the sense that they supported the idea of training women as physicians. The practice of obstetrics by women physicians promised an eventual end to the obnoxious man midwifery, against which reactionaries had battled unsuccessfully for so long. The restoration of obstetrics to women—as either midwives or physicians—carried with it the prospect that "greedy" and "licentious" men could be eliminated from the field. "Woman's sphere" could then be redefined along reactionary lines, that is, to include control of obstetrics as it once had in the eighteenth century. This accomplished, the nation presumably would resume its proper moral course, each of the sexes functioning with propriety untarnished, and the special spheres of man and woman intact.[7]

The overwhelming majority of male physicians were unalterably opposed to permitting women to enter medicine, even with the understanding that the women would concentrate on obstetrics and gynecology. The belief that the profession was overcrowded was partly, but not entirely, responsible. Physicians reflected the social norms of society; most men and probably most women found the idea of women physicians incongruous. Woman's place was said to be naturally and divinely ordained. Her "innate" physiological, intellectual, and emotional characteristics were deemed insurmountable obstacles to successful medical study and subsequent professional practice. Some doctors chose to ignore women's efforts hoping that eventually the notion would founder and disappear. A considerable number, however, did feel somehow compelled to justify their exclusion of women.

Before the polemic over women physicians had taken shape, however, an event occurred in western New York State that for many threatened (or promised) prompt restoration of all obstetrical practice to women. The ramifications of the incident were felt throughout the profession and vividly illustrate not only the concerns of physicians caught up in early Victorian prudishness, but the way in which doctors effectively met the challenge to their medical monopoly.

Early in January 1850 Dr. James Platt White, Professor of Obstetrics at Buffalo Medical College, introduced to American medicine a highly controversial teaching variation that soon became known as "demonstrative midwifery." In order to give his students practical knowledge of the birth process, White arranged to have his entire class attend an actual delivery. Before taking action, he shared his plan with colleagues on the faculty and received their unqualified approval, as the *Buffalo Medical Journal* reported in March 1850. Mary Watson, a twenty-six-year-old Irish immigrant then an inmate of the Erie County Poor House, unwed and pregnant with her second child, agreed to serve as the professor's subject. Subsequently she received ten dollars from White, although this had not been part of the original agreement.[8]

Shortly before her confinement, Mary Watson was housed in the basement of the college, adjacent to the janitor's apartment. In the days immediately prior to the onset of labor, Dr. White permitted students to make abdominal stethoscopic examinations of the fully clothed patient to hear intrauterine sounds. During the labor, students under White's supervision also made tactile vaginal examinations.[9] As the fetal head was about to emerge from under the pubic arch, the class of twenty students and several invited physicians entered the room to observe. Dr. White then partially removed the patient's clothing to demonstrate the correct technique of applying support to the perineum. Students later testified that although the patient had been exposed for two to five minutes, they were not aware of any exposure of the genital organs, since the professor had covered the perineum with napkins while applying support. Mary Watson's labor and delivery were natural, and at no time did she complain of her treatment.[10]

Following the delivery, White's students expressed gratitude to their professor and pride in the fact that the University of Buffalo had been the first American medical school to introduce clinical instruction in midwifery.[11] On February 19 the *Buffalo Commercial Advertiser* carried an editorial supporting the innovation. On February 27, however, the *Buffalo Courier* published an anonymous article criticizing Dr. White for demonstrating the process of childbirth on a live subject. Dr. White had admittedly been present during the labor, but, commented the author, "Delicacy forbids me to touch upon the manner in which these [eight] hours were passed. Suffice it to say that the tedium was relieved by such methods, as a congregation of boys would know well how to employ." The experiment had permitted students "their salacious stare" to satisfy a "meretricious curiosity" at Mary Watson's expense. He pronounced the whole episode irregular and an outrage to public decency.[12]

Horatio N. Loomis, a Buffalo physician, agreed so completely with this assessment that he paid for the printing of additional copies of the article, which he distributed to patients and friends. In response, White and his colleagues sued Loomis for libel. In April the Buffalo Grand Jury handed down an indictment, and in June the case of *The People* versus *Doctor Horatio N. Loomis* was tried before the Court of Oyer and Terminer. The jury eventually returned a verdict of not guilty.[13]

The Buffalo experiment and the attendant notoriety provoked bitter controversy within the profession. In March 1850 John Hanenstein and sixteen other doctors from the Buffalo area sent a letter to the editor of the *Buffalo Medical Journal* challenging the need for demonstrative midwifery. White's experiment merited severe rebuke, they contended, because it was "wholly unnecessary for the purpose of teaching, unprofessional in manner, and grossly offensive alike to morality and common decency." They hoped for the sake of the medical profession that such an "exhibition" would not be repeated in Buffalo "or in any civilized community."[14]

Reaction to such criticism was prompt. Austin Flint, Professor of Theory and Practice of Medicine at Buffalo and editor of the *Buffalo Medical Journal,* replied that the demonstration "commend[ed] itself to the cordial approbation of the medical profession." The *Boston Medical and Surgical Journal* agreed, applauding the innovation and pointing out that clinical instruction in obstetrics, although new to American medical schools, was common in the lying-in hospitals of Europe. It was regrettable, commented the editor, that some doctors had objected. Similar sentiments were expressed by the editor of the *New York Journal of Medicine,* who pronounced Dr. White's course of action "honorable, high-minded, and judicious." In the past, he recalled, physicians had opposed innovation. The use of the stethoscope and the speculum had been disputed, and there had been "more than bitter persecution" visited upon the early accoucheurs. "We regret to learn," he continued, "that among the members of our own profession there is even one who retains a mite of the semblance of bygone days in this respect." The *Louisville Medical Journal* took a dim view of the "prudish Miss Nancies of Buffalo." Commented that publication: "We can easily imagine a childlike simplicity that would put pantelets upon the legs of a piano and that would screen with a veil every thing capable of exciting prurient ideas, but we do not like to see this excessive flirtation with modesty, introduced into medical teaching."[15]

During the course of the Loomis libel trial, presiding Judge Mullett attempted to put the question in perspective. He acknowledged the propriety of all legitimate means employed by practitioners, even when their use might suggest an offense to modesty and moral delicacy. To safeguard her health and preserve the happiness of those dependent upon her, he observed, a woman must turn to her physician. In doing so, however, she did not surrender her claims to modesty, delicacy, or sensibility. "These guardians of female virtue may be compelled to step back for the occasion," he noted, "but they stand around her like Diana's Nymphs while she is bathing; let the practitioner make one significant manifestation of an unholy thought, and they rally around the insulted one." Surely the defendant, as an honorable member of the profession, must realize that those who stood at the bedside of a woman in the agonizing throes of parturition did not harbor libidinous thoughts. They could feel only pity and sympathy for those who faced danger and often death in childbirth. If the imputations of impure thought were in fact true, he pointed out, they would be as true of students the day after graduation as they were the day before. "Miserable indeed would be the relations between the public and that highly useful profession," he concluded, "if such suspicion had any foundation in truth."[16]

The conclusion of the Loomis trial did not put an end to the debate. Chandler Gilman expressed alarm over the effects of the public controversy on the profession. He believed that demonstrative midwifery had merit and was as important to students as clinical instruction in surgery. The principal question was whether physicians could win acceptance of any innovation without offending public opinion. Recalling the charges of indelicacy and impropriety raised against physicians who introduced the vaginal speculum, and noting the continued criticism of men in the fields of obstetrics and gynecology, he insisted that every physician needed to prove to the public that his motives were above reproach. He warned:

It is the motive with which he acts that is to be his defence; and if this defence will not avail demonstrative midwifery, neither will it avail the use of the speculum, the attendance of a male obstetrician, or in fact any prescribing by a man for the sexual diseases of females. All must stand or fall together.[17]

In the *New York Medical Gazette,* the editor noted his sympathy for Gilman's uneasiness. If any impropriety had been involved in the Buffalo situation, the writer said, the public spotlight would soon provide a remedy. "If not," he predicted, "it will be a God-send to the project of transferring obstetric practice to the other sex, for whom medical schools are now *in limine* at Boston and Philadelphia."[18]

As expected, the critics of man midwifery found support for their cause in the Buffalo experiment. William Hosmer charged in the August 14, 1850, issue of the *Northern Christian Advocate* that the incident was only one specific abuse in a long list of objectionable practices that should result in returning obstetrical practice to women. Both groups of physicians, those who favored demonstrative midwifery and those who argued vehemently against it, were agreed on one point: The glare of publicity growing out of the Buffalo episode threatened the continuance of man midwifery.

A number of physicians critical of the Buffalo experiment admitted that some form of clinical instruction in obstetrics was desirable. Perhaps, observed the editor of the *New York Medical Gazette,* some of White's critics would have been disarmed had the adjective "clinical" been applied to his instruction rather than the unfortunate "demonstrative." He saw value in the teaching device, provided that instructors and students observed decorum and maintained correct attitudes. It was certain that any student who entertained the notion that "levity or any unworthy associations" were connected with childbirth would soon have them dispelled by what he witnessed when actually present in a lying-in chamber![19] Another physician, who preferred to remain anonymous, write to the *Buffalo Medical Journal* in support of the continuation of clinical teaching. Alluding to the "embarrassment and fright" experienced by young physicians on their first obstetrics cases, he detailed his own baptism:

I was left alone with a poor Irish woman and one crony, to deliver her child . . . and I thought it necessary to call up before me every circumstance I had learned from books. . . . I must examine, and I did—but whether it was head or breech, hand or foot, man or monkey, that was defended from my uninstructed finger, by the distended membranes, I was as uncomfortably ignorant, with all my learning, as the foetus itself that was making all this fuss. [20]

Fortunately, the woman's labor was a normal one, and the doctor was showered with praise for his part in it. As he sat grinning, happy to have "escaped commission of murder," however, new complications arose. The placenta did not come away by itself; although he cautiously attempted its removal, he failed. Luckily for his patient, the doctor's former preceptor dropped by, "and with five words of *clinical demonstrative* instruction, every difficulty was removed." [21]

"C. M." took still a different view. The proliferation of medical schools had created such keen competition that in their efforts to survive, some schools lured students with "specious exhibitions *miscalled* 'Clinical Instruction.'" Genuine clinical instruction was indispensable, he maintained, but could only be obtained at a patient's bedside. This was best acquired when students attended the hospital wards or worked in the practice of a good preceptor. The aspect of the White demonstration most damaging to the profession was that the so-called "*improvement* . . . consisted in subjecting the process of parturition to ocular inspection in one of its stages." Although he did not feel that the demonstration had incited "libidinous emotions" in White's students, this was really beside the point. Dr. White should not have exposed his patient at all. In practice, physicians almost never resorted to ocular assistance in cases of parturition; when they conducted vaginal examinations, they "instinctively" closed their eyes, both out of feelings of delicacy and to improve their powers of concentration. It was therefore very wrong to teach students to employ vision in such cases, for they would be likely to carry this over into their own practices. American women, he warned, would never tolerate this impropriety, and he reminded readers of the not too distant past "when the very presence of a male practitioner in the house was scarce endured." [22]

Equally distressing was Chandler Gilman's testimony at the Loomis trial, continued this critic. Gilman had admitted that when he was required to turn a fetus in utero, it was his custom "to expose the woman entirely." A practice such as this, particularly when performed in the presence of students, "might well result in a public reaction against accoucheurs," he predicted.[23] The *New York Medical Gazette* agreed that exposure of the patient was "*never* necessary" and could not be condoned. "Catheterism, vaginal exploration, manipulations . . . whether manual or instrumental, delivery by the forceps and embryotomy itself, can all be performed by a competent man as well without the eye as with it." If this were not so, remarked the editor, "then should we hail the new project of educating female accoucheurs, and transferring all such practice to the other sex, as the dictate of propriety and good sense."[24]

In view of the furor demonstrative midwifery created and the dire forecasts of practitioners regarding the future of male-dominated obstetrical practice, it is not surprising that the American Medical Association addressed itself to the innovation. At its third annual meeting in Cincinnati in 1850, the association adopted a resolution calling for an investigation to ascertain whether "any practicable scheme" might be devised "to render instruction in midwifery more practical than it has hitherto been in the medical schools."[25]

The next annual meeting, held in Charleston in the spring of 1851, was evidently a stormy one. The resolution calling for an investigation of the merits of demonstrative midwifery had been referred to the Committee on Medical Education rather than to the Committee on Obstetrics. This caused ill feeling. Members of the latter committee concluded their report by observing that they had omitted discussion of the issue. After noting that the medical journals had reviewed the Buffalo experiment "in a very able manner," they added with some bitterness that "however desirous your committee may have felt to express their views upon a subject of so much interest, the fact that its consideration was referred, by a vote of this Association, to another committee, reminded them that their opinion was not only not asked for, but cannot be desired."[26]

For its part, the Committee on Medical Education chose to submit a separate report on demonstrative midwifery, which it appended to its regular report. After making the observation that this topic, if discussed at all, should more properly have been considered by the Committee on Obstetrics, the education committee proceeded to review the facts surrounding the Buffalo controversy. The patient had freely consented to the demonstration. Witnesses differed on the amount of exposure to which she had been subjected as the fetal head emerged from the os externum, but the committee felt this was unimportant. The real issue, which warranted discussion in a "calm, considerate and dignified manner," was whether any exposure of a woman patient was ever necessary.[27]

The committee outlined the four major contentions of the advocates of demonstrative midwifery: (1) the student witnessed the child emerge from under the pubic arch; (2) he was visually impressed with the need to support the perineum; (3) he could have immediately demonstrated to him the exact manner in which this support was to be given; and (4) the student received visual verification of the professor's diagnosis relative to type of presentation. In essence, the committee rejected all of these. There was no need for students to use a live subject, for the manner in which the fetus emerged from the os externum could easily be demonstrated on mannequins and was thoroughly pictured on plates. Any student who failed to be convinced by his preceptor of the importance of supporting the perineum was too dull and irresponsible to become a doctor. Inasmuch as this support normally was given without utilizing vision, there was no point in permitting the student to observe the procedure. And finally, verification of the professor's diagnosis of presentation could be accomplished by touch, or the student could take the professor's word for it. When one compared true clinical instruction under the supervision of a preceptor with demonstrative midwifery, continued the report, it was obvious that the former provided instruction that the latter could not. Demonstrative midwifery, pronounced the committee, was "unnecessary" and "incompetent."[28]

It was unfortunate, observed the committee, that there existed an erroneous but widespread belief that women were asked to sacrifice their modesty in order to be treated for gynecological ailments. It was woman's duty to submit to proper treatment when necessary, and no necessary treatment could be considered immodest. There had been cases, acknowledged the report, where doctors had employed the vaginal speculum without justification. Such instances had tended to embarrass honorable physicians and their patients,

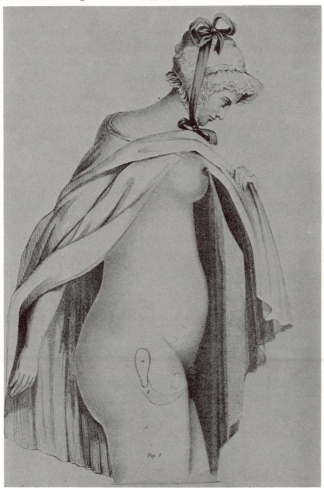

These plates, taken from a medical text widely used in the nineteenth century, depict the various stages of pregnancy utilizing cutaway sections superimposed on the main model. In the absence of clinical instruction, young physicians often were forced to rely upon illustrations such as these to fill the gaps in their obstetrical education.—From G. Spratt, *Obstetric Tables*, London, 1848. (Courtesy of the State University of New York Upstate Medical Center Library.)

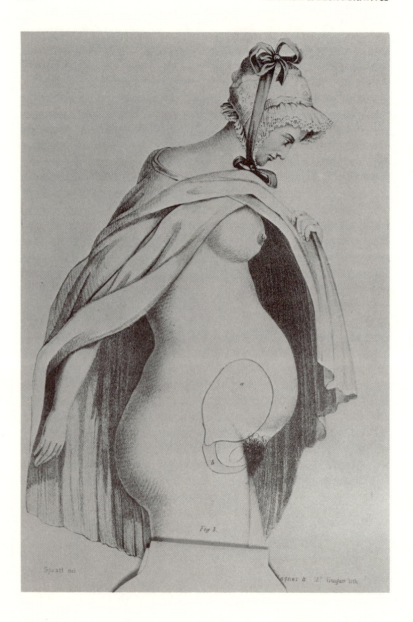

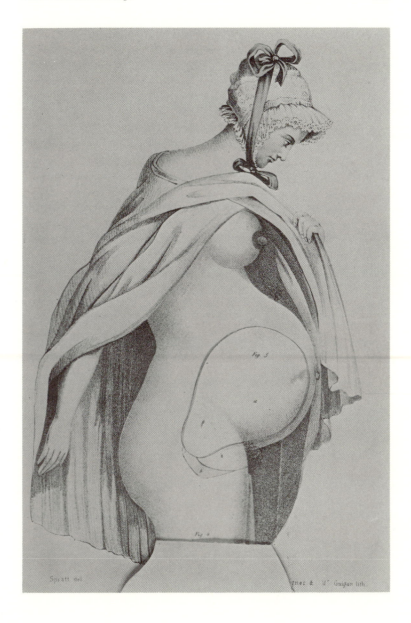

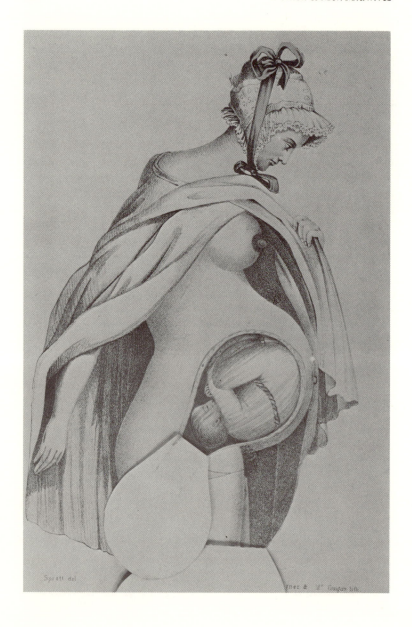

for unnecessary treatment was always immodest. Nor could the committee countenance the lecture-room practice of making "indecent allusions" about the relations between physicians and their female patients. This pandering to the "depraved taste" of students did serious injury to the profession. It was of the utmost importance, cautioned the committee, that the confidential relationship between patient and doctor remain unimpaired. "The object both of the individual practitioner and of the profession, should be to meet most fully the demands of science and humanity, and yet not offend a sensitive, but rational delicacy, nor give countenance to an unblushing shamelessness."[29]

Unnecessary treatment, demonstrative midwifery, and failure on the part of physicians to observe the proprieties were all responsible for the prevailing public prejudice against employing men in obstetrics and gynecology, warned the committee.

Indelicate practices had given rise to the project for training female practitioners of medicine. The project will for obvious reasons, be unsuccessful . . . chiefly because the community generally will be convinced that, although some physicians are guilty of transgressing the rules of propriety and modesty in their intercourse with their patients, medical men, as a body are pure-minded men, and . . . their honour, as well as their skill, is worthy of the public.[30]

Regrettably, it is not possible to learn what was said during the debate that followed presentation of the committee's report. On June 15, 1851, the *New York Medical Gazette* informed its readers that the committee's comments were "discussed with some degree of ardor and sensitiveness." In any case, the delegates to the Fourth Annual Meeting adopted unanimously a resolution approving the opinions expressed in the report.

Demonstrative midwifery had provoked "a warfare in medical journals in newspaper style," and the profession's central body had rejected the innovation. In doing so, doctors had recognized that the controversy threatened the reputation of the entire profession at a time when its claim to the practice of obstetrics and gynecology was being challenged publicly. The position of the American Medical Association in 1851 served as a portent for the future. In the ensuing decade physicians, conscious of a fully mounted attack in the form of projects to educate women physicians, mustered their forces in a successful effort to preserve their domain. This need not imply that physicians acted solely out of selfish motives, although self-interest did play a large part. Given the idealized picture of nineteenth-century woman, doctors could advance many culturally acceptable arguments in support of their contention that there was no place for women in medical practice.

In 1847 Elizabeth Blackwell's admission to medical school focused attention not only on this extraordinary young woman but also on Geneva Medical College. By enrolling a woman, Geneva had earned title, as the *Buffalo Medical Journal* pointed out, "to the distinction, meritorious or otherwise, of first practically exemplifying the experiment of opening the door of medical instruction to a female." Sensitive to criticism and unwilling to perpetuate the example, the school did not admit another woman until 1863.[31] Blackwell's conduct had not created a scandal. From the journal kept during her residence in the small rural community, it is evident that she was conscious of the importance of her precedent-setting study. Determined to keep her personal behavior above reproach, she succeeded by keeping very much to herself when not attending classes, finally winning the admiration of teachers and classmates. So many doctors had dismissed her venture as mere caprice, assuming that she would fail to complete the course once the novelty had worn thin, that Blackwell's graduation in January 1849 occasioned great interest. Geneva's president called her up alone to the platform and conferred the doctor of medicine upon "domina Blackwell." After thanking him for his remarks, she replied, "It shall be the effort of my life . . . to shed honour on my diploma."[32]

Writing to the editor of the *Boston Medical and Surgical Journal,* "D. K." termed the ceremony a farce. "If a clique of pseudo-reformers, or some mushroom Thomsonian or hydropathic association had conferred this degree," it would have come as no great surprise. It was lamentable that Geneva Medical College, an orthodox school, had been "the first to commence the nefarious process of amalgamation," which disregarded that "intuitive sense of propriety" inducing "all civilized nations to regard the professions of law, medicine and divinity as masculine duties." Blackwell's course in seeking "laurels in forbidden paths" could not be justified "by any urgent necessity." Added the writer candidly, "The profession was quite too full before, and could well dispense with her services."[33] The *Ohio Medical and Surgical Journal* was equally antagonistic. A door had been opened and a precedent set. What would hinder other women from "unsexing" themselves in a similar manner, wondered the editor? Possibly no harm had been done in this particular instance, but he hoped fervently "that this, the first, will be the last case of the kind we shall have to record."[34]

In November 1850 Harriot K. Hunt, who had continued her medical practice in Boston after Harvard's refusal to admit her to its medical lectures, tried again to gain admittance. Her new letter of application addressed to the "Gentlemen of the Medical Faculty" asked them to consider the "progress of the age" in reaching their decision. Asserting that public sentiment in favor of women physicians was on the increase, she asked pointedly whether it should be "mind, or sex" that determined the issue. She denied the validity of a sexist discrimination that would prevent "the perception of woman" from being joined "with the reflection of man." "*Sex,*" she insisted, "will never be felt where science leads, for the atmosphere of thought will be around every lecture." Less than a month later she received the welcome reply. Oliver Wendell Holmes, Dean of the Faculty, communicated the faculty's decision to admit Hunt to the medical lectures, indicating however that there was no commitment to grant a degree.[35]

Shortly thereafter, the medical students intervened "to preserve the dignity" of Harvard by presenting the faculty with six resolutions of protest. No "woman of true delicacy" would subject herself to the embarrassment of attending medical lectures in the company of men. They claimed that they were not opposed to permitting woman to exercise her rights but could not sanction any woman to appear "in places where her presence is calculated to destroy our respect for the modesty and delicacy of the sex." Calling upon their professors to rescind the decision, they warned that the innovation was not only detrimental to the college but threatening to its very existence.[36] In the face of such resistance, Hunt withdrew her application. The *Boston Medical and Surgical Journal* approved the students' position: Women who wished to become doctors or to assume other "masculine professions" should attend separate colleges.[37]

Various other obstacles faced women who sought careers in medicine. Professional opposition made it difficult to find registered physicians willing to act as preceptors. The wives or daughters of physicians were fortunate in this regard. Elizabeth Blackwell was encouraged by Quaker physicians, and the Friends remained sympathetic to women. Some women who earned the medical degree and went into practice took on private students, as Dr. Martha A. Sawin did in Boston. Sectarian physicians, reflecting the liberal attitudes of their reform theories, were amenable to accepting women students. The nine women matriculants at the Syracuse Medical College from 1854 to 1855 had studied with a total of six different preceptors.[38] Probably most of these were eclectics.

When Elizabeth Blackwell returned from Europe and attempted to establish a practice on University Place in New York City, she encountered opposition on all sides. She worried constantly about money; the medical profession shunned her; society suspected her; and she sometimes received insolent letters. When she applied for a physician's place in the women's department of the New York Dispensary, she was refused and advised to form her own.[39]

Unable to prevent entirely the education of women as physicians, the medical societies refused to admit them to membership. In 1853 Dr. Nancy Talbot Clark, then practicing in Boston, applied for admission to the Suffolk County Medical Society. The members were thrown into "dreadful consternation," particularly as one of the society's by-laws imposed a fine of $400 upon any censor who refused to admit a qualified applicant. The Massachusetts Medical Society, to which the problem was referred, inserted "male" before the word "applicant," and Dr. Clark was denied admission. Not until 1881 did the Massachusetts Medical Society admit a woman.[40]

In 1858 the censors of the Philadelphia County Medical Society, replying to introduced resolutions that proposed the admission of women, recommended that the members of the regular profession "withhold from the faculties and graduates of the female medical colleges, all countenance and support; . . . they cannot, consistently with sound medical ethics, consult or hold professional medical intercourse with their professors or alumnae." Attempts by the Montgomery County and Lancaster Medical societies to have the censors' action repealed were unsuccessful.[41] The New York-based *American Medical Gazette* protested that such advertised ostracism was unwise, claiming that it created additional support for women doctors and their teachers. The New York Medical Society had not "declared war upon the windmill" nor would it, observed the *Gazette.*[42] All the same, this society admitted no women as members.

The antagonism persisted into the postbellum era. In 1872 D. W. Yandell, president of the American Medical Association, defended the right of women to practice medicine if limited to certain specialties. It was up to the public to decide whether or not women should practice, he maintained.

If they want women doctors, such will be found ready to meet the demand. If those now pressing forward in their studies so eagerly, find their services are not wanted, they will take down their signs, get married—if they can— or turn to lecturers, or to some more lucrative employment. I hope they will never embarrass us by a personal application for seats in this Association. I could not vote for that.[43]

In 1859 the *American Medical Gazette,* noting a vacancy in the surgery chair at the Female Medical College of Philadelphia, sarcastically proposed the candidacy of a Mrs. Lodge, M.D. The Brooklyn woman, charged the *Gazette,* "has proved her surgical skill, by destroying a mother and her unborn twins, by female doctoring, a few days since."[44] The implication is clear and suggests another obstacle that faced women physicians of the period. Abortionists advertised openly in the press, usually styling themselves "female physicians." Among the most notorious was Madame Restell, of whom Elizabeth Blackwell observed:

She was a woman of great ability and defended her course in public papers. She made a large fortune, drove a fine carriage, had a pew in a fashionable church and though often arrested, was always bailed out by her patrons. She was always known distinctively as a 'female physician,' a term exclusively applied at the time to those women who carried on her vile occupation.[45]

To Blackwell it seemed "a horror" that the term, which she hoped would "become a noble position for women," had been so corrupted.[46] Both the *New York Sun* and the *New York Herald* accepted advertisements from abortionists, although Horace Greeley's *Tribune* did not. In 1841 Greeley took his rivals to task for accepting "blood-money," but the practice continued.[47] The *New York Journal of Medicine,* reporting in 1845 an increase in the percentage of stillbirths and premature births in New York spanning a decade, implied that the rise was due to "the operations of Madam Restell, Costello, and their collaborators." At mid-century the *New York Medical Gazette,* under the heading "Female Doctors," observed that a woman lecturer and her husband [Mary Gove Nichols and Thomas L. Nichols] had begun to conduct a "hydropathic establishment" in the city. New York, commented the *Gazette,* until recently had not heard much about female physicians, except for " 'Madam Restell' and other abortionists."[48]

In Boston Abby Crocker, described as "a female physician [who] studied in Boston but did not graduate," was implicated in a case of suspected abortion. Although the charges against her were dismissed for lack of evidence, Samuel Gregory was quick to inform readers of the *Boston Medical and Surgical Journal* that Crocker had never attended New England Female Medical College.[49]

Nor was it any easier for women doctors to escape the taint in Philadelphia. A physician who supported medical education for women that would give them exclusive control over obstetrics claimed that critics had leveled abortionist charges against the graduates of the Female Medical College of Philadelphia. He personally doubted the validity of the accusations but pointed out that even if they were true, they would merely be illustrative of "a good cause misrepresented and abused."[50]

When Dr. Horatio R. Storer published his book on criminal abortion in 1860, he pointedly disclaimed any intention of inciting prejudice against either midwives or "female physicians" or of advocating their general suppression. He noted, nevertheless, that women attendants were in a favored position to act as abortionists, owing to "their relations to women at large, their immunities in practice, the profit of this trade, [and] the difficulty, especially from the fact that they are women, of insuring their conviction."[51]

To what extent the graduates of medical colleges conducted abortions cannot be documented. Both sexes appear to have had their share of illegal practitioners to whom leisure-class women suffering from the "female complaint" of unwanted pregnancy could resort when the popularly advertised abortion-inducing drugs, uterine probes, and spring catheters failed to resolve their "female problem." The medical profession, by concentrating its charges on women, of course, cast suspicion upon the entire movement to train them in medicine. Once thrown out, accusations and insinuations such as those made by Augustus K. Gardner, Professor of Obstetrics at New York's College of Physicians and Surgeons, were impossible to refute. In an introductory lecture touching on the flourishing business of quackery in 1851, he revealed the growing sensitivity of the medical establishment to the inseparable issues of feminism and women in medicine.

We have lecturers and lecturesses, and female colleges, where the very large and highly intelligent classes are taught how to get children, and especially how not to get them. The Women's Rights Convention cannot see why women should bear children more than men, and while waiting some plan to equalize the matter, they refuse to bear them themselves.[52]

The physicians' economic interests played a part in their attempt to keep women out of medicine. The men who controlled the profession were unwilling to suffer a loss of income by surrendering to women the very branches that promised the greatest rewards. Dr. John Van Pelt Quackenbush reminded his students how profitable obstetrics was for the young physician. Acknowledging that all wished to acquire "a fair share of patronage, and receive a proper remuneration" for services rendered, he asked, "What better mode presents itself, than to become good obstetricians? Who holds the key, that opens a large practice to the general practitioner, if the accoucheur does not?" When Samuel Gregory began his project to educate midwives in Boston, the local medical journal called attention to the fact that women were being prepared for a "department of practice considered quite lucrative." Elizabeth Blackwell recalled that when she was making the rounds of various medical schools in an attempt to gain admission, one professor whom she encountered believed that a woman doctor would be immediately successful. He was so convinced of this that he proposed entering into partnership with her, sharing any profits of over five thousand dollars on her first year's practice.[53]

Harvard's John Ware, Professor of the Theory and Practice of Medicine, cautioned students that their objections to women physicians, couched in terms of "truthfulness and usefulness," must not reflect "a mean jealousy of encroachment on a profitable field of labor."[54] When women began to seek membership in the medical societies, the *Boston Medical and Surgical Journal* referred to the "serious inroads made by female physicians in the obstetrical business, one of the essential branches of income to a majority of all well-established practitioners." Raising the question of the best course of action, the editor warned his male readers that they would be "denounced as a band of jealous monopolists" were they to deny women membership.[55]

Fear of financial loss was only one among many reasons for men's opposition, and it is important to remember that physicians were not immune to the social imperatives then prevalent. To the doctors, woman's sphere was natural. Charles Meigs contended not only that she found her rewards "within the narrow circle of her domestic reign" but also that exceptions "surprise us and are unnatural." Women, insisted another physician, properly inhabited the "gay world of dance, and song, and flowers, and dress, to which their nature adapt[ed] them, and in which they [were] beautiful." It was essential, insisted practitioners, that any one practicing obstetrics be given thorough medical training. Women could not properly submit to the rigors of medical education, for if they did they would divest themselves of those very qualities that enabled men to hold them in such high esteem.[56]

Within woman's sphere her special duties, no less important than those of man, but different, more "refined" and "delicate" were performed. Although governed by the same moral and physical laws, insisted another writer, man and woman were not identical, and neither were their worlds. Any woman who moved beyond her ordained environment "unsexed" herself. In stooping from her "angelic eminence" to the humiliating tasks of medicine, she at once became "denaturalized" and could no longer be "a woman in all that makes a woman lovable and valuable." By undertaking to obtain that thorough preparation requisite for medical practice, woman would impair those "higher characteristics" for which man honored and loved her.[57]

Modest and refined women, doctors asserted, would not subject themselves to the embarrassments of the medical lecture or the dissecting room. The *Buffalo Medical Journal* quoted with relish reports that the graduates of the Boston Female Medical College were vulgar and coarse creatures; one woman attended by some "female doctors" in New York reportedly found that none of them "had . . . the slightest claim to the title of lady," claiming that they indulged in vulgar street talk and gossip. Genuine ladies were known to prefer "gentlemen" physicians, far more delicate in their approach and a great deal more courteous than the women. None of this surprised the editor, for he agreed that the "real lady" was as out of place in medicine as in a regiment of dragoons. Another physician saw the plan to educate women as doctors as nothing more than a plea for the return of the midwives, and he maintained that the "grannies" had spoken and committed more vulgarity than had ever been charged to medical men.[58]

Physicians found another affront to modesty in the instruction of women by men. Those women who could not be dissuaded from the folly of seeking medical training should at least be taught by members of their own sex, protested one critic. To do otherwise was to engage in deplorable behavior offending propriety, morality, the canons of good taste, and even woman's comeliness itself. He suggested that lecturers be imported from abroad and cited the successful careers of Mme. Louise Lachapelle (1769-1821) and Mme. Marie Boivin (1773-1841) to illustrate that a few, extraordinary women might be found to do the job. Earlier in the decade a New York journal had voiced similar criticism. Commented the editor after a visit to the Female Medical College in Philadelphia:

We cannot envy the task self-imposed by these [male] teachers, and we cannot refrain from the expression of pity for their infatuated pupils. We opine that both . . . will become heartily ashamed of their imbecility and folly, and repent hereafter for their misspent time and labor. . . . We saw in their [medical] museum, objects upon which no modest woman can look without a blush, in the presence of the other sex; nor any virtuous maiden study under the teacher of men, without mental impurity and moral deterioration.[59]

Included in the male physicians' attack upon the movement were writers who supported women's efforts. One critic charged that William Hosmer, who had defended the cause of the woman physician in *The Young Lady's Book,* had written a work that no "lady" would read. One could deduce from reading this work the character of the students attending the New England Female Medical College, concluded this judge. The pamphlet by an anonymous author who appealed to the Rhode Island Medical Society to educate women and restore obstetrics to them elicited this unconditional condemnation: "We must say that we have never read a more indelicate, immoral, indecent, filthy and calumnious publication. . . . We doubt whether any woman, worthy of the name, will withhold it from the flames, a moment after reading it, lest her sex should be polluted by its presence."[60]

In response to the allegation that male physicians offended propriety when treating women patients, the doctors fell back on their argument of necessity. In Europe, where midwives still monopolized obstetrics, they explained, the practice stemmed from necessities imposed by poverty and a scattered population, and definitely not from any superior sense of modesty or elevated morality among European women. American ladies furthermore did not libel physicians with charges of indelicate behavior, insisted one physician. They had learned the correctness of placing considerations of safety beyond those of false delicacy, discovering in the process that the physicians' conduct on the whole was "irreproachable." Allegations to the contrary came from the pens of men, "whose grossly indelicate works" and perversions of truth unfairly perpetuated these false notions.[61] "Shrinking delicacy," set forth another doctor, was nothing more than a "myth" that "sensible" women dismissed because they knew better than to permit such nonsense to interfere with their health. "Those who are not sensible can usually be brought to see the necessity for setting aside an artificial modesty and doing what is fit and necessary to be done," he confidently concluded. Commented still another, "the gratuitous services so freely afforded by medical men" in large cities, combined with available "means of relieving the sick poor by dispensaries and other institutions," obviated the midwives' services even to poor urban women who only "rarely" employed them.[62]

The profession advanced other pragmatic reasons as proof that medicine and women were incompatible. Marriage, "a divine and natural institution," was the proper goal of women; to avoid it was wrong morally, naturally, socially, and religiously. It was hardly possible for any woman "to run a household, rear a family, and also practice medicine," explained the *Boston Medicial and Surgical Journal.* One man dismissed the question entirely by saying that "the bare mention of the thought of married females engaging in the medical profession, is too palpably absurd to require any exposition. It carries along with it, a sense of shame, vulgarity and disgust." The practice of medicine carried with it many inconveniences that women were not in a position to overcome, ran the argument. A man called upon for a night call could rush to his patient at once; a woman would first need to call a groom to prepare her carriage. Such a delay might prove crucial. The tale of the woman doctor on a night call who informed the gentleman of the household that she expected him to see her home was merely one illustration of the "problem." Furthermore, it was "self-evident" that the physical structure of the female made her unfit at all times for strenuous occupations, and especially so during a portion of each month. One glance at woman's slender bones and tender muscles revealed sufficient "reason to conclude that God made *male-man* in strength, wisdom and beauty, but female-man his counterpart . . . in beauty, wisdom and strength."[63]

Law and the ministry, the two other professions of the day, were closed to women and properly so, insisted the doctors. All three occupations demanded that its practitioners exercise great intelligence. Woman's intellectual capacity, although not necessarily inferior to man's, was said to be very different. As Charles Meigs explained, both woman's intellectual powers and her moral perceptivity were "as feminine as her organs." Woman lacked strength of mind, correct judgment, coolness in the face of difficulty, and the courage to meet danger; she was "rash, impulsive, easily swayed by circumstances and importunity . . . [and] yield[ed] to the feelings of the breast, rather than to the commands of . . . intellect." It followed that she was incapable of reaching those prompt decisions so essential in the practice of medicine. Neither habit nor education, claimed Dr. N. Williams, could provide her with the nerve and self-possession needed to meet the challenges of the profession. In spite of her "perceptive faculties," woman was not known to excel in logic, and as one medical journal pointed out, she rarely stopped to reason. That woman was impulsive and learned "all she ever knows of a subject at first glance" was "a beautiful element in her character."

This "childlike element" sometimes produced "really wonderful results, but something more than all this," insisted Williams, was "necessary to the physician." Exceptions to this composite picture of woman might be admitted, but as John Ware of Harvard explained, "a profession cannot be filled by exceptions."[64]

European *accoucheuses* such as Marie Boivin and Louise Lachapelle had demonstrated exceptional ability, and the doctors did not deny it. Utilizing the reasoning in which sexists and racists have historically taken refuge, doctors explained that they were exceptions: When compared with the thousands of distinguished male physicians Europe had produced, the number of European women who excelled in medicine was paltry indeed. Even with their extensive training, observed a physician, *accoucheuses* still were forced to call for male assistance in difficult cases. In obstetrics particularly, the nature of the work conflicted with woman's gentle nature. "The forceps, the murderous perforator, and the blunt hook, are neither tender, refined, nor graceful; and though we might respect the woman who could use them well and manfully," commented the *Buffalo Medical Journal,* "it would be the same very distant respect which we cherish for an accomplished female tight-rope dancer."[65]

When the Boston Female Medical College opened in 1849, their journal had taken the position that physicians would not object greatly to the "new-made midwives." Wrote the editor, "we have no thought of crying out for revenge, or for assistance in putting down a daring rebellion, but are rather disposed to have people accommodated in such matters," provided it did not affect their safety. The patronizing tone persisted: "Women have brains, and when cultivated, show themselves, in many circumstances and conditions, equal to those who are technically denominated their lords and masters," was a later comment, wishing "success to the female medical schools and prosperity to the fair pupils." The Boston journal's attitude was more liberal than most, out of the belief that blatant criticism would backfire. In an obvious swipe at Samuel Gregory's school, the editor counseled at one point that inasmuch as institutions to train women had been chartered and were receiving public support, the best course for male physicians was to try to make them as "respectable as possible," thereby preventing them from becoming the mere instruments of selfish "knaves." As long as some respectable members of society supported the women's projects, it was unwise to engage in conduct that would exasperate them. "To fulminate anathemas, or work ourselves into a rage" about women physicians would produce the unwelcome result of having the men "laughed at for a senseless display of ill will." Professor John Ware held a similar view. In voicing opposition the men, regardless of their own convictions, must refrain from displaying hostility and defiance. No woman doctor, he warned, was "a subject for ridicule," and no honorable gentleman could ever make any "respectable female practitioner the object of a heartless jest or a cold-blooded sarcasm."[66]

Writing from New York, another physician commented that if women were to be trained in medicine at all, the profession must take the lead in assuring that they were taught science and not quackery. An obstetrics professor from that city sounded the alarm that rampant quackery was creating a situation whereby the "province of midwifery threaten[ed] to secede from the union by which she is bound to medicine and surgery."[67] The proposed remedy was to insure that male students were so thoroughly educated that they could eliminate abuses. By allowing "dolts" to graduate from the medical schools, the profession itself was responsible for the general decline in medical prestige, charged a colleague. Another was convinced that a growing tendency among doctors to advertise themselves in secular newspaper as specialists in female complaints had opened the way to the ladies. The *New York Medical Gazette* agreed that the profession was to blame for creating the conditions that swayed public opinion in favor of women practicing obstetrics and gynecology. "It is high time," observed the editor, "that midwifery and the peculiar diseases of females should be rescued from the whole tribe of *specialists* of our sex, whose false pretensions to exclusive skill in these departments is fast becoming a public nuisance." The claims of these "advertising gentry," he continued, affected all doctors. He singled out for special attack such "abuses" as demonstrative midwifery in Buffalo and the "obstetrical clinique" in New York. Were these and similar outrages permitted to continue, the inevitable result, he warned, would be to transfer the practice of obstetrics into the hands of properly educated women.[68]

Although scattered records and incomplete files make accurate calculations impossible at this writing, the total number of women who held the medical degree by 1860 probably fell within the range of two to three hundred.[69] Elizabeth Blackwell's graduation from Geneva in 1849, followed by that of Nancy Talbot Clark, Emily Blackwell, and Marie Zakrzewska from Cleveland Medical College in 1852, 1854, and 1856, respectively, were the sole instances in which women succeeded in gaining admission to and graduating from orthodox medical schools in the decade. As late as 1870, a total of only ten women were graduates of the men's medical colleges teaching regular therapeutics.[70]

The lone alternative for women who insisted on pursuing orthodox medical study was to attend one of the two women's colleges, both of which had an association with eclectic medicine in their early years. After 1852 the Female Medical College of Pennsylvania was successful in obtaining the services of orthodox physicians, thus moving into the regular column in fact, if not always in the eyes of male detractors. Once women instructors were available, they continued the orthodox policy. The New England Female Medical College claimed regular status after temporarily sharing some Eclectic professors with Philadelphia. Despite Marie Zakrzewska's efforts to upgrade the school's quality during her brief association with it, its program remained inferior to that of the other woman's medical college.

With the possible exception of the four women graduates of Geneva and Cleveland, the preponderance of men in the profession was inclined to classify all women physicians indiscriminately as "irregulars." Typical was the report of the New Jersey State Medical Society for 1866, which listed 596 "regular" and 151 "irregulars." Typical was the report of the New Jersey State women physicians, "all of them of the class known as the progressive bloomer kind, spiritualists and infidels."[71]

The great majority of women who earned the medical degree in this period did so by attending sectarian colleges willing to admit them. It is not clear how many women studied sectarian medicine as a last resort. It has generally been assumed that women attended these schools because they were barred from orthodox men's colleges. This certainly was true of some. The woman who was adamently opposed to sectarian principles and/or unwilling to add the "disability" of "irregular" to that of sex did have the alternative of the women's colleges. Graduates from these colleges did encounter greater resistance from the profession than did women who attended men's schools, but the numbers comprising the latter were so few in the early years that comparisons break down. Still, one cannot summarily reject the hypothesis that just as some men chose to study sectarian medicine because they rejected the "allopathic" or heroic procedures of the regulars, some women deliberately chose eclectic and later homeopathic systems out of preference. The choice for those who identified with the goals of the women's movement might have been influenced, too, by the fact that the eclectic colleges not only established a policy that welcomed women, but freely acknowledged the validity of the claim that women added important positive dimensions to medical practice.

Frederick Waite was able to locate sufficient data on fifty-four women in this decade who fell into the regular category. Forty-one of these remained regular practitioners, but thirteen, slightly more than one-fifth, eventually moved into eclectic or homeopathic practice.[72] To what degree such decisions to study or practice a particular system were influenced by financial considerations is not clear. Those who could afford the cost of medical education generally were drawn from the economically privileged.[73] Even so, women who wished to develop successful practices would have found it advantageous to seek patronage among reformers in sectarian strongholds.

Records left by students and practitioners indicate that a wide variety of motivating elements influenced their decisions to enter medicine. Yet, these women shared a feminist orientation in the general sense of that term. By studying medicine and planning to utilize their knowledge, they were moving beyond traditional strictures and actively redefining woman's role. This was so even when they pointedly rejected all identification with the goals articulated by hard-core feminists. In its present phase, feminism encompasses women and men whose views reflect many nuances; the same was true in the earlier period. The opposition early medical women encountered sometimes radicalized them to the point where they demanded equality, but even when it failed to do so, their actions and their rhetoric demonstrated a shared desire to improve the quality of life for themselves and for their sisters. By using medical information and imparting it to others who accepted a more restrictive view of woman's sphere, they were working to widen woman's world and developing a sense of sisterhood as well.[74]

Women physicians and their supporters at times echoed the arguments of anti-man midwifery critics by insisting that propriety would be restored if obstetrics was once again controlled by women. In 1849 a student at the Boston Female Medical College explained that a proper sense of decorum "*should* proclaim" that obstetrics belonged exclusively to women's province. If men persisted in raising the question of propriety, insisted "Harmony" in 1850, they might soon find that women would take the matter into their own hands. It was woman's place to care for her own sex, and "when society is timed aright, this will be her place, and it will be man's 'peculiar' province not to interfere, unless in cases of dire necessity."[75]

Mrs. E. L. Willis, writing for an eclectic journal, asserted the public demand for educated women physicians that arose from need.

Modesty must be shielded from outrage; and that loveliness which is inherent in every true Woman, preserved in all its freshness to make them happy whom she holds dear. This is difficult if her hours of peril are not sacred from persons of the other sex. Purity seems tarnished, virtue of less value, and beauty too little removed from the charms of the meretricious.[76]

Women physicians would become "paragons for their sex," continued Mrs. Willis, elevating the "tone of the female character," diminishing human suffering, decreasing the ranks of "the unfortunate, the shameless and abandoned." Pleading for "many sisters in this cause of Humanity," she promised they would be "ministers of mercy to a suffering and abused sex."[77] This comparison of the male physician's woman patient with the prostitute brings to mind the argument against men midwives a century earlier and illustrates the continuity of this theme. "Whenever I see a married woman nice in sentiments, and delicate in her expressions, and find she is attended by a male midwife," wrote a critic in 1764,

"I consider her a pretender to both: I look on her with contempt; and I consider that, if she had the authority of custom to support it, she would permit me, or any other man to take the same liberty."[78]

Shortly after she had earned her doctor of medicine, Margaretta Gleason pointed out that man midwifery was of modern origin. Nowhere in the Bible, she reminded her readers, was there any mention of men attending women in childbirth, yet Christian men spoke of "innovation and the impropriety of educating women as physicians." The historical summary of obstetrics spanning five thousand years that Dr. Gleason had addressed "in particular to . . . [her] sisters" reminded them of the "annals of sacred and profane history," which united in recording woman's "deeds and services in the Profession."[79]

Mary Baum Hanchett, attending her second course of lectures at Syracuse Medical College in 1851, called attention to the "peculiar and admirable feature" that characterized eclectic reform: "the freedom of its institutions." She credited Reform Medicine with opening the "portals of medical science . . . for the admission of women." To avail themselves of the privileges thus granted, "a few noble-hearted and persevering females" had "dared to brave the tide of public opinion, aye, even the sneers" of their own sex, to whose "pitiable condition" and "welfare" they had dedicated themselves. They would be amply recompensed, assured Hanchett, if they received nothing more than "the consciousness of having done their duty, in endeavoring to prepare themselves to rightly discharge the highly responsible duties devolving upon them."[80]

Sarah J. Hale did not see how really good doctors could possibly object to women practitioners who restricted their services to women and children. Marie Boivin was an admitted asset to French medicine, reminded Hale, and American women could make similar contributions in an area already acknowledged as theirs— the preservation of health. Properly instructed and recognized by men practitioners, women could join with them in combatting disease, advancing medicine, and enhancing the prestige of the profession.[81]

To the men's argument that women were most useful when performing the auxilliary role of nurse, one woman doctor replied in a feminist vein:

Woman may nurse the sick man in all diseases . . . but she may not *prescribe* even among the diseases of her own sex. Our *gallant* young disciples of Galen, together with our veteran hoary headed and conservative followers of Esculapius are the only ones *they think* qualified to take *fee.* As long as woman may be contented to perform the drudgery for these *lords* of the Profession, to wait upon them, to nurse and cure their patients, and let *them* take the *fee,* it is all right; but the moment that she thinks her services are justly entitled to remuneration, then she is getting out of her *sphere.* Away with such selfishness which would throw obstacles in her path of duty and usefulness.[82]

Society, misjudging woman's "true character . . . had yet to learn her proper sphere," insisted another medical student, "for the idea that woman's mind was capable of scientific investigation had not [yet] shed its genial influence upon the superstitious views of ignorance." Woman could not heal the ills of her family on love, continued this writer appealing for the dissemination of medical knowledge. Crediting "Medical Reform" with granting women the liberty to learn, she importuned: "Say not woman transgresses the bounds of *propriety* when seeking to acquaint herself of that knowledge designed for *all,* though in the *halls of Medical Science.*"[83]

Among the resolutions adopted unanimously at the fifth annual meeting of the New York State Eclectic Medical Society in 1854 were those reported by the seven-woman Committee on Female Medical Education. A new age of progress had dawned in America, stated the committee, and the public was sympathetic now to women who aspired to play a significant role in improving society. Medical practice was a means by which they could achieve this goal, and the treatment of women and children fell within the proper orbit of the woman doctor. In the interest of enabling women effectively to discharge their duties as wives and mothers, the woman physician had an obligation to transmit health laws and a knowledge of anatomy and physiology.[84]

Dr. Lydia Folger Fowler reiterated this theme. Now that there was a college that admitted men and women equally to medical study, the day was passing when "if a woman could knit, spin and sew, she was considered a perfect paragon of excellence [and] all heaven-born aspirations of the soul were checked." Every woman, insisted Fidelia Warren, had a duty to learn something about medicine. Not everyone would become a practicing physician, but each could play an important part in reducing suffering and disease.[85]

Dr. Mary Walker, the only woman ever awarded the Congressional Medal of Honor, received her degree from Syracuse Medical College. In 1855 her commencement address struck a dramatic note: Woman, declared Walker, cried out for liberty, even as had Patrick Henry. "Her language is—my chains of circumscribed thought *must be sundered.* 'Give me liberty of thought or give me death!' Let me pursue the studies for which I have the greatest taste—theology, law, medicine, or whatever it may be."[86]

Although it is evident that women with the temerity to attempt careers in medicine represented the harvest of reforming impulses, many carefully avoided the appearance of allying themselves with extreme feminist doctrines. "Harmony," arguing the case for giving women the "privilege" of studying medicine, disassociated herself from more radical sisters. "I would not be understood as holding the least fellowship with that infatuated class of females who are clamoring for equal civil and political rights," she wrote. "They are truly and surely stepping beyond the boundary distinctly marked out by the Creator."[87] Hila Reeves took much the same position. It was not woman's function to rival man, but rather to serve as his ally. In order to do this, she needed scientific medical knowledge. Admitting that women were ignorant because they had been forced to live in a "crushed condition," Reeves still did not advocate equality of the sexes. "I do not say make her your senator, your judge or magistrate. I do not say make her the orator, the patriot or philanthropist. It is enough that woman bear her own burdens; let those having been instructed by her to perform do their part." Similar sentiments were expressed anonymously by "Mrs. F.___" in a letter to the editor of the *American Medical and Surgical Journal.* Young women should be instructed in physiology so that they can maintain their health, she pointed out. Lest she be mistaken for a radical, she quickly added:

I do not claim any sympathy with that class denominated 'Woman's Rights,' for I now enjoy all the freedom necessary, and am content with moving in the sphere God designed for woman—but as regards female physicians, 'tis right and proper, that there should be such.[88]

Who else but woman, asked Mrs. F., was "so well calculated to cheer and sympathize, as she who had a like nature" and was subject to the same disorders? There was no more "noble cause" than medicine for women.[89]

Delivering the valedictory at her medical college, M. Jane Averell discussed the usefulness of the woman physician. Although she might not be "up to braving raging storms or attacks of midnight assassins," she could play the valuable and socially acceptable role of teacher and in so doing provide woman with vital information on health and medical reform. Lydia Folger Fowler observed that if woman's mental faculties were not equal to those of man, when properly cultivated they were sufficient to enable her to be a "*lesser luminary* and to shine in her sphere as brilliantly as he in his."[90]

Sarah J. Hale explained that when woman prescribed for the sick, she was not trespassing in man's forbidden territory. Studying medicine harmonized with the duties society expected woman to perform. In fact, these duties must be carried out "by the fireside, the bedside, in the 'inner chamber' where her true place is," Hale reasoned, concluding that when man appeared there he was "out of his sphere." Even so staunch a feminist as Harriot K. Hunt based one of her defending arguments on the claims of modesty. She and her sister had treated women with diseases that "few male practitioners" could have managed, because the latter "could not have drawn their diagnosis, without that confession from the patient which could not be given . . . with delicacy" to any man. Women of "refinement and purity" generally reserved their confidences for other women. "No male practitioner can proclaim as his right," objected Hunt, "that a woman shall make him her father-confessor; nor is it his office to probe wounds in a nature with which his is not sexually identified."[91]

The transitional decade of the 1850s is a microcosm in which are found the major elements that dominated the debate over women's place in medicine and women's health care for the next hundred years. Vestiges linger today. They are revealed, for example, in the pitifully small percentage of women who earn the medical degree and in the profession-inflicted insults reported by women medical students and interns. They linger, too, in the embarrassments and discomfit of patients who, in spite of stated personal preferences, frequently can find no alternative in their communities to the male gynecologist or obstetrician.[92]

The patronizing comment of the *New York Medical Gazette* in 1853 that the profession would "gladly herald a capable Faculty qualified to impart a thorough medical education to every female in the land . . . who should choose to practice our profession among her own sex"[93] was misleading. It carried with it a suggestion of acceptance that rarely materialized in the period. Instead, the profession assiduously resisted the threatened invasion of the lucrative fields of obstetrics and the diseases of women and children that men had brought under their control. By defining woman's nature and by attributing to her sexually unique, "innate" emotional and physical characteristics, the profession was able to reason that woman's very nature disqualified her for the medical life. Any woman who steadfastly resisted these restrictive definitions and persisted in seeking the forbidden place could then be accused of unsexing herself and acting unnaturally. By keeping its medical colleges closed to all but a few women applicants and barring them from hospital practice and membership in medical societies, the profession hoped to halt the drive to train women. When women turned to alternative facilities for training, many men in the profession then protested that women were not properly "qualified" to go forth and practice.

All of this is not to suggest that male physicians bore the exclusive responsibility for creating the boundaries and definitions that restricted the sphere of leisure-class women. Doctors were products of their age and reflected its values. Raised in the cultural milieu of middle-class morality, they accepted society's assumptions about women and men and felt compelled to function professionally within a framework that revered modesty and the "delicacy of the sexes." Always vulnerable to charges that male attendants threatened to undermine morality, doctors devised male solutions for women's problems as well as for their own. It was they who articulated what constituted offenses to modesty and what did not by contending that "necessary" treatment was never immodest and then determining what was "necessary." Digital examinations and deliveries without "ocular assistance," official rejection of "demonstrative mid-wifery," and the distinctions between "genuine" and "false" modesty all are examples of male solutions devised to permit continued domination of the field.

Initially, the men had been the intruders. The "new obstetrics" of the eighteenth century was the contribution of male surgeons, and it enabled men to achieve prominence in a previously woman-controlled domain. With a better understanding of the anatomy and physiology of the gravid female, the mechanics of parturition itself, and the improved obstetrical instruments men developed, cases of abnormal childbirth could be less hazardous and were frequently of shorter duration. Once this was established, occasional charges of immodest procedures and "meddlesome midwifery" were woefully inadequate weapons with which to repel the male invaders, who finally excluded the midwives from the lying-in chambers of the urban leisure class.

The arrival of the new obstetrics brought reactionary protest against the immorality of man midwifery. Some critics argued against the value of instruments, and very few sought to give women the thorough training they needed in order to compete. Most critics shared a sex-biased view that denied woman's ability to learn the procedures requisite to becoming the man midwife's technical equal. Reactionary criticism persisted but made little headway into the 1800s. In the Age of Reform, however, egalitarian impulses, attacks upon orthodox medicine, and emergent feminism all joined with the reactionary forces to produce a threat more potent than any the doctors had encountered previously. The men reacted accordingly and succeeded in preserving their control.

Anti-man midwifery critics never realized their goal of returning obstetrics to the exclusive practice of women, but their arguments had served the useful purpose of perpetuating the idea that it was incongruous to expect women to observe the dictates of a rigid moral code and at the same time require them to set modesty aside when in need of medical assistance. The new wave of reformers looked forward, focusing directly on opening the medical profession to women as a matter of right, even while agreeing that modesty was best served by the woman physician. Despite the many formidable obstacles, a small band of women did manage to enter the profession before the onset of the War Between the States. Among these avant-garde were a few women who gave the lie to predictions for immediate failure by remaining active in medicine for many years. These small successes heartened those who followed by demonstrating that woman's sphere was not immutable.

NOTES

1. Mary Putnam Jacobi, "Woman in Medicine," in Annie Nathan Meyer, ed., *Woman's Work in America* (New York: Holt, 1891), p. 160.

2. Harriot K. Hunt, *Glances and Glimpses; or Fifty Years Social, Including Twenty Years Professional Life* (Boston: John P. Jewett & Co., 1856), p. 267.

3. Elizabeth Blackwell, "An Appeal in Behalf of the Medical Education of Women," (New York, 1856), quoted in Jacobi, "Woman in Medicine," p. 161. In the late nineteenth century a "remarkable increase" in the number of women physicians reduced this sense of anomaly. See Mary Roth Walsh, *"Doctors Wanted: No Women Need Apply": Sexual Barriers in the Medical Profession, 1835-1975* (New Haven and London: Yale University Press, 1977), p. xvi.

4. "Declaration of Sentiments" and "Resolutions" adopted at the Seneca Falls Convention, 1848, in Judith Papachristou, *Women Together: A History in Documents of the Women's Movement in the United States* (New York: Alfred A. Knopf, 1976), p. 25; "Rochester Resolutions," in ibid., p. 26.

5. *Proceedings of the Woman's Rights Convention, Held at Syracuse, September 8th, 9th, and 10th, 1852* (Syracuse: J. E. Masters, 1852), p. 51; The *New York Daily Times,* September 7, 1853.

6. Dr. Mary Putnam Jacobi insisted that women should not be limited to obstetrics and gynecology yet admitted that these services presented the best opportunities for women to move into general practice. See Jacobi, "Woman in Medicine," p. 154. Even in these branches opposition to women remained strong well into the late nineteenth century. In 1879 James R. Chadwick, Professor of Obstetrics at Harvard, commented that of all branches of medicine, obstetrics was the "one branch . . . in which women, owing to their physical and mental characteristics, are least likely to succeed." See James R. Chadwick, "The Study and Practice of Medicine by Women," *International Review* 7 (October 1879):446. One recent study shows that obstetrics and gynecology, as medical specialties dealing exclusively with women, might be expected to recruit and attract women physicians but fails to do so. The proportion of women who elect this service is only slightly higher than a random sampling would produce. See

Barbara L. Kaiser and Irwin H. Kaiser, "The Challenge of the Women's Movement to American Gynecology," *American Journal of Obstetrics and Gynecology* 120 (November 1, 1974):657. Additional information on contemporary trends is found in Maryland Y. Pennell and Josephine E. Renshaw, "Distribution of Women Physicians, 1971," *Journal of the American Medical Women's Association* 28 (April 1973):181-186 and Esther Harr, et al., "Factors Related to the Preference for a Female Gynecologist," *Medical Care* 13 (September 1975):782-790.

7. For an introduction to the diversity of feminist ideology see: Aileen S. Kraditor, *Up From the Pedestal: Selected Writings in the History of American Feminism* (New York: Quadrangle Books, 1968), especially pp. 3-24; Gerda Lerner, "Placing Women in History: Definitions and Challenges," *Feminist Studies* 3 (Fall 1975):5-14; William O'Neill, *The Woman Movement: Feminism in the United States and England* (Chicago: Quadrangle Books, 1971); William H. Chafe, *The American Woman: Her Changing Social, Economic and Political Roles, 1920-1970* (New York: Oxford University Press, 1972); Eleanor Flexner, *Century of Struggle: The Women's Rights Movement in the United States* (Cambridge: Harvard University Press, 1975).

8. The portion of this chapter dealing with demonstrative midwifery, slightly expanded, appeared originally in Jane B. Donegan, "Man-Midwifery and the Delicacy of the Sexes," in Carol V. R. George, ed., *"Remember the Ladies": New Perspectives on Women in American History* (Syracuse, N.Y.: Syracuse University Press, 1975) and is reprinted with permission of Syracuse University Press. *Report of the Trial, The People versus Dr. Horatio N. Loomis, for Libel,* reported by Frederick T. Parsons, Stenographer (Buffalo: Jewett, Thomas & Co., 1850), p. 21.

9. *Report of the Loomis Trial,* pp. 10-11; 20; *American Journal of the Medical Sciences* 21 (January 1851):270; *Buffalo Medical Journal* 5 (March 1850):624.

10. *Report of the Loomis Trial,* pp. 9-11, 18-21.

11. *Buffalo Medical Journal* 5 (February 1850):565.

12. *Buffalo Courier,* February 27, 1850, reprinted in *Report of The Loomis Trial,* pp. 44-45.

13. As the editor of the *Buffalo Medical Journal* pointed out, the verdict did not necessarily indicate disapproval of demonstrative midwifery, inasmuch as the jury did not decide on this matter. *Buffalo Medical Journal* 6 (July 1850):115. On July 5, 1851, the (Boston) *Daily Evening Transcript* reported that the Reverend John C. Robie, editor of the *Buffalo Christian Advocate,* was also under indictment for publishing "a similar article" criticizing demonstrative midwifery.

14. *Buffalo Medical Journal* 5 (March 1850):621.

15. *Buffalo Medical Journal* 5 (February 1850):564; *Boston Medical and Surgical Journal* (hereinafter referred to as *B.M.S.J.*) 42 (April 24, 1850): 257; *New York Journal of Medicine and the Collateral Sciences* 4 (May 1850):395-396; *Louisville Medical Journal* (June 1850), quoted in Herbert Thoms, *Our Obstetric Heritage* (Hamden, Conn.: The Shoe String Press, 1960), p. 133.

16. *Report of the Loomis Trial,* pp. 34-35.

17. C. R. G., "Demonstrative Midwifery," *New York Medical Gazette* 1 (July 6, 1850):5-6.

18. Ibid., p. 6.

19. *New York Medical Gazette* 1 (September 14, 1850): 166-168.

20. *Buffalo Medical Journal* 6 (September 1850):250.

21. Ibid., p. 251.

22. *American Journal of the Medical Sciences* 20 (October 1850):446-449.

23. Ibid., pp. 450-451. *Report of the Loomis Trial,* p. 23. "C. M." may have been the Philadelphia obstetrician, Charles D. Meigs, listed as a contributor to this volume. Austin Flint ascribed authorship to Caspar Morris, another Philadelphia practitioner. See *Buffalo Medical Journal* 6 (November 1850): 380.

24. "Observations on Clinical Obstetrics," *New York Medical Gazette,* reprinted in *Medical News and Library* 8 (October 1850):83-84.

25. "Minutes of the Third Annual Meeting of the American Medical Association," *Transactions of the American Medical Association,* Vol. 3 (Philadelphia: Collins, 1850), p. 42.

26. "Report of the Committee on Obstetrics," submitted at the fourth annual meeting of the American Medical Association, *Transactions of the American Medical Association,* Vol. 4 (Philadelphia: Collins, 1851), pp. 406-407.

27. "Report of the Committee on Medical Education in relation to 'Demonstrative Midwifery,' " submitted at the fourth annual meeting of the American Medical Association, *Transactions of the American Medical Association,* Vol. 4, pp. 436-437.

28. Ibid., pp. 439-440.

29. Ibid., p. 440.

30. Ibid., p. 441.

31. *Buffalo Medical Journal,* quoted in *B.M.S.J.* 37 (January 1858):507; Frederick C. Waite, "American Sectarian Medical Colleges Before the Civil War," *Bulletin of the History of Medicine* 19 (February 1946):158. This was Martha Rogers, who graduated in 1865. [Kate Campbell Hurd-Mead, *Medical Women of America* (New York: Froben Press, 1933), p. 41.]

32. Elizabeth Blackwell, *Pioneer Work for Women* (London: J. M. Dent & Sons Ltd.; New York: E. P. Dutton, 1915), p. 70. The faculty at Geneva had been kind and encouraging. Dr. Webster, Professor of Anatomy, told Blackwell that her plan for studying medicine was "capital," and Dr. Lee, Professor of Materia Medica, said the experiment would be a good advertisement for the college. He added that he would bring the matter to the attention of the medical journals, predicting that within a decade, one third of the medical students in the country would be women. (pp. 54-56) Blackwell's career has retained interest for historians and biographers. See, for example, the recent scholarly account by Nancy Sahli, "Elizabeth Blackwell, M.D. (1821-1910): A Biography," Ph.D. Dissertation, University of Pennsylvania, 1974; Hurd-Mead, *Medical Women*; Jacobi, "Woman in Medicine"; Wendell Tripp, "Dr. Elizabeth Blackwell's Graduation—An Eye-Witness Account by Margaret Munro Delancey," *New York History* 43 (April 1962):182-185; E. P. Link, "Elizabeth Blackwell, Citizen and Humanitarian," *Woman Physician* 26 (September 1971):451-458; as well as popular accounts such as Dorothy Clarke Wilson, *Lone Woman: The Story of Elizabeth Blackwell, The First Woman Doctor* (Boston: Little, Brown, 1970), and Ishbel Ross, *Child of Destiny: The Life Story of the First Woman Doctor* (New York: Harper, 1949).

33. D. K., "The Late Medical Degree to a Female," *B.M.S.J.* 40 (February 21, 1849):58-59. Geneva Medical College, founded in 1835, was an orthodox or regular school. In 1872 it was absorbed by Syracuse University, which continued to teach orthodox medicine. From its inception Syracuse admitted women students, graduating 34 women doctors by 1900. [Hurd-Mead, *Medical Women*, p. 41.) In 1950 the College of Medicine became part of the State University of New York Upstate Medical Center at Syracuse. There was no connection between Geneva Medical College-Syracuse University College of Medicine-Upstate Medical Center and the eclectic Central Medical College, or Syracuse Medical College discussed in Chapter 7, although the two are often confused. [H. G. Weiskotten, "A History of Syracuse University College of Medicine," *Onondaga County Medical Society Sequicentennial Book* (Syracuse, N.Y.: Onondaga County Medical Society, 1957); Harvey Cushing, "The Pioneer Medical Schools of Central New York: An Address at the Centenary Celebration of the College of Medicine of Syracuse University, June 4, 1934" in the Archives of SUNY Upstate Medical Center.] A generally unknown fact that would not have pleased "D. K." is that in 1847 another orthodox medical school, Castleton Medical College in Vermont, had also agreed to admit Blackwell. See the correspondence between Blackwell and Dr. Perkins in Frederick C. Waite,

"Two Early Letters by Elizabeth Blackwell," *Bulletin of the History of Medicine* 21 (January-February 1947):110-112.

34. *Ohio Medical and Surgical Journal* 1 (March 1849):380. Not all of the comment was adverse, however. The *Boston Medical and Surgical Journal* followed Blackwell's progress with interest and objectivity in the years immediately following her graduation, publishing letters she mailed to America while pursuing further study abroad. See Elizabeth Blackwell to Professor James Webster, Paris, June 23, 1849, in *B.M.S.J.* 42 (February 20, 1850):60-63; Elizabeth Blackwell, Letter to a Friend, Paris, 1850 in *B.M.S.J.* (May 29, 1850):351-354.

35. Harriot K. Hunt to the Gentlemen of the Medical Faculty of Harvard College, Boston, November 12, 1850, in Hunt, *Glances,* pp. 265-267; O. W. Holmes to Harriot K. Hunt, Boston, December 5, 1850 in Hunt, *Glances,* p. 268.

36. These resolutions are quoted in Hunt, *Glances,* p. 270, and Chadwick, "The Study and Practice of Medicine," pp. 463-464.

37. *B.M.S.J.* 43 (December 18, 1850):406. Hunt's application was not the only one that the students considered objectionable. Three black men, sponsored by the American Colonization Society, were also excluded after being termed "socially repulsive." According to the account given in the *Boston Medical and Surgical Journal,* the majority of students present at a morning meeting held that the faculty was entitled to admit whom it chose. Unaware that resolutions of protest would be introduced at an afternoon session, they failed to attend, and the resolutions "respectfully remonstrating against the admission of *colored* men and white women" passed. For a brief discussion of the black men, see Walsh, *"Doctors Wanted,"* p. 32n. Rebecca Lee, who graduated from the New England Female Medical College in March 1864, was the first black woman to earn the medical degree in the United States, and probably in the world. See Frederick C. Waite, *History of the New England Female Medical College, 1848-1874* (Boston: Boston University School of Medicine, 1950), p. 56.

38. *Northern Christian Advocate,* April 18, 1849; Blackwell, *Pioneer Work,* p. 47; Waite, *History of the New England Medical College,* p. 83; *Syracuse Medical and Surgical Journal* 6 (July 1854), 190-191.

39. Blackwell, *Pioneer Work,* p. 154.

40. Frederick C. Waite, "Dr. Nancy E. (Talbot) Clark, The Second Woman Graduate in Medicine to Practice in Boston," *New England Medical Journal* 205 (December 17, 1931):1195; Hurd-Mead, *Medical Women,* p. 57. Dr. Clark was a graduate of the orthodox Cleveland Medical College.

41. Guilielma Fell Alsop, *History of the Women's Medical College,*

Philadelphia, Pennsylvania, 1850-1950 (Philadelphia: Lippincott, 1950), pp. 61; 63-64. Martin Kaufman, "The Admission of Women to Nineteenth-Century American Medical Societies," *Bulletin of the History of Medicine* 50 (Summer 1976):251-260, discusses later nineteenth-century developments.

42. *American Medical Gazette* 10 (August 1859):622-624.

43. Quoted in Morris Fishbein, *A History of the American Medical Association, 1847-1947* (Philadelphia: W. B. Saunders, 1947), p. 85. Four years later, Dr. Sarah Hackett Stevenson, a graduate of the Women's College of Northwestern University, became the first woman delegate to a meeting of the American Medical Association. (p. 91)

44. *American Medical Gazette* 10 (August 1859):623.

45. Blackwell, *Pioneer Work,* p. 24.

46. Ibid.

47. James H. Young, *The Toadstool Millionaires: A Social History of Patent Medicines in America Before Federal Regulation* (Princeton: Princeton University Press, 1961), p. 84.

48. *New York Journal of Medicine,* o.s. 5 (July 1845):141; *New York Medical Gazette* 1 (July 13, 1850):23.

49. *B.M.S.J.* 54 (February 21, 1856):68; 54 (February 28, 1856):87.

50. S. C. Young, "Obstetrical Reflections, Suggested by Passages in the First Chapter of Exodus," *New Orleans Medical and Surgical Journal* 17 (September 1860):836.

51. Horatio R. Storer, *On Criminal Abortion in America* (Philadelphia: J. B. Lippincott & Co., 1860), pp. 56-57. It is interesting to see the persistence of the historical association between midwifery and abortion discussed in Chapter 1.

52. John S. Haller, Jr., and Robin M. Haller, *The Physician and Sexuality in Victorian America* (New York: W. W. Norton & Company, Inc., 1977), p. 117 lists some of the advertised medicines used in the first half of the century. Augustus K. Gardner, *A History of the Art of Midwifery: A Lecture Delivered at the College of Physicians and Surgeons, November 11, 1851 . . .* (New York: Stringer and Townsend, 1852), p. 31. Two recent studies that demonstrate the continuing relationship between women's attempts to control unwanted pregnancy and the social tension this produces are Carroll Smith-Rosenberg and Charles Rosenberg, "The Female Animal: Medical and Biological Views of Woman and Her Role in Nineteenth-Century America," *Journal of American History* 60 (September 1973): 332-356, and Linda Gordon, *Woman's Body, Woman's Right: A Social History of Birth Control in America* (New York: Grossman Publishers, 1976).

53. John Van Pelt Quackenbush, *An Address Delivered Before the Students of the Albany Medical College, Introductory to the Course on Obstetrics, November 5, 1855* (Albany: B. Taylor, 1855), p. 14; *B.M.S.J.* 40 (July 25, 1849):505; Blackwell, *Pioneer Work,* p. 49.

54. John Ware, "Success in the Medical Profession, An Introductory Lecture delivered at the Massachusetts Medical College, November 6, 1850," *B.M.S.J.* 43 (January 22, 1851):520.

55. *B.M.S.J.* 48 (February 16, 1853):66.

56. Charles D. Meigs, *Lecture on some of the Distinctive Characteristics of the Female, Delivered Before the Class of the Jefferson Medical College, January 5, 1847* (Philadelphia: Collins, 1847), pp. 10-11; *Buffalo Medical Journal* 12 (July 1856):115; [Walter Channing], *Remarks on the Employment of Females as Practitioners in Midwifery,* By a physician (Boston: Cummings and Hilliard, 1820), p. 7.

57. D. K., "Late Medical Degree," p. 58; N. Williams, "A Dissertation on 'Female Physicians'," *B.M.S.J.* 43 (August 28, 1850):70; *Ohio Medical and Surgical Journal* 1 (March 1849):380; *New York Medical Gazette* 1 (July 13, 1850):23; Gardner, *History of Midwifery,* p. 7.

58. Daniel Holmes, "An Essay on Medical Education," *Transactions of the Medical Association of Southern Central New York, 1854* (Auburn: W. J. Moses, 1854):51; *Buffalo Medical Journal* 13 (August 1857):191; John Holston to D. M. Reese, Zanesville, November 10, 1853, *New York Medical Gazette* 5 (May 1854):225.

59. *American Medical Gazette* 10 (August 1859):622-624; *New York Medical Gazette* 9 (October 19, 1850):247.

60. *B.M.S.J.* 53 (November 1, 1855):294; *New York Medical Gazette and Journal of Health* 2 (January 1, 1851):12.

61. *B.M.S.J.* 54 (April 3, 1856):169, 173.

62. *Buffalo Medical Journal* 12 (July 1856):114; *B.M.S.J.* 53 (November 1, 1855):293.

63. *B.M.S.J.* 53 (November 1, 1855):294; Williams, "Female Physicians," pp. 70-71. The ways in which medical men defined menstruation and argued its supposed effects upon women's physical and intellectual development are examined in Vern L. Bullough and Martha Vought, "Women, Menstruation and Nineteenth-Century Medicine," *Bulletin of the History of Medicine* 47 (January-February 1973):66-82.

64. *B.M.S.J.* 54 (April 3, 1856):169; Williams, "Female Physicians," pp. 71-73; *B.M.S.J.* 53 (November 1, 1855):292-293; Meigs, *Lecture on Physical Characteristics,* p. 6; Gardner, *History of Midwifery,* p. 8; *Buffalo Medical Journal* 12 (July 1856):113; Ware, "Success in the Medical Profession," p. 519. As late as 1891 the editor of the *Journal of the American*

Medical Association asked whether "unfortunate, pain-inflicted woman
[could] ever occupy a sphere of unquestioned usefulness in medicine where
physical and mental vigor, fortitude, and endurance" were regarded as
prime requisites to successful practice. That women could offer sympathy
and understanding to patients he did not dispute. Yet he concluded that
because women lacked other requisite characteristics, they might "be
useful in the medical world," but would never "be great" as practitioners.
["The Province of Woman in Medicine," *Journal of the American
Medical Association* (June 1891):893.

65. *B.M.S.J.* 53 (November 1, 1855):293; 54 (April 3, 1856):172; *Buffalo
Medical Journal* 12 (July 1856):113.

66. *B.M.S.J.* 40 (July 25, 1849):506; 51 (October 25, 1854):263; 45 (December 10, 1851):398; Ware, "Success in the Medical Profession," p. 530.

67. *New York Medical Journal* 4 (November 1853):519; Gardner, *History of Midwifery,* p. 31.

68. James H. Stuart, "Medical Reform," *New Jersey Medical Reporter,*
in *New York Medical Gazette* 2 (September 1, 1851):200; "Letter to the
Editor," *New York Medical Gazette* 4 (May 1853):232-233. The author was
objecting to such advertisements as that placed by a Dr. Ramsay, who
called himself a Professor of Obstetrics and the Diseases of Women and
Children. Recently arrived from Great Britain, Ramsay claimed knowledge
of "specific Remedies and new Inventions of the highest value," used
chloroform in obstetrical cases, and stood ready to supply patients with
"really efficacious Female Pills or other *established* remedies" at prices
lower than those charged by "quacks" for their pernicious nostrums.
[*Daily Evening Transcript,* July 31, 1850; *New York Medical Gazette* 4
(November 1853):519.]

69. Elizabeth Blackwell estimated that there were roughly three hundred
women physicians by 1859. See Jacobi, "Women in Medicine," p. 162.
Early in the 1860s Samuel Gregory claimed the figure was in excess of two
hundred. [Samuel Gregory, "Female Physicians," *Living Age* 73 (May 3,
1862):248.]

70. Waite, "American Sectarian Medical Colleges," p. 158.

71. David L. Cowen, *Medicine and Health in New Jersey: A History*
(Princeton: D. Van Nostrand Company, Inc., 1964), p. 71.

72. Waite, *History of the New England Female Medical College,* p. 82.

73. Walsh, *"Doctors Wanted,"* p. 62.

74. I have used feminism in the general sense of the movement to expand
opportunities for women. In the literature dealing with this term, I have
found William O'Neill's distinctions between hard-core and social feminists
and Aileen Kraditor's discussion of the feminists' search for autonomy

helpful. See William F. O'Neill, "Feminism as a Radical Ideology," in *Dissent: Explorations in the History of American Radicalism,* ed. Alfred F. Young (De Kalb, Ill.: Northern Illinois University Press, 1968), pp. 275-300, and Aileen Kraditor, ed., *Up From the Pedestal: Selected Writings in the History of American Feminism* (New York: Quadrangle, 1968), pp. 3-24.

Carroll Smith-Rosenberg's essay, "Beauty, the Beast, and the Militant Woman: A Case Study in Sex Roles and Social Stress in Jacksonian America," *American Quarterly* 23 (October 1971):562-584, shows how women active in moral reform developed a sense of sisterhood while aggressing against the sex-role stereotyping that permitted the double standard. Women participants in other reform movements of the nineteenth century seem to have developed similar perspectives. Regina Morantz, "The Lady and Her Physician," *Clio's Consciousness Raised: New Perspectives on the History of Women,* eds. Mary Hartman and Lois W. Banner (New York, Evanston, San Francisco, London: Harper and Row, 1974), p. 50, suggests that women physicians working to "refine and purify Victorian society" used an argument that was self-defeating because it reinforced the separation of female and male spheres. It should be noted, however, that there was virtually no way a woman could have attracted patients in the 1850s unless she limited her practice to members of her own sex and their children. Early women physicians realized this and may have put a good face on the matter by emphasizing the positive effects of their work. Mary Roth Walsh, *"Doctors Wanted,"* p. 84, points to the need for a thorough analysis of the irregular practitioners to enhance our understanding of feminist ideology. My research to date on sectarian physicians indicates that some of them were much more radical than the women who choose the orthodox system eventually taught at the women's medical colleges.

75. "Letter to the Editor on the Practice of Midwifery by Females," *B.M.S.J.* 41 (August 22, 1849):61; "Letter to the Editor from 'Harmony'," *Northern Christian Advocate* (August 28, 1850).

76. Mrs. E. L. Willis, "Female Medical Education," *American Medical and Surgical Journal* 1 (September 1851):182.

77. Ibid., pp. 182-183.

78. [Philip Thicknesse], *Man-Midwifery Analysed: and the Tendency of That Practice Detected and Exposed* (London: R. Davis, 1764), p. 20.

79. Margaretta Gleason, "Medical Education of Women," *American Medical and Surgical Journal* (hereinafter referred to as *A.M.S.J.*) 1 (May 1851):81-82.

80. Mary E. Hanchett, "Medical Reform," *A.M.S.J.* 1 (December 1851):238-239.

81. Sarah J. Hale, *New York Medical Gazette* 4 (November 1853):520.

82. See, for example, Holston to Reese, *New York Medical Gazette* 5 (May 1854):226; *Reveille* (Syracuse, New York) November 2, 1849; Gleason, "Medical Education," p. 169.

83. Mrs. E. Noteman, "Woman and Her Relation to Medical Science," *A.M.S.J.* (June 1851):107-109.

84. "Transactions of the New York State Eclectic Medical Society, Fifth Annual Meeting, January 10, 1854," in *Syracuse Medical and Surgical Journal* 6 (March 1854):41.

85. Lydia Folger Fowler, "Medical Progression," *Syracuse Medical and Surgical Journal* 6 (August 1854):201; Fidelia Warren, "Medical Education of Women," *Syracuse Medical and Surgical Journal* 6 (November 1854):294.

86. Mary E. Walker, "Address Delivered at Commencement of the Syracuse Medical College, February 22, 1855, *American Medical and Surgical Journal* 7 (April 1855):149. Walker received the Medal of Honor for meritorious service during the Civil War, during which time she served as a surgeon. An act of Congress in 1917 rescinded the award, but it was restored on July 4, 1977. A bibliography of Walker is found in Edward James, ed., *Notable American Women, 1607-1950: A Biographical Dictionary* (Cambridge, Mass.: Belknap Press, 1971), pp. 532-533.

87. "Letter to the Editor," *Northern Christian Advocate,* (August 28, 1850).

88. Hila Reeves, "Woman's Sphere and Influence," *Syracuse Medical and Surgical Journal* 6 (December 1854):315-316. "Letter to the Editor," *A.M.S.J.* 7 (March 1855):99-100.

89. "Letter to the Editor," *A.M.S.J.* 7 (March 1855): 100.

90. M. Jane Averell, "Valedictory Address Delivered at the Fourth Annual Commencement of Syracuse Medical College, February 6, 1854," *Syracuse Medical and Surgical Journal* 6 (March 1854):45; Fowler, "Medical Progression," p. 201.

91. Sarah J. Hale, "An Appeal to American Christians on Behalf of the Ladies' Medical Missionary Society," *Godey's Magazine and Lady's Book* 64 (March 1852):187; Hunt, *Glances,* pp. 155-156.

92. One outgrowth of modern feminism has been a renewed attack upon sexist attitudes within the medical profession. In addition to the works cited throughout this book, some current titles dealing with this theme include: Suzanne Arms, *Immaculate Deception: A New Look at Women and Childbirth in America* (Boston: Houghton Mifflin, 1975); Gena Corea, *The Hidden Malpractice: How American Medicine Treats Women as Patients and Professionals* (New York: William Morrow and Company, Inc., 1977); Margaret A. Campbell [Mary Howell], *Why Would a Girl Go Into*

Medicine? (Old Westbury, N.Y.: The Feminist Press, 1974); Diane Scully and Pauline Bart, "A Funny Thing Happened on the Way to the Orifice: Women in Gynecology Textbooks," *American Journal of Sociology* 78 (January 1973):1045-1049; Bonnie Bullough and Vern L. Bullough, "Sex Discrimination in Health Care," *Nursing Outlook* (January 1975):40-45; G. J. Barker-Benfield, *The Horrors of the Half-Known Life: Male Attitudes Toward Women and Sexuality in Nineteenth-Century America* (New York, San Francisco, and London: Harper and Row, 1976).

93. *New York Medical Gazette* 4 (September, 1853):411-412.

Selected Bibliography

PRIMARY SOURCES

Manuscripts

Bard, Samuel. Remarks on the Constitution, Government, Discipline and Expenses of Medical Schools; submitted to the Regents of the University of New York, in obedience to their requisition for such information, April 3, 1819. New-York Historical Society.

Bardiana Collection. Bard College, Annandale-on-Hudson, New York.

Rates of Medical Charges in New York City, 1790s. New-York Historical Society.

Official Documents

The Colonial Laws of New York from the year 1664 to the Revolution. 5 vols. Albany: Lyon, 1894-1896.

Laws and Ordinances of the . . . City of Albany. Albany, N.Y.: Robertson, 1773.

Laws, Orders and Ordinances of the City of New York. New York: Bradford, 1731.

Laws, Statutes, Ordinances and Constitutions . . . of the City of New York. New York: Parker, 1749.

Laws, Statutes, Ordinances and Constitutions . . . of the City of New York. New York: Holt, 1763.

Minutes of the Common Council of the City of New York, 1765-1776. 8 vols. New York: Dodd, Mead & Co., 1905.

Newspapers

Boston Daily Evening Transcript. 1850-1851.
Boston Weekly News-Letter. 1730-32.
New York Daily Times. 1851-53.
New York Gazette and Weekly Mercury. 1768-83.
New York Herald. 1848-50.
New York Mercury. 1762-68.
New York Tribune. 1850-53.
New York Weekly Post-Boy. 1765-69.
Northern Christian Advocate. 1847-51.
Pennsylvania Gazette. 1730-66.
Royal American Gazette. 1777-80. New York.
Syracuse Daily Standard. 1850-51. Syracuse, N.Y.

Organizational Records

Proceedings of the Woman's Rights Convention, Held at Syracuse, September 8th, 9th, and 10th, 1852. Syracuse, N.Y.: J. E. Masters, 1852.
Transactions of the American Medical Association, 1848-1860. 13 vols. Philadelphia: Collins, 1848-60.
Transactions of the American Medical Association of Southern Central New York, 1847-1857. 11 vols. Binghamton, N.Y.: Binghamton Democrat; Ithaca, N.Y.: Mack, Andrus & Co., et al., 1847-57.
Transactions of the Medical Society of the State of New York, 1832-1860. 14 vols. Albany: Munsell & Tanner, 1832-60.
Transactions of the Medical Society of the State of New York, from its organization in 1807 up to and including 1831. 2 vols. Albany, N.Y.: C. Van Benthuysen & Sons, 1868.

Medical Periodicals

Aesculapian Register. 1 vol. Philadelphia: Robert Desilver, 1824.
American Journal of the Medical Sciences. 26 vols. Philadelphia: Carey, Lea & Carey, 1827-40; n.s., 39 vols. Philadelphia: Lea & Blanchard, 1840-60.
American Medical and Philosophical Register. 4 vols. New York: Van Winkle, 1810-14. (Volume 3 is missing.)
Boston Medical and Surgical Journal. 59 vols. Boston: Clapp, 1833-60.
Buffalo Medical Journal and Monthly Review. 15 vols. Buffalo: Jewett, Thomas & Co., 1845-60.

Bulletin of Medical Science. 4 vols. Philadelphia: Ed Barrington and George D. Haswell, 1843-46.

Eclectic Journal of Medicine. 4 vols. Philadelphia: Haswell, Barrington & Haswell, 1836-40.

Eclectic Repertory and American Critical Review, Medical and Philosophical. 10 vols. Philadelphia: Anthony Finley, 1810-1820.

Medical News and Library. 18 vols. Philadelphia: Lea & Blanchard, 1843-60.

Medical Repository. 23 vols. New York: T. & J. Swords, 1797-1823.

New York Journal of Medicine and the Collateral Sciences. 9 vols. New York: J. & H. G. Langley, 1843-48; n.s., 16 vols. New York: R. F. Hudson, 1848-56.

New York Journal of Medicine and Surgery. 4 vols. New York: George Adlard et al., 1839-41.

New York Lancet. 1 vol. New York: J. G. Bennett & J. A. Houston, 1842.

New York Medical Gazette and Journal of Health. 4 vols. New York: J. Crowen et al., 1850-54. (Volume 3 is missing.)

Ohio Medical and Surgical Journal. 12 vols. Columbus: J. H. Riley & Co., 1849-60.

Syracuse Medical and Surgical Journal. 8 vols. Syracuse, N.Y.: J. N. Betts & Jesse Watson, 1851-56. (Individual volumes bear different titles: *American Medical and Surgical Journal, American Journal of Medicine, Eclectic and American Journal of Medicine, Union Journal of Medicine.*)

Books and Pamphlets

Adams, M. *Man-Midwifery Exposed! or What it is, and What it Ought to be: Proving the practice to be injurious and disgraceful to Society; the frequent cause of jealousy and disgust; and of serious mischief to delicate and modest females: With Broad Hints to New Married People, and Young Men & Women.* London: S. W. Fores, 1830.

An Appeal to the Medical Society of Rhode Island, In Behalf of Woman to be Restored to her Natural Rights as "Midwife," and elevated by education to be the Physician of her own sex., Printed for the author, 1851.

Bard, Samuel. *An Attempt to Explain and Justify the Use of Cold in Uterine Hemorrhages with a View to Remove the Prejudices which Prevail among the Women of this City against the Use of this Safe and Necessary Remedy.* New York: Gaine, 1788.

————. *A Compendium of the Theory and Practice of Midwifery, Containing Practical Instructions for the Management of Women During*

Pregnancy in Labour, and in Child-bed, 5th ed. New York: Collins, 1819.

Beach, W[ooster]. *An Improved System of Midwifery adapted to the Reformed Practice of Medicine . . . with Remarks on Physiological and Moral Elevation.* New York: Scribner, 1851.

Blackwell, Elizabeth. *Medicine as a Profession for Women.* New York: Trustees of the New York Infirmary for Women, 1859.

――――. *Pioneer Work for Women.* London: J. M. Dent & Sons Ltd.; New York: E. P. Dutton, 1915.

Buchan, William. *Domestic Medicine: or a Treatise on the Prevention and Cure of Diseases by Regimen and Simple Medicines.* Fairhaven, Vt.: James Lyon, 1798.

Burns, John. *The Anatomy of the Gravid Uterus, with practical inferences relative to Pregnancy and Labour . . .* New York: Collins & Perkins, 1809.

[Channing, Walter]. *Remarks on the Employment of Females as Practitioners in Midwifery,* By a physician. Boston: Cummings and Hilliard, 1820.

Chapman, Edmund. *A Treatise on the Improvement of Midwifery; Chiefly with Regard to the Operation. To which are added Fifty-seven Cases, Selected from upwards of Twenty-seven Years Practice. A Work particularly adapted to improve such, of either Sex, whose Profession has already led them to make some Progress in this Science,* 3rd ed. London: L. Davis and C. Reymers, 1759.

Culpeper, Nicholas. *A Directory for Midwives: Or, A Guide for Women, In their Conception, Bearing, and Suckling their Children. . .* London: Norris, Bettesworth, Ballard and Batley, 1724.

Curtis, A. *Lectures on Midwifery and the Forms of Disease Peculiar to Women and Children, Delivered to the Members of the Botanico-Medical College of Ohio,* 2nd ed. Columbus, Ohio: Jonathan Phillips, 1841.

Cutbush, Edward. *A Discourse Delivered at the Opening of the Medical Institution of Geneva College, State of New York, February 10, 1835.* Geneva, N.Y.: Greves, 1835.

Denman, Thomas. *Aphorisms on the Application and Use of the Forceps and Vectis; on preternatural Labours, on Labours attended with Hemorrhage, and with Convulsions,* 1st American ed. Philadelphia: Benjamin Johnson, 1803.

――――. *An Introduction to the Practice of Midwifery,* 2 vols. New York: James Oram, 1802.

Dewees, William Potts. *A Compendious System of Midwifery, Chiefly designed to facilitate the Inquiries of those who may be pursuing this branch of study,* 1st ed. Philadelphia: Carey and Lea, 1824.

Dewees, William P. *A Compendium of Midwifery, Chiefly designed to facilitate the Inquiries of those who may be pursuing this branch of study,* 2d ed. Philadelphia: Carey & Lea, 1826.

Dewees, William [Potts]. *An Essay on the Means of Lessening Pain, and Facilitating Certain Cases of Difficult Parturition.* Philadelphia: John Oswald, 1806.

Drake, Daniel. *Practical Essays on Medical Education, and the Medical Profession, in the United States.* Cincinnati: Roff & Young, 1832.

Ewell, James. *The Medical Companion.* Philadelphia: Anderson & Meehan, 1816.

Ewell, Thomas. *Letters to Ladies, Detailing Important Information Concerning Themselves and Infants.* Philadelphia: W. Brown, 1817.

Fores, S. W. [pseud. John Blunt]. *Man-midwifery Dissected; or the Obstetric Family-Instructor. For the use of Married Couples, and Single Adults of both Sexes. Containing a Display of the Management of every Class of Labours by Men and Boy-Midwives; also of their cunning, indecent and cruel Practices. Instructions to Husbands how to counteract them. A Plan for the complete instruction of Women who possess promising talents, in order to supersede Male practice. Various arguments and Quotations, proving that Man-Midwifery is a personal, a domestic, and a national Evil. In Fourteen Letters. Addressed to Alexander Hamilton, M.D., F.R.S., &c. Edinburgh. Occasioned by Certain Doctrines contained in his letters to Dr. W. Osborn.* By John Blunt, Formerly a student under various teachers, but not a practitioner of the art. London: S. W. Fores, 1793.

Gardner, Augustus K. *A History of the Art of Midwifery: A Lecture Delivered at the College of Physicians and Surgeons, November 11, 1851, Introductory to a Course of Private Instruction on Operative Midwifery; Showing the Past Inefficiency and Present Natural Incapacity of Females in the Practice of Obstetrics.* New York: Stringer and Townsend, 1852.

Gassett, Helen M. *Categorical Account of the Female Medical College to the People of the New England States.* Boston: Printed for the author, 1855.

Gregory, George. *Medical Morals, Illustrated with Plates and Extracts from Medical Works; Designed to Show the Pernicious Social and Moral Influence of the Present System of Medical Practice, and the*

Importance of Establishing Female Medical Colleges, and Educating and Employing Female Physicians for Their Own Sex. New York: Published by the author, 1853.

Gregory, Samuel. *Letter to Ladies in Favor of Female Physicians.* New York: Fowler and Wells, 1850.

Guy's Hospital, London. *Syllabus of Lectures on Midwifery Delivered at Guy's Hospital & at Dr. Lowder's & Dr. Haighton's Theatre, Southwark.* London: Guy's Hospital, 1799.

Hamilton, Alexander. *Outlines of the Theory and Practice of Midwifery.* Worcester, Mass.; Isaiah Thomas, 1794.

Hodge, Hugh L. *Introductory Lecture to the Course on Obstetrics and the Diseases of Women and Children, Delivered in the University of Pennsylvania, November 7, 1838.* Philadelphia: J. G. Auner, 1838.

Hosack, David. *Syllabus of the Courses of Lectures on the Theory and Practice of Physic and on Obstetrics and the Diseases of Women and Children delivered in the University of New York.* New York: Van Winkle, Wiley & Co., 1816.

Hosmer, William. *Appeal to Husbands and Wives in Favor of Female Physicians.* New York: G. Gregory, 1853.

_____. *The Young Lady's Book; or Principles of Female Education.* Auburn and Buffalo, N.Y.: Miller, Orton & Mulligan, 1855.

Hunt, Harriot K. *Glances and Glimpses; or Fifty Years Social, Including Twenty Years Professional Life.* Boston: John P. Jewett & Co., 1856.

Hunter, William. *Hunter's Lectures of Anatomy.* Amsterdam: Elsevier Publishing Company, 1972.

_____. *Two Introductory Lectures Delivered by William Hunter To His Last Course of Anatomical Lectures, at His Theatre in Windmill-Street: As they were left corrected for the Press by himself.* London: J. Johnson, 1784.

Jex-Blake, Sophia. *Medical Women: A Thesis and a History.* Edinburgh: Oliphant, Anderson & Ferrier, 1886; London: Hamilton, Adams and Co., 1886; New York: Source Book Press Reprint, 1970.

Manning, Henry. *A Treatise on Female Diseases,* 2nd ed. London: R. Baldwin, 1775.

Mauriceau, François. *The Diseases of Women with Child, and in Childbed,* 2nd ed., trans. Hugh Chamberlen. London: John Darby, 1683.

Maygrier, Jacques Pierre. *Midwifery Illustrated,* 3rd ed., trans. A. Sidney Doane. New York: Harper, 1834. Facsimile edition, Skokie, Ill., Medical Heritage Press, 1969.

Meigs, Charles D. *Females and Their Diseases.* Philadelphia: Lea & Blanchard, 1848.

_____. *Introductory Lecture to a Course on Obstetrics Delivered in Jefferson Medical College, November 4, 1841.* Philadelphia: Merrihew & Thompson, 1841.

_____. *Lecture on some of the Distinctive Characteristics of the Female, Delivered Before the Class of the Jefferson Medical College, January 5, 1847.* Philadelphia: Collins, 1847.

Memis, John. *The Midwife's Pocket-Companion: or a Practical Treatise of Midwifery on a New Plan . . . adapted to the Use of the Female as well as the Male Practitioner in that Art.* London: Edward and Charles Dilly, 1765.

Miller, Peter. *An Essay on the Means of Lessening the Pains of Parturition.* Philadelphia: Maxwell, 1804.

Mitchell, Samuel L. *A Discourse on the Life and Character of Samuel Bard . . .* New York: Fanshaw, 1821.

M'Vickar, John. *A Domestic Narrative of the Life of Samuel Bard.* New York: A. Paul, 1822.

Nicholson, William. *The British Encyclopedia or Dictionary of Arts & Sciences* 8, 3rd American ed. Philadelphia: Mitchell, Ames and White, 1821.

Nihell, Elizabeth. *A Treatise on the Art of Midwifery. Setting Forth Various abuses therein, especially as to the practice with instruments: the Whole serving to put all Rational Inquirers in a fair way of very safely forming their own Judgment upon the Question; which it is best to employ, In cases of Pregnancy and Lying-In, a Man-Midwife or, a Midwife.* London: Morley, 1760.

Parr, Bartholomew. *The London Medical Dictionary.* 2 vols. Philadelphia: Mitchell, Ames and White, 1819.

Pugh, Benjamin. *A Treatise of Midwifery, chiefly with regard to the operation, with several improvements in that ART. To which is added some Cases, and Descriptions with Plates of several new Instruments both in Midwifery and Surgery.* London: J. Buckland, 1754.

Quackenbush, John Van Pelt. *An Address Delivered Before the Students of the Albany Medical College, Introductory to the Course on Obstetrics, November 5, 1855.* Albany, N.Y.: B. Taylor, 1855.

Report of the Trial, "The People versus Dr. Horatio N. Loomis, for Libel," reported by Frederick T. Parsons, Stenographer. Buffalo, N.Y. Jewett, Thomas & Co., 1850.

Rush, Benjamin. *The Autobiography of Benjamin Rush: His "Travels Through Life" together with his Commonplace Book for 1789-1813,* ed. George W. Corner. Princeton, N.J.: For the American Philosophical Society by Princeton University Press, 1948.

_____. *Medical Inquiries and Observations,* 2nd ed. 4 vols. Philadelphia: J. Conrad, 1805.

_____. *Sixteen Introductory Lectures, To Courses of Lectures Upon the Institutes and Practice of Medicine . . . delivered in the University of Pennsylvania.* Philadelphia: Bradford and Innskeep, 1811.

Seaman, Valentine. *The Midwives Monitor, and Mothers Mirror: Being three Concluding Lectures of a Course of Instruction on Midwifery. Containing Directions for Pregnant Women; Rules for the Management of Natural Births, and for early discovering when the Aid of a Physician is necessary; AND CAUTIONS FOR NURSES, RESPECTING Both the MOTHER AND CHILD.* New York: Isaac Collins, 1800.

Sims, J. Marion. *The Story of My Life.* New York: D. Appleton and Co., 1884; New York: Da Capo Press, 1968.

Smellie, William. *A Collection of Cases and Observations in Midwifery to illustrate His Former Treatise, or First Volume on that Subject.* London: D. Wilson and T. Durham, 1754.

_____. *A Collection of Preternatural Cases and Observations in Midwifery,* 2nd ed. London: D. Wilson and T. Durham, 1766.

_____. *A Set of Anatomical Tables, with Explanations, and an Abridgment of the Practice of Midwifery, with a view to illustrate a Treatise on that Subject, and Collection of Cases,* notes by A. Hamilton. Worcester, Mass.: Isaiah Thomas, 1793.

_____. *A Treatise on the Theory and Practice of Midwifery*, 3rd ed. London: D. Wilson & T. Durham, 1756.

Smith, Elisha. *The Botanic Physician, Being a Compendium of the Practice of Medicine, upon Botanic Principles.* New York: Daniel Adee, 1844.

Smith, Hugh. *Letters to Married Ladies,* 2nd ed. New York: G. & C. Carvill et al., 1829.

Smith, William. *The History of the Late Province of New York, from Its Discovery to the Appointment of Governor Colden in 1762.* 2 vols. New York: The New-York Historical Society, 1829.

Spratt, G. *Obstetric Tables: Comprising Graphic Illustrations, with Descriptions and Practical Remarks: Exhibiting on Dissected Plates Many Important Subjects in Midwifery.* London: S. Highly, 1848.

[Stevens, John]. *An Important Address to Wives and Mothers on the Dangers and Immorality of Man-Midwifery, By a Medical Practitioner.* London: O. Hodgson, 1830.

_____. *Man-Midwifery Exposed, or the Danger and Immorality of Employing Men in Midwifery Proved; and the Remedy for the Evil Found.* London: William Horsell, 1850.

Storer, Horatio R. *On Criminal Abortion in America*. Philadelphia: J. B. Lippincott & Co., 1860.

[Thicknesse, Philip]. *A Letter to a Young Lady*. London: R. Davis et al., 1764.

_____. *Man-Midwifery Analysed: and the Tendency of That Practice Detected and Exposed*. London: R. Davis, 1764.

_____. *Man-Midwifery Analysed: and the Tendency of That Practice Detected and Exposed. With a Copper-Plate Representing An Exact Drawing, taken from the Death, of a MONSTER that was born in the Year 1745; with a Description at Large of the said Lusus Naturae*, 2nd ed. London: R. Davis and T. Caslon, 1765.

Thornton, Alice. "The Autobiography of Mrs. Alice Thornton, of East Newton, Co. of York," in Joan Goulianos, ed. *by a Woman Writt, Literature from Six Centuries By and About Women*. Baltimore: Penguin Books, 1974, pp. 31-53.

Whiteford, Hugh. *An Inaugural Dissertation on the Catamenia*. Philadelphia: Benjamin Johnson, 1802.

Wistar, Caspar. *Eulogium on William Shippen, M.D. &c., delivered before the College of Physicians of Philadelphia, March, 1809*. Philadelphia: Dobson, 1818.

Wollstonecraft, Mary. *A Vindication of the Rights of Woman* (London, 1792), ed. Carol H. Poston. New York: W. W. Norton & Co., Inc., 1975.

Wood, George B. *An Oration Delivered Before the Philadelphia Medical Society, February 14, 1824*. No place: J. Harding, for the Society, 1824.

Yates, William, and MacLean, Charles. *A View of [the] Science of Life; on the Principles established in the Elements of Medicine of the late . . . John Brown, M.D.* Philadelphia: William Young 1797.

Contemporary Articles: Signed

Adams, Joseph. "On Midwives and Accoucheurs," *London Medical and Physical Journal* 35 (February 1816):84-88.

Atkinson, J. "Remarks on Dr. Kinglake's Observations on the Obstetric Practice," *London Medical and Physical Journal* 35 (January 1816):3-7.

Averell, M. Jane. "Valedictory Address Delivered at the Fourth Annual Commencement of the Syracuse Medical College, February 6, 1854," *Syracuse Medical and Surgical Journal* 6 (March 1854):44-49.

Chadwick, James R. "The Study and Practice of Medicine by Women," *International Review* 7 (October 1879):444-471.

Clark, Peter H. "An Address to the Students of Syracuse Medical College, N. Y.," *American Medical and Surgical Journal* 1 (May 1851): 90-94.

Coventry, Charles B. "History of Medical Licensing in the State of New York," *New York Journal of Medicine,* o. s. 4 (March 1845):151-161.

Darlington, Thomas. "The Present Status of the Midwife," *American Journal of Obstetrics and Diseases of Women and Children* 63 (April 1911):870-876.

Fowler, L. N. "Medical Progression," *Syracuse Medical and Surgical Journal* 6 (August 1854):200-202.

Gilman, C. R. "The Use and Abuse of the Speculum," *New York Journal of Medicine and the Collateral Sciences,* n.s. 6 (January 1851):2-15.

Gleason, Margaretta. "Medical Education of Women," *American Medical and Surgical Journal* 1 (May 1851):81-84; 1 (October 1851):189-191. Reprinted in *Syracuse Medical and Surgical Journal* 6 (June 1854): 136-138; 6 (July 1854):167-169.

Gregory, Samuel. "Female Physicians," *Living Age* 73 (May 3, 1862): 243-249.

Hale, Sarah J. "An Appeal to American Christians on Behalf of the Ladies' Medical Missionary Society," *Godey's Magazine and Lady's Book* 64 (March 1852):185-188.

Hanchett, Mary E. "Medical Reform," *American Medical and Surgical Journal* 1 (December 1851):238-239.

Heath, B. S. "What is the Eclectic Medical System of Practice?" *American Medical and Surgical Journal* 1 (February 1851):32-34.

Holmes, Daniel. "An Essay on Medical Education," *Transactions of the Medical Association of Southern Central New York, 1854.* Auburn, N. Y.: W. J. Moses, 1854, pp. 36-52.

Jacobi, Mary Putnam. "Woman in Medicine," in Annie Nathan Meyer, ed., *Woman's Work in America.* New York: Holt, 1891, pp. 139-205.

Kinglake, R. "In Reply to Messrs. Wayte and Atkinson, on Obstetric Practice," *London Medical and Physical Journal* 35 (March 1816): 174-182.

_____. "On Obstetric Practice," *London Medical and Physical Journal* 34 (October 1815):290-292.

_____. "On Obstetric Practice, in Reply to Dr. Merriman," *London Medical and Physical Journal* 35 (May 1816):363-367.

Leland, P. W. "Empiricism and its Causes," *Boston Medical and Surgical Journal* 47 (November 3, 1852):283-294.

Manley, Thomas H. "Women as Midwives," *Transactions of the New York State Medical Association for the Year 1884.* New York: Appleton, 1885, pp. 370-375.

Marsh, Horatio, M.D., "Moral Development a Requisition of Medical Men," *American Medical and Surgical Jurnal* 1 (February 1851):35-37.

McClintoch, A. H. "Memoir of William Smellie, M.D.," in A. H. McClintoch ed., *Smellie's Treatise on the Theory and Practice of Midwifery,* Vol. 1. London: The New Sydenham Society, 1876, pp. 1-23.

Merriman, Samuel. "On the Art of Midwifery as exercised by Medical Practitioners in Reply to Dr. Kinglake," *London Medical and Physical Journal* 35 (April 1816):282-291.

Metcalf, John G. "Statistics in Midwifery," *American Journal of the Medical Sciences,* n.s. 6 (October 1843):327-344.

Mitchell, J. T. "On the Necessity of Adopting Laws by which the Wives of the Labouring Classes and the Poor Shall Have Secured to them In their Labours the Attendance of Qualified Accoucheurs, Female as Well as Male," *Transactions of the Obstetrical Society of London for the Year 1873.* (London: Longmans, Green & Co., 1874), pp. 3-9.

Noteman, Mrs. E. "Woman and Her Relation to Medical Science," *American Medical and Surgical Journal* 1 (June 1851):107-109.

Potter, S. H. "Commencement Remarks, February 22, 1855," *American Medical and Surgical Journal* 7 (April 1855):151-153.

Reeves, Hila. "Woman's Sphere and Influence," *Syracuse Medical and Surgical Journal* 6 (December 1854):315-317.

Rodgers, John R. B. "Annual Address to the New York State Medical Society, 1815," *Transactions of the Medical Society of the State of New York, from its organization in 1807 up to and including 1831,* Vol. 1. Albany, N.Y.: C. Van Benthuysen & Sons, 1868.

Rush, Benjamin. "A Defence of Blood-Letting as a Remedy for Certain Diseases," *Medical Inquiries and Observations* 4, 2nd ed. (Philadelphia: J. Conrad & Co., 1805) pp. 275-361.

_____. "An Inquiry into the Comparative State of Medicine in Philadelphia, Between the Years 1760 and 1765, and the Year 1805," *Medical Inquiries and Observations* 4, 2nd ed., Philadelphia: J. Conrad & Co., 1805, pp. 365-405.

_____. "On the Means of Acquiring Business and the Causes Which Prevent the Acquisition, and Occasion the Loss of It, In the Profession of Medicine," *Sixteen Introductory Lectures, To Courses of Lectures Upon the Institutes and Practice of Medicine . . . delivered in the University of Pennsylvania.* Philadelphia: Bradford and Innskeep, 1811, pp. 232-255.

_____. "On the Means of lessening the Pains and Danger of Child-Bearing and of Preventing its Consequent Diseases," *Medical Repository* 6 (1803):26-30.

Stuart, James H. "Medical Reform," *New Jersey Reporter,* reprinted in *New York Medical Gazette* 2 (September 1, 1851):200-201.

Vaughan, John. "An Inquiry into the Utility of Occasional Blood-Letting in the Pregnant State of Disease . . ." *Medical Repository* 6 (1803):31-37.

Walker, Mary E. "Address Delivered at Commencement of the Syracuse Medical College, February 22, 1855," *American Medical and Surgical Journal* 7 (April 1855):148-150.

Ware, John. "Success in the Medical Profession, An Introductory Lecture delivered at the Massachusetts Medical College, November 6, 1850, *Boston Medical and Surgical Journal* 43 (January 22, 1851):496-504;43 (January 29, 1851):509-522.

Warren, Fidelia. "Medical Education of Women," *Syracuse Medical and Surgical Journal* 6 (November 1854):293-295.

Wayte, John. "On the Necessity of Accoucheurs," *London Medical and Physical Journal* 34 (December 1815):450-452.

————. "Remarks on Dr. Kinglake's Opinions Concerning the Obstetric Art," *London Medical and Physical Journal* 35 (May 1816):359-363.

Williams, N. "A Dissertation on 'Female Physicians'," *Boston Medical and Surgical Journal* 43 (August 28, 1850):69-75.

Willis, Mrs. E. L. "Female Medical Education," *American Medical and Surgical Journal* 1 (September 1851):181-183.

Wing, Joel A. "On Spinal Irritation," *Transactions of the Medical Society of the State of New York, 1845,* Vol. 6. Albany, N.Y.: Munsell and Tanner, 1845, pp. 73-76.

Young, S. C. "Obstetrical Reflections, Suggested by Passages in the First Chapter of Exodus," *New Orleans Medical and Surgical Journal* 17 (September 1860):834-838.

Contemporary Articles: Unsigned

A. "The Use and Importance of the Practice of PHYSIC; together with the Difficulty of the Science, and the dismal Havock made by Quacks and Pretenders," *The Independent Reflector* (February 15, 1753): 47-50.

"Additional Letter on Corsets," by the American editor, in Hugh Smith, *Letters to Married Ladies.* New York: G. & C. Carvill et al., 1829, pp. 200-206.

C. M. "Review of Report of the Trial, *The People* v. *Dr. Horatio N. Loomis* for Libel . . .", *American Journal of the Medical Sciences,* n.s. 20 (October 1850):441-451.

C. R. G. "Demonstrative Midwifery," *New York Medical Gazette* 1 (July 6, 1850):5-6.

"Case of Her Royal Highness the late Princess CHARLOTTE of Wales," *London Medical Repository* 8 (December 1, 1817): 534-537.

"Clerical Encouragement of Empiricism," *Boston Medical and Surgical Journal* 41 (August 8, 1849):9-11.

D. K. "The Late Medical Degree to a Female," *Boston Medical and Surgical Journal* 40 (February 21, 1849):58-59.

"Demonstrative Midwifery Libel Trial," *Boston Medical and Surgical Journal* 43 (August 21, 1850):53-57.

"Doctress in Medicine," *Boston Medical and Surgical Journal* 40 (February 7, 1849):25-26.

"Early Practitioners of Midwifery in England," *London Medical and Physical Journal* 27 (February 1812):117-118.

"Female Doctors," *Aesculapian Register* 1 (August 12, 1824):79.

"Female Doctors," *New York Medical Gazette* 1 (July 13, 1850):23.

"Feminine Doctors," *American Medical Gazette* 10 (July 1859):622-624.

"Instruction of Midwives in Paris," *Boston Medical and Surgical Journal* 32 (July 9, 1845):467.

L. S. M. "Woman and Her Needs," *De Bow's Commercial Review* 13 (November 13, 1851-52):267-291.

"Lady Abettors of Quackery," *Boston Medical and Surgical Journal* 36 (March 10, 1847):128.

"Letter to the Editor on the Practice of Midwifery by Females, written by a member of the class of the Boston Female Medical College," *Boston Medical and Surgical Journal* 41 (August 22, 1849):61.

"Memoir of the Late Doctor John Bard," *American Medical and Philosophical Register* 1 (July 1810):61-65.

"Observations on Clinical Obstetrics," *New York Medical Gazette,* reprinted in *Medical News and Library* 8 (October 1850):83-84.

"Obstetrics," *Eclectic Journal of Medicine* 1 (November 1836):27-30.

"The Practice of Midwifery by Females," *Boston Medical and Surgical Journal* 41 (August 22, 1849):59-61.

"Presidential Address, June, 1854," *Transactions of the Medical Association of Southern Central New York* (Auburn, N.Y.: W. J. Moses, 1854), pp. 3-24.

"Resolutions of the New York State Eclectic Medical Society Meeting, Syracuse, New York, June 16, 1851," *American Medical and Surgical Journal* 1 (July 1851):132-133.

W. "On Modesty," *The Ladies Magazine and Repository of Entertaining Knowledge* 1 (June 1793):36.

"Women Physicians," *Macmillan's Magazine* 18 (September 1868):369-380.

SECONDARY SOURCES

Books

Alsop, Gulielma Fall. *History of the Women's Medical College, Philadelphia, Pennsylvania, 1850-1950.* Philadelphia: Lippincott, 1950.

Arms, Suzanne. *Immaculate Deception: A New Look at Women and Childbirth in America.* Boston: Houghton Mifflin, 1975.

Aveling, J. H. *English Midwives: Their History and Their Prospects.* London: Churchill, 1872.

Barker-Benfield, G. J. *The Horrors of the Half-Known Life: Male Attitudes Toward Women and Sexuality in Nineteenth-Century America.* New York, San Francisco, and London: Harper and Row, 1976.

Bell, Whitfield J., Jr. *The Colonial Physician & Other Essays.* New York: Science History Publications, 1975.

_____. *John Morgan, Continental Doctor.* Philadelphia: University of Pennsylvania Press, 1965.

Boorstin, Daniel. *The Americans: The Colonial Experience.* New York: Random House (Vintage Books), 1964.

Brennan, Barbara, and Heilman, Joan Rattner. *The Complete Book of Midwifery.* New York: E. P. Dutton, 1977.

Bridenbaugh, Carl, and Bridenbaugh, Jessica. *Rebels and Gentlemen: Philadelphia in the Age of Franklin.* New York: Oxford University Press, 1962. (Originally published by Reynal & Hitchcock, 1942.)

Campbell, Margaret A. [Mary Howell] *Why Would a Girl Go Into Medicine?* Old Westbury, N.Y.: The Feminist Press, 1974.

Carroll, Berenice A. *Liberating Women's History: Theoretical and Critical Essays.* Urbana, Chicago, and London: University of Illinois Press, 1976.

Castiglioni, Arturo. *A History of Medicine,* 2nd ed., trans. E. B. Krumbhaar. New York: Knopf, 1958.

Corea, Gena. *The Hidden Malpractice: How American Medicine Treats Women as Patients and Professionals.* New York: William Morrow & Co., Inc., 1977.

Corner, Betsy Copping. *William Shippen, Jr., Pioneer in American Medical Education.* Philadelphia: American Philosophical Society, 1951.

Cowen, David. *Medicine and Health in New Jersey: A History.* Princeton, N.J.: D. Van Nostrand Company, Inc., 1964.

Cutter, Irving S., and Viets, Henry R. *A Short History of Midwifery,* 1st ed. (reprinted). Philadelphia and London: W. B. Saunders, 1964.

Dexter, Elisabeth A. *Career Women of America, 1776-1840.* Francestown, N.H.: M. Jones, 1950.

_____. *Colonial Women of Affairs: A Study of Women in Business and the Professions in America Before 1776.* Boston and New York: Houghton Mifflin, 1924.

Donnison, Jean. *Midwives and Medical Men: A History of Inter-Professional Rivalries and Women's Rights.* New York: Schocken Books, 1977.

Drinker, Cecil K. *Not So Long Ago: A Chronicle of Medicine and Doctors in Colonial Philadelphia.* New York: Oxford University Press, 1937.

Duffy, John. *A History of Public Health in New York City, 1625-1866.* New York: Russell Sage Foundation, 1968.

Ehrenreich, Barbara, and English, Dierdre. *Complaints and Disorders: The Sexual Politics of Sickness.* Old Westbury, N.Y.: The Feminist Press, 1973.

_____. *Witches, Midwives and Nurses: A History of Women Healers.* Old Westbury, N.Y.: The Feminist Press, 1973.

Fishbein, Morris. *A History of the American Medical Association, 1847-1947.* Philadelphia: W. B. Saunders, 1947.

Forbes, Thomas R. *The Midwife and the Witch.* New Haven and London: Yale University Press, 1966.

Fothergill, John. *Chain of Friendship: Selected Letters of Dr. John Fothergill of London, 1735-1780,* Introduction and Notes by Betsy C. Corner and Christopher C. Booth. Cambridge, Mass.: The Belknap Press of Harvard University Press, 1971.

Fox, R. Hingston. *Dr. John Fothergill and His Friends: Chapters in Eighteenth Century Life.* London: MacMillan and Co., Limited, 1919.

Freeman, Jo. *Women: A Feminist Perspective.* Palo Alto, Calif.: Mayfield Publishing Co., 1975.

Friedson, Elliot, and Lorber, Judith. *Medical Men and Their Work.* New York: Aldine-Atherton, 1972.

Garrison, Fielding H. *An Introduction to the History of Medicine,* 4th ed. Philadelphia: W. B. Saunders, 1929.

George, Carol V. R., ed. *"Remember the Ladies": New Perspectives on Women in American History.* Syracuse, N.Y.: Syracuse University Press, 1975.

George, M. Dorothy. *London Life in the Eighteenth Century.* New York: Harper and Row, 1965.

Gordon, Maurice Bear. *Aesculapius Comes to the Colonies.* Ventnor, N.J.: Ventnor Publishers, Inc., 1949.

Graham, Harvey [I. Harvey Flack]. *Eternal Eve.* London: W. Heinemann, 1950.

Guerra, Francisco. *American Medical Bibliography.* New York: Lathrop Harper, 1962.

Guttmacher, Alan. *Pregnancy and Birth.* New York: New American Library, 1962.

Haggard, Howard W. *Devils, Drugs and Doctors,* 4th ed. New York: Pocket Books, Inc., 1959.

Haller, John S., Jr., and Haller, Robin M. *The Physician and Sexuality in Victorian America.* New York: W. W. Norton & Company, Inc., 1977; Urbana, Chicago, and London: University of Illinois Press, 1974.

Hurd-Mead, Kate Campbell. *Medical Women of America.* New York: Froben Press, 1933.

James, Edward, ed. *Notable American Women, 1607-1950: A Biographical Dictionary.* Cambridge, Mass.: Belknap Press, 1971.

Johnstone, Robert W. *William Smellie: The Master of British Midwifery.* Edinburgh and London: E. & S. Livingstone Ltd., 1952.

Kaufman, Martin. *American Medical Education: The Formative Years, 1765-1910.* Westport, Conn.: Greenwood Press, 1976.

———. *Homeopathy in America. The Rise and Fall of a Medical Heresy.* Baltimore and London: The Johns Hopkins Press, 1971.

Kerr, J. M. Munro; Johnstone, R. W.; and Phillips, Miles H. *Historical Review of British Obstetrics and Gynaecology.* Edinburgh & London: E. & S. Livingstone, 1954.

Kett, Joseph F. *The Formation of the American Medical Profession: The Role of Institutions, 1780-1860.* New Haven and London: Yale University Press, 1968.

Klein, Viola. *The Feminine Character: History of an Ideology.* New York: International University Press, 1949.

Kobler, John. *The Reluctant Surgeon.* London: W. Heinemann, 1960.

Kraditor, Aileen, ed., *Up From the Pedestal: Selected Writings in the History of American Feminism* (New York: Quadrangle, 1968), pp. 3-24.

Langstaff, J. Brett. *Dr. Bard of Hyde Park.* New York: E. P. Dutton, 1942.

Lause, Leonard. *Obstetrical Forceps.* New York: Harper, 1968.

Lerner, Gerda. *The Female Experience: An American Documentary.* Indianapolis: The Bobbs-Merrill Company, Inc., 1977.

Litoff, Judy Barrett. *American Midwives: 1860 to the Present.* Westport, Conn.: Greenwood Press, 1978.

Macalpine, Ida, and Hunter, Richard. *George III and the Mad-business.* New York: Pantheon Books, 1970.

Marlow, H. Carlton, and Davis, Harrison M., *The American Search for Woman.* Santa Barbara, Calif.: Clio Books, 1976.

Marshall, Clara. *The Woman's Medical College of Pennsylvania: An Historical Outline.* Philadelphia: Blakiston & Son, 1897.

The Midwife in the United States: Report of a Macy Conference. New York: Josiah Macy Jr. Foundation, 1968.

Norwood, William Frederick. *Medical Education in the United States Before the Civil War.* Philadelphia: University of Pennsylvania Press, 1944.

Notestein, Wallace. *The English People on the Eve of Colonization, 1603-1630.* New York: Harper & Brothers, 1954.

O'Neill, William. *The Woman Movement: Feminism in the United States and England.* Chicago: Quadrangle Books, 1971.

Packard, Francis R. *History of Medicine in the United States.* 2 vols. New York: Hafner, 1963. (Originally published by Paul B. Hoeber, 1931).

Papachristou, Judith. *Women Together: A History in Documents of the Women's Movement in the United States.* New York: Alfred A. Knopf, 1976.

Peachey, George C. *A Memoir of William and John Hunter.* Plymouth, Eng.: William Brendon and Son Ltd., 1924.

Poynter, F. N. L., ed. *The Evolution of Medical Practice in Britain.* London: Pitman Publishing Co., Ltd., 1961.

Ricci, James V. *The Development of Gynaecological Surgery and Instruments.* Philadelphia: Blakiston, 1949.

Rich, Adrienne. *Of Woman Born: Motherhood as Experience and Institution.* New York: W. W. Norton & Company, Inc., 1976.

Riegel, Robert. *American Feminists.* Lawrence, Kansas: University of Kansas Press, 1963.

Sahli, Nancy. "Elizabeth Blackwell, M.D. (1821-1910): A Biography." Ph.D. Dissertation, University of Pennsylvania, 1974.

Shade, William. *Our American Sisters,* 2nd ed. Boston: Allyn and Bacon, 1976.

Shafer, Henry B. *The American Medical Profession, 1783-1850.* New York: Columbia University Press, 1936.

Shryock, Richard H. *The Development of Modern Medicine.* New York: Knopf, 1947.

_____. *Medical Licensing in America, 1650-1965.* Baltimore: Johns Hopkins Press, 1967.

_____. *Medicine in America: Historical Essays.* Baltimore: Johns Hopkins Press, 1966.

_____. *Medicine and Society in America, 1660-1860.* Ithaca, N.Y.: Cornell University Press, 1962.

Spencer, Herbert R. *The History of British Midwifery from 1650 to 1800.* London: John Bale Sons & Danielsson, 1927.

Stokes, I. N. Phelps. *The Iconography of Manhattan, 1498-1909.* 6 vols. New York: Robert H. Dodd, 1915-1928.

Stookey, Byron. *A History of Colonial Medical Education: In the Province of New York, with its Subsequent Development, 1767-1830.* Springfield, Ill.: Charles C. Thomas, 1962.

Thomas, K. Bryn. *James Douglas of the Pouch and His Pupil William Hunter.* Springfield, Ill.: Charles C. Thomas, 1964.

Thoms, Herbert. *Chapters in American Obstetrics.* Springfield, Ill.: Charles C. Thomas, 1933.

―――. *Our Obstetric Heritage.* Hamden, Conn.: The Shoe String Press, 1960.

Truax, Rhoda. *The Doctors Warren of Boston: First Family of Surgery.* Boston: Houghton Mifflin, 1968.

Vietor, Agnes C., ed. *A Woman's Quest: The Life of Marie E. Zakrzewska, M.D.* New York and London: D. Appleton and Company, 1924; New York: Arno Press, 1972.

Waite, Frederick C. *History of the New England Female Medical College, 1848-1874.* Boston: Boston University School of Medicine, 1950.

Walsh, Mary Roth. *"Doctors Wanted. No Women Need Apply": Sexual Barriers in the Medical Profession, 1835-1975.* New Haven and London: Yale University Press, 1977.

Wilson, Dorothy Clarke. *Lone Woman: The Story of Elizabeth Blackwell, The First Woman Doctor.* Boston: Little, Brown, 1970.

Young, James H. *The Toadstool Millionaires: A Social History of Patent Medicines in America Before Federal Regulation.* Princeton: Princeton University Press, 1961.

Articles

Baer, Joseph L. "A Century of Obstetrics and Gynecology," *Illinois Medical Journal* 77 (May 1940):468-470.

Bancroft-Livingston, George. "Louise de la Vallière and the Birth of the Man Midwife," *Journal of Obstetrics and Gynaecology of the British Commonwealth,* n.s. 63 (April 1956): 261-267.

Bell, Whitfield J., Jr. "Medical Practice in Colonial America," *Bulletin of the History of Medicine* 31 (September-October 1957):442-453.

―――. "Philadelphia Medical Students in Europe, 1750-1800," *The Pennsylvania Magazine of History and Biography* 67 (January 1943):1-29.

Blake, John B. "The Compleat Housewife," *Bulletin of the History of Medicine* 49 (Spring 1975):30-42.

_____. "Mary Gove Nichols, Prophetess of Health," *Proceedings of the American Philosophical Society* 106, no. 3 (June 1962):219-234.

_____. "Women and Medicine in Ante-Bellum America," *Bulletin of the History of Medicine* 39 (March-April 1965):99-123.

Bullough, Bonnie, and Bullough, Vern L. "Sex Discrimination in Health Care," *Nursing Outlook* (January 1975):40-45.

Bullough, Vern L., and Vought, Martha. "Women, Menstruation and Nineteenth-Century Medicine," *Bulletin of the History of Medicine* 47 (January-February 1973):66-82.

Goodell, W. "When and Why Were Male Physicians Employed as Accoucheurs?" *American Journal of Obstetrics and Diseases of Women and Children* 9 (August 1876):381-390.

Harr, Esther, et al. "Factors Related to the Preference for a Female Gynecologist," *Medical Care* 13 (September 1975):782-790.

Heaton, Claude E. "Medicine in New York during the English Colonial Period, 1664-1775," *Bulletin of the History of Medicine* 17 (January-February 1945):9-37.

_____. "Obstetrics at the New York Almshouse and at Bellevue Hospital," *Bulletin of the New York Academy of Medicine,* n.s. 16 (January 1940):38-47.

_____. "Obstetrics in Colonial America," *American Journal of Surgery,* n.s. 45 (September 1939):606-610.

Kaiser, Barbara L., and Kaiser, Irwin H. "The Challenge of the Women's Movement to American Gynecology," *American Journal of Obstetrics and Gynecology* 120 (November 1, 1974):652-665.

Kaufman, Martin. "The Admission of Women to Nineteenth-Century American Medical Societies," *Bulletin of the History of Medicine* 50 (Summer 1976):251-260.

Kett, Joseph F. "Provincial Medical Practice in England, 1730-1815," *Journal of the History of Medicine and Allied Sciences* 19 (January 1964):17-29.

King, H. D. "The Evolution of the Male Midwife with Some Remarks on the Obstetrical Literature of Other Ages," *American Journal of Obstetrics and Gynecology* 77 (February 1918):177-186.

Klukoff, Philip J. "Smollet's Defence of Dr. Smellie in 'The Critical Review'," *Medical History* 14 (January 1970):31-41.

Kobrin, Frances E. "The American Midwife Controversy: A Crisis of Professionalization," *Bulletin of the History of Medicine* 40 (July-August 1966):350-363.

Lerner, Gerda. "Placing Women in History: Definitions and Challenges," *Feminist Studies* 3 (Fall 1975):1-14.

Link, E. P. "Elizabeth Blackwell, Citizen and Humanitarian," *Woman Physician* 26 (September 1971):451-458.

Macalpine, Ida, et al. "Porphyria in the Royal Houses of Stuart, Hanover, and Russia. A Follow-Up Study of George III's Illness," *British Medical Journal* 1 (January 6, 1968):7-18.

Mangert, William F. "The Origin of the Male Midwife," *Annals of Medical History,* n.s. 4 (September 1932):453-465.

Morantz, Regina. "The Lady and Her Physician," in *Clio's Consciousness Raised: New Perspectives on the History of Women.* New York, Evanston, San Francisco, and London: Harper and Row, 1974, pp. 38-53.

Morgan, Edmund. "The Puritans and Sex," in Jean Friedman and William Shade, *Our American Sisters,* 2nd ed. (Boston: Allyn and Bacon, 1976), 11-23.

Naylor, Mildred V. "Sylvester Graham, 1794-1851," *Annals of Medical History* 4, 3rd series (May 1942):236-240.

Nelson, Mary. "Why Witches Were Women," in *Women: A Feminist Perspective,* ed. Jo Freeman. Palo Alto, Calif.: Mayfield Publishing Company, 1975, pp. 335-350.

O'Neill, William F. "Feminism as a Radical Ideology," in *Dissent: Explorations in the History of American Radicalism,* ed. Alfred F. Young. De Kalb, Ill.: Northern Illinois University Press, 1968, pp. 275-300.

Packard, Francis R. "How London and Edinburgh Influenced Medicine in Philadelphia in the Eighteenth Century," *Annals of Medical History,* n.s. 4 (May 1932):219-244.

_____. "The Practice of Medicine in Philadelphia in the Eighteenth Century," *Annals of Medical History,* n.s. 5 (March 1933):135-150.

Peachey, George C. "William Hunter's Obstetrical Career," *Annals of Medical History,* n.s. 2 (September 1930):476-479.

Penman, W. R. "The Public Practice of Midwifery in Philadelphia," *Transactions of the College of Physicians of Philadelphia, 1869* (October 1869):124-132.

Pennell, Maryland Y., and Renshaw, Josephine E. "Distribution of Women Physicians, 1971," *Journal of the American Medical Women's Association* 28 (April 1973):181-186.

Reed, Amy Louise. "Female Delicacy in the Sixties," *Century* 90 (October 1915):855-864.

Rucker, M. Pierce. "Benjamin Rush, Obstetrician," *Annals of Medical History* 3rd series 3 (November 1941):487-500.

Sablowsky, Ann H. "The Power of the Forceps: A Comparative Analysis of the Midwife—Historically and Today," *Women and Health* 1 (January-February 1976):10-13.

Scheffey, Lewis C. "The Earlier History and the Transition Period of

Obstetrics and Gynecology in Philadelphia," *Annals of Medical History,* 2, 3rd series (May 1940):215-224.

Scully, Diane, and Bart, Pauline. "A Funny Thing Happened on the Way to the Orifice: Women in Gynecology Textbooks," *American Journal of Sociology* 78 (January 1973):1045-1049.

Smith, Hilda. "Feminism and the Methodology of Women's History," in Berenice A. Carroll, *Liberating Women's History: Theoretical and Critical Essays* (Urbana, Chicago, London: University of Illinois Press, 1976), pp. 368-384.

_____. "Gynecology and Ideology in Seventeenth-Century England," in ibid., pp. 97-114.

Smith-Rosenberg, Carroll. "Beauty, the Beast, and the Militant Woman: A Case Study in Sex Roles and Social Stress in Jacksonian America," *American Quarterly* 23 (October 1971):562-584.

_____. "The Hysterical Woman: Sex Roles and Role Conflict in Nineteenth-Century America," *Social Research* 39 (Winter 1972):652-678.

_____, and Rosenberg, Charles. "The Female Animal: Medical and Biological Views of Woman and Her Role in Nineteenth-Century America," *Journal of American History* 60 (September 1973):332-356.

Snapper, I. "Midwifery, Past and Present," *Bulletin of the New York Academy of Medicine,* n.s. 39 (August 1963):503-532.

Stern, Madeline B. "Lydia Folger Fowler, M.D.: First American Woman Professor of Medicine," *New York State Journal of Medicine* 77 (June 1977):1137-1140.

Storer, Horatio R. "The Medals of Benjamin Rush, Obstetrician," *Journal of the American Medical Association* 13 (September 7, 1889):330-335.

Thomas, T. Gaillard. "A Century of American Medicine, 1776-1876; Obstetrics and Gynaecology," *The American Journal of the Medical Sciences* 72 (July 1876):133-170.

Thoms, Herbert. "Thomas Chalkey James, A Pioneer in the Teaching of Obstetrics in America," *American Journal of Obstetrics and Gynecology* 29 (February 1935):289-294.

_____. "William Shippen, Jr., The Great Pioneer of American Obstetrics," *American Journal of Obstetrics and Gynecology* 37 (March 1939):512-517.

Thornton, John L., and Want, Patricia C. "William Hunter's 'The Anatomy of the Gravid Uterus 1774-1974'," *Journal of Obstetrics and Gynaecology of the British Commonwealth,* n.s. 81 (January 1974):1-10.

Tripp, Wendell. "Dr. Elizabeth Blackwell's Graduation—An Eye-Witness Account by Margaret Munroe DeLancey," *New York History* 43 (April 1962): 182-185.

Valle, Rosemary Keupper. "The Cesarean Operation in Alta California

During the Franciscan Mission Period (1769-1833)," *Bulletin of the History of Medicine* 48 (Summer 1974):265-275.

Viets, Henry R. "The Medical Education of James Lloyd in Colonial America," *Yale Journal of Biology and Medicine* 31 (September 1958):1-13.

Wager, A. E. "Women as Physicians," *The Galaxy* 6 (December 1868): 774-786.

Waite, Frederick C. "American Sectarian Medical Colleges Before the Civil War," *Bulletin of the History of Medicine* 19 (February 1946):148-166.

_____. "Dr. Lucinda Susannah (Capen) Hall, The First Woman Doctor to Receive a Medical Degree from a New England Institution," *New England Journal of Medicine* 210 (March 22, 1934):644-647.

_____. "Dr. Lydia (Folger) Fowler, The Second Woman to Receive the Degree of Doctor of Medicine in the United States," *Annals of Medical History,* n.s. 4 (May 1932):290-297.

_____. "Dr. Martha A. (Hayden) Sawin, The First Woman Graduate in Medicine to Practice in Boston," *New England Journal of Medicine* 205 (November 26, 1931):1053-1055.

_____. "Dr. Nancy E. (Talbot) Clark, The Second Woman Graduate in Medicine to Practice in Boston," *New England Medical Journal* 205 (December 17, 1931):1195-1198.

_____. "Medical Education of Women at Penn Medical University," *Medical Review of Reviews* 39 (June 1933):255-260.

_____. "Two Early Letters by Elizabeth Blackwell," *Bulletin of the History of Medicine* 21 (January-February 1947):110-112.

Welter, Barbara. "The Cult of True Womanhood: 1820-1860," *American Quarterly* 18 (Summer 1966):162-184.

_____. "Female Complaints," *Dimity Convictions: The American Woman in the Nineteenth Century.* Athens, Ohio: Ohio University Press, 1976, pp. 57-70.

Wright-St. Clair, R. E. "Early Essays at Regulating Midwives," *New Zealand Medical Journal* 63 (November 1964):724-728.

Index

ABOUT THE AUTHOR

Jane B. Donegan is a Professor of American History at Onondaga Community College, Syracuse, New York. Her articles have appeared in the *Onondaga County Medical Society Bulletin* and *"Remember the Ladies."*